DAT

Children's health and the environment

A global perspective

A RESOURCE MANUAL
FOR THE HEALTH SECTOR

J. Pronczuk-Garbino, MD
Editor-in-Chief

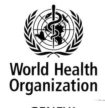

**World Health
Organization**

GENEVA

2005

WHO Library Cataloguing-in-Publication Data

Children's health and the environment : a global perspective : a resource manual
for the health sector / J. Pronczuk-Garbino, editor-in-chief.

1.Child welfare   2.Environmental health   3.Environmental pollution
4.Manuals   I.Pronczuk-Garbino, Jenny.

ISBN 92 4 156292 7   (NLM classsification: WA 320)

Contents

Acknowledgements

The World Health Organization gratefully acknowledges the contributions of many experts from around the world who framed the concept of this resource manual, authored the various chapters, reviewed text, edited and designed the publication, and provided invaluable advice during the long preparation process.

The inspiration provided by the "green book" (Handbook of pediatric environmental health) of the American Academy of Pediatrics (AAP) was pivotal for this initiative, which was indeed strongly supported by AAP members, especially by Dr Ruth Etzel, Dr Sophie Balk and Dr Kathy Shea. The advice provided by WHO colleagues dealing with different aspects of human environmental health was crucial in the initial conception of this manual, and is deeply appreciated. We are very thankful to Dr Terri Damstra, who was always ready to provide new ideas, inspiration and support. Ms Martha Shimkin worked with enthusiasm on this manual, dealing with problems and always finding a solution. Thanks to her encouragement and support, this project became a reality. We are especially grateful to Dr Sonja Junge, who managed to recruit potential authors and follow up until their manuscripts were produced and received in WHO and who supported this initiative up to its culmination. Ms Eva Rehfuess collected and collated all the case studies in record time and her contribution is highly appreciated. We are thankful to Ms Anne Marie Pfister for compiling the rough first manuscripts; to Ms Caron Gibson who formatted texts and prepared vignettes, and to Dr Cesar Chelala who reviewed the text. Ms Maya Kanetsuka helped with enthusiasm during the final stages of preparation, and Dr Pat Butler provided substantial editorial input, with great insight and personal dedication.

The support provided by the United States Environmental Protection Agency (US EPA) to the preparation and publication of this manual is deeply appreciated. Our thanks go to Ms Martha Berger, who envisioned the need for such materials and for transferring knowledge and experience across the world.

We appreciate the efforts of all those who in one way or another contributed to the production of the manual, and regret any omissions that may have occurred. Our deep thanks go to all the authors, co-authors and reviewers from different parts of the world who freely offered their precious time, work, experience and effort for the benefit of colleagues in the health sector, and overall for the benefit of children everywhere.

Jenny Pronczuk de Garbino, MD
Editor-in-Chief

Preface

Children face the excitement of a changing world, with many opportunities and challenges; but they also encounter formidable barriers to their health, development and well-being in the form of environmental threats. During recent decades, new knowledge has emerged about the special vulnerability of children to environmental risks in the places where they live, learn and grow. Children's and adolescents' exposure to chemical, physical, and biological risks at home, in school, in the playground, at work and elsewhere deserves our immediate attention and needs to be recognized as an important threat to their development and survival. Action to reduce the risks is required at global, regional and national levels.

In 1999, a Task Force on Children's Environmental Health was set up by the World Health Organization (WHO). Its activities culminated at the International Conference on Children's Environmental Health: Hazards and Vulnerability, in March 2002, with a pledge to promote action enunciated in the Bangkok Statement. WHO was urged to *"incorporate children's environmental health into the training for health care providers and other professionals"*. At the World Summit on Sustainable Development in September 2002, WHO called for a global movement to create healthy environments for children. The proposal of a global alliance was backed by many countries, as well as by representatives of non-governmental organizations, the private sector, academia and international organizations. This worldwide call to action was the first of its kind, recognizing children, both girls and boys, as the essence of sustainable development and binding nations together in the search for healthy and safe lives for children.

As one of the action steps towards the protection of children's health and environments, WHO has produced this resource manual for health care practitioners. The manual, inspired by the American Academy of Pediatrics *Handbook of pediatric environmental health* (1999 and 2003), is intended as an introductory resource tool for health care professionals around the world, and especially in developing countries, who aim to increase their knowledge and understanding of children and environmental health.

Health professionals in the "front line", dealing with children and adolescents, and interacting with their families and communities, are well positioned to recognize, investigate and help prevent environmentally related diseases. They are in a strategic position to collect data, undertake research, stimulate decision-makers to take action, and promote the education of family members and the general public. This resource manual will enable health care providers to play a proactive and preventive role and to assume their responsibilities, expanding their horizons in the area of paediatrics, family and community medicine.

While the design, content and compilation of the manual was coordinated by WHO, the chapters have been contributed by experts in the field of paediatric health and the environment. In most cases, the co-authors are from different parts of the world, sharing insights and expertise gained from their professions, research activities and personal experiences. Each chapter was reviewed by one or more experts in the field, as well as by WHO staff. Authors verified their sources, made available at the end of each chapter, to provide readers with additional sources of information. When possible, electronic access has been encouraged, by provision of World Wide Web sites. WHO also makes this publication available on its web site at www.who.int/ceh.

With deepest appreciation of the many professionals who freely contributed to this book in numerous ways, WHO is pleased to offer *Children's health and the environment* as part of a concerted effort to increase the health, happiness, and quality of life of our world's children.

Introduction 1

CHAPTER 1

Children are not little adults[1]

P. J. Landrigan
A. Garg
Center for Children's Health and the Environment,
Department of Community and Preventative Medicine,
Mount Sinai School of Medicine, New York, USA

Introduction

Children around the world today confront environmental hazards that were neither known nor suspected a few decades ago. More than 80 000 new synthetic chemical compounds have been developed over the past 50 years. Children are especially at risk of exposure to the 15 000 of these chemicals produced in quantities of 4500 kg or more per year, and to the more than 2800 chemicals produced in quantities greater than 450 000 kg per year. These high-production-volume (HPV) chemicals are those most widely dispersed in air, water, food crops, communities, waste sites and homes (1). Worldwide many thousands of deaths occur as a result of poisoning, with the vast majority being among children and adolescents after accidental exposure. Many hundreds of HPV chemicals have been tested for their potential human toxicity, but fewer than 20% have been examined for their potential to cause developmental toxicity to fetuses, infants, and children (1, 2).

Until about ten years ago, chemical exposure was principally a problem for children in the developed countries. However, it is becoming a problem in developing countries as hazardous industries relocate there as a consequence of globalization and in an effort to escape ever stricter labour and environmental laws in the developed countries.

In addition to the hazards of new chemicals, children worldwide confront traditional environmental hazards, including poor water quality and sanitation, ambient and indoor air pollution, vector-borne diseases, unintentional injuries, inadequate housing, and effects of climate variability and change.

Children's unique susceptibility

Children are highly vulnerable to environmental hazards for several reasons (3, 4). Children have disproportionately heavy exposures to environmental toxicants. In relation to body weight, children drink more water, eat more food, and breathe more air than adults. Children in the first 6 months of life drink seven

---

[1]Reviewed by **I. Makalinao**, Department of Pharmacology and Toxicology, University of the Philippines, College of Medicine, Manila, Philippines.

times as much water per kg of body weight and 1–5-year-old children eat 3–4 times more food per kg than the average adult. The air intake of a resting infant is proportionally twice that of an adult. As a result, children will have substantially heavier exposures than adults to any toxicants that are present in water, food, or air. Two additional characteristics of children further magnify their exposures: their hand-to-mouth behaviour, and the fact that they live and play close to the ground.

Children's metabolic pathways, especially in the first months after birth, are immature. Children's ability to metabolize, detoxify, and excrete many toxicants is different from that of adults. In some cases, children may actually be better able than adults to deal with some toxicants, e.g. paracetamol. Commonly, however, they are less well able to deal with toxic chemicals and thus are more vulnerable to them.

Children undergo rapid growth and development, and their developmental processes are easily disrupted. The organ systems of infants and children change very rapidly before birth, as well as in the first months and years of life. These developing systems are very delicate and are not able to repair adequately damage caused by environmental toxicants. Thus, if cells in an infant's brain are destroyed by chemicals such as lead, mercury, or solvents, or if false signals are sent to the developing reproductive organs by endocrine disruptors, there is a high risk that the resulting dysfunction will be permanent and irreversible.

Because children generally have more future years of life than adults, they have more time to develop chronic diseases triggered by early exposures. Many diseases that are caused by toxicants in the environment require decades to develop. Many such diseases, including cancer and neurodegenerative diseases, are now thought to arise through a series of stages that require years or even decades from initiation to actual manifestation of disease. Carcinogenic and toxic exposures sustained early in life, including prenatal exposures, appear more likely to lead to disease than similar exposures encountered later.

Diseases in children possibly linked to environmental exposures

Children are exposed to a series of health risks from environmental hazards. Environment-related illnesses are responsible for more than 4.7 million deaths annually in children under the age of five (5). Both "basic" and traditional risks, such as unsafe water, poor sanitation, indoor air pollution, poor food hygiene, poor quality housing, inadequate waste disposal, vector-borne diseases and hazards that cause accidents and injuries, as well as "modern" environmental risks endanger children's health. Newly emerging environmental threats to the health of children derive from high levels of natural or man-made toxic substances in the air, water, soil and food chain, global climate change and ozone depletion, electromagnetic radiation and contamination by persistent organic pollutants and chemicals that disrupt endocrine functions.

Environmental health hazards

The risks to children in their everyday environments are numerous. But there are six groups of environmental health hazards that cause the bulk of environmentally related deaths and disease among children (12), as outlined below.

Household water security

Contaminated water is the cause of many life-threatening diseases including diarrhoea, the second biggest child-killer in the world. Diarrhoea is estimated to cause 1.3 million child deaths per year—about 12% of total deaths of children under five in developing countries. Around the world, both biological disease agents and chemical pollutants are compromising the quality of drinking-water. Water contamination can spread diseases such as hepatitis B, dysentery, cholera and typhoid fever. High levels of arsenic, lead or fluoride may lead to both acute and chronic diseases in children.

Subclinical toxicity

A critically important intellectual step in the development of understanding of children's special susceptibility to chemical toxins has been the recognition that environmental toxins can cause a range of adverse effects in children. Some of these effects are clinically evident, but others can be discerned only through special testing and are not evident on the standard examination—hence the term "subclinical toxicity". The underlying concept is that there is a dose-dependent continuum of toxic effects, in which clinically obvious effects have their subclinical counterparts (6, 7).

The concept of subclinical toxicity has its origins in the pioneering studies of lead toxicity in clinically asymptomatic children undertaken by Herbert Needleman and colleagues (8). Needleman et al. showed that children's exposure to lead could cause decreased intelligence and altered behaviour, even in the absence of clinical symptoms of lead toxicity. The subclinical toxicity of lead in children has subsequently been confirmed in prospective epidemiological studies (9). Similar subclinical neurotoxic effects have been documented in children exposed in the womb to polychlorinated biphenyls (PCBs) (10) and to methylmercury (11).

Hygiene and sanitation

Globally, 2.4 billion people, most of them living in periurban or rural areas in developing countries, do not have access to any type of sanitation facilities. Coverage estimates for 1990–2000 show that little progress was made during this period in improving coverage. The lowest levels of service coverage are found in Africa and Asia, where 48% and 31% of the rural populations, respectively, do not have these services. Examples of sanitation-related diseases include cholera, typhoid, schistosomiasis, and trachoma—a disease that causes irreversible blindness, and currently affects about 6 million people, with another 500 million at risk of the disease.

Air pollution

Air pollution is a major environment-related health threat to children and a risk factor for both acute and chronic respiratory disease as well as a range of other diseases. Around 2 million children under five die every year from acute respiratory infections (ARI) aggravated by environmental hazards. Indoor air pollution is a major causal factor for ARI deaths in rural and urban areas of developing countries. Outdoor air pollution, mainly from traffic and industrial processes, remains a serious problem in cities throughout the world, particularly in the ever-expanding megacities of developing countries. A major problem is the continuing use of lead in petrol (13). It is estimated that a quarter of the world's population is exposed to unhealthy concentrations of air pollutants such as particulate matter, sulfur dioxide, and other chemicals.

Disease vectors

Numerous vector-borne diseases affect children's health. Their impact varies in severity. Malaria is particularly widespread and dangerous, existing in 100 countries and accounting for more than 800 000 deaths annually, mostly in children under five. Schistosomiasis is a water-borne disease that mainly affects children and adolescents, and is endemic in 74 developing countries. Japanese encephalitis occurs only in south and south-east Asia, where it is linked with irrigated rice production ecosystems. The annual number of clinical cases is estimated at about 40 000. Some 90% of cases are in children in rural areas, and 1 in 5 of these children dies. Annual mortality due to dengue is estimated at around 13 000; more than 80% of these deaths occur in children.

Chemical hazards

As a result of the increased production and use of chemicals, myriad chemical hazards are nowadays present in children's homes, schools, playgrounds and communities. Chemical pollutants are released into the environment by uncontrolled industries or through leakage from toxic waste sites. In 2002 about 350 000 people died as a result of poisoning, and 46 000 were children and adolescents exposed accidentally (www.who.int/evidence/bod). Pesticides, cleaners, kerosene, solvents, pharmaceuticals and other products unsafely stored or used at home are the most common causes of acute toxic exposure. Some result in life-threatening poisoning. Chronic exposure to a number of persistent environmental pollutants is linked to damage to the nervous and immune systems and to effects on reproductive function and development, as exposure occurs during periods of special susceptibility in the growing child or adolescent. Children are quite vulnerable to the neurotoxic effects of lead in paint and air, which may reduce their intelligence and cause learning disabilities and behavioural problems, in particular reduced attentiveness. They are also vulnerable to the developmental effects of mercury released into the environment or present as a food contaminant. Another problem is asbestos, which is used extensively as an insulator in the construction industry (14).

Injuries and accidents

In 2000 an estimated 685 000 children under the age of 15 were killed by an unintentional injury, accounting for approximately 20% of all such deaths worldwide. Unintentional injuries are among the ten leading causes of death for this age group. Worldwide, the leading causes of death from unintentional injury among children are road traffic injuries and drowning, accounting for 21% and 19%, respectively. Unintentional injuries among children are a global problem, but children and adolescents in certain regions of the world are disproportionately affected. It is estimated that 98% of all unintentional injuries in children occur in low- and middle-income countries, and 80% of all childhood deaths from unintentional injuries occur in the African, South-East Asian and Western Pacific regions.

Chronic effects of environmental hazards

Exposure to environmental hazards is known or suspected to be responsible for a series of acute and chronic diseases that, in the industrialized countries, have replaced infectious diseases as the principal causes of illness and death in childhood.

Urbanization and pervasive poverty in developing countries aggravate both "basic" and "modern" health risks. Developing countries therefore face a double burden in paediatric environmental health.

The chronic diseases represent a "new paediatric morbidity", and include the following.

Asthma

Asthma prevalence among children under 18 years of age has more than doubled over the past decade in many industrialized and developed countries. This increase is particularly evident in urban centres, where asthma has become the leading cause of children's admissions to hospital and of school absenteeism (15, 16).

Ambient air pollutants, especially ground-level ozone and fine particulates from automobile exhausts, appear to be important triggers of asthma. Asthma incidence declines when levels of these pollutants drop (17). Indoor air pollution, including use of open fires for cooking and heating, insect dust, mites, moulds and environmental tobacco smoke are additional triggers.

Sharp discrepancies in asthma by socioeconomic and racial or ethnic status have been noted in certain countries. In New York City, hospital admission rates for asthma are 21 times higher in the poorest communities than in the wealthiest ones (18). Globally, the International Study of Asthma and Allergies in Childhood (ISAAC) demonstrated a wide range in rates for symptoms of asthma. Up to 15-fold differences were found between countries, with a range of 2.1% to 4.4% in Albania, China, Greece, Indonesia, Romania and the Russian Federation, and 29.1% to 32.2% in Australia, New Zealand, Ireland and the United Kingdom (19).

Childhood cancer

The reported incidence of cancer among children under 18 years of age in the United States has increased substantially in the past 20 years (20). Indeed, childhood cancer incidences around the world are on the rise. Industrialized countries have succeeded in bringing the death rates from childhood cancer down, thanks to improved treatment. Still, in the United States, the incidence of acute lymphoblastic leukaemia (ALL), the most common childhood cancer, increased by 27.4% from 1973 to 1990, from 2.8 cases per 100 000 children to 3.5 per 100 000. Since 1990, ALL incidence has declined in boys in the United States, but continues to rise in girls. Between 1973 and 1994, incidence of primary brain cancer (glioma) increased by 39.6%, with nearly equal increases in boys and girls (21). In young white men, 20–39 years of age, although not in black men, incidence of testicular cancer increased by 68%. The causes of these increases are not known. In tropical Africa, Burkitt lymphoma is the most common childhood malignancy. However, in Nigeria there was a marked decrease in the relative frequency of Burkitt lymphoma from 37.1% in the period 1973 to 1990 to 19.4% between 1991 and 1999 which was seen partly as a consequence of improved living conditions and greater control of malaria (22). The risk of liver cancer is influenced by a number of factors; persistent infection with the hepatitis B or C virus is strongly associated with this kind of malignancy. Aflatoxins, one of the most potent mutagenic and carcinogenic mycotoxins, also represent a major risk factor for hepatocellular carcinoma, especially in high-incidence areas, i.e. south-east Asia and parts of Africa. Immunization against hepatitis B or protection against hepatitis C and reduced aflatoxin exposure would reduce the risk for liver cancer in these populations (23, 24).

Lead poisoning

Countries that have succeeded in removing lead from petrol have accomplished a major public health goal that greatly benefits all citizens, especially children. There have been significant studies of lead in blood before and after elimination of lead from petrol in a number of industrialized countries. These studies show conclusively a direct relationship between lead in petrol and lead levels in children's blood. Still, even with the tremendous improvement in blood lead levels in countries that have removed lead from petrol, there are other sources of lead exposure. For example, in the USA, despite a 94% decline in blood lead levels since 1976, an estimated 930 000 preschool children in the United States still have elevated blood lead levels (10 µg/dl or above) and suffer from lead toxicity (25). These children are at risk of diminished intelligence, behavioural disorders, failure at school, delinquency, and diminished achievement (9). Rates of lead poisoning are highest in poor children from disadvantaged groups in urban centres. New immigrants to the United States are often at high risk, because they tend to live in poor-quality housing, are not aware of the dangers of lead-based paint, and may bring medications or cosmetics containing lead from their home countries (25).

In the industrially developed countries, consumption of lead has decreased sharply in the past two decades. This reduction reflects the phasing out of leaded petrol and decreases in industrial use of lead (26). Major reductions in human exposure and in population blood lead levels have resulted. By contrast, in countries undergoing transition to industrialization, lead use in petrol as well as in industry remains widespread, environmental contamination may be intense, and blood lead levels in workers as well as in residents of communities near polluting industries have been reported to be dangerously elevated (27–30). A study conducted in Romania examined lead levels in children from a polluted municipality: only six children out of 42 had blood lead levels below 10 µg/dl (27). A devastating experience in Trinidad and Tobago demonstrated the impact of lead exposure on child health, in this case from battery recycling. A six-year-old boy died from acute lead poisoning, with a blood lead level above 140 µg/dl, and many children had to undergo chelating therapy and suffered permanent damage from exposure to extremely high lead levels.

Developmental disorders

Developmental disorders, including autism, attention deficit disorder, dyslexia and mental retardation affect 5–8% of the 4 million children born each year in the United States (31). The causes are largely unknown, but exposure to lead, mercury, PCBs, certain pesticides and other environmental neurotoxicants are thought to contribute. An expert committee convened by the US National Academy of Sciences concluded in July 2000 that 3% of all developmental disorders in American children are the direct consequence of toxic environmental exposures, and that another 25% are the result of interactions between environmental factors and individual children's susceptibility (32).

Endocrine disruption

Endocrine disruptors are chemicals in the environment that have the capacity to interfere with the body's hormonal signalling system. The effects of these chemicals have been well documented in experimental animals exposed in the laboratory as well as in wildlife populations in contaminated ecosystems such as the Great Lakes in North America.

While data on the human health effects of endocrine disruptors are still scant, it would appear that the embryo, fetus and young child are at greatest risk of adverse consequences following exposure to these chemicals, because the human reproductive and endocrine systems undergo complex development in fetal life and thus are highly vulnerable to toxic influences. It is hypothesized, but not proven, that endocrine-disrupting compounds may be responsible, at least in part, for an increased incidence of testicular cancer, a reported doubling in incidence of hypospadias (33) and the increasingly early onset of puberty in young girls.

The international response to children's environmental health

The first major international development in children's environmental health was the Declaration of the Environment Leaders of the Eight on Children's Environmental Health, issued in Miami in 1997 by the group of highly industrialized nations, the so-called G-8 (34). The Miami Declaration expressed the commitment of these nations to children's environmental health and included specific commitments to remove lead from petrol, to improve air quality, and to improve the quality of drinking-water. The Declaration also called for improvements in the scientific risk assessments that underpin environmental regulations to explicitly incorporate children, and set forth international cooperation to do further research on endocrine-disrupting chemicals. This Declaration has catalysed developments in many international organizations and nongovernmental organizations (NGOs).

In 2002, the World Health Organization (WHO) launched an initiative to improve environmental protection of children, reflecting its major thrust at the World Summit on Sustainable Development, which took place in Johannesburg, South Africa. "Our top priority in health and development must be investing in the future—in children and the young—a group that is particularly vulnerable to environmental hazards," stated WHO's then Director-General, Dr Gro Harlem Brundtland. She set forth the Healthy Environments for Children Alliance which many international organizations, nations, NGOs and businesses have responded to and have begun to put into action.

A WHO working group on children's environmental health has been active in bringing together participants from developed as well as developing countries since early 2000. The United Nations Environment Programme (UNEP), the World Bank, and the United Nations Children's Fund (UNICEF) have joined in partnership with WHO in these efforts.

The international community of NGOs is becoming active in children's environmental health. An umbrella organization, the International Network of Children's Environmental Health & Safety (INCHES), was formed to link grassroots organizations in various countries. INCHES, in conjunction with a US NGO, the Children's Environmental Health Network (CEHN) hosted a global conference on children's environmental health in Washington in September 2001 to raise international interest in children's environmental health. This was followed by a WHO conference in Bangkok, Thailand, which considered environmental threats to the health of children in South-East Asia and the Western Pacific (see resulting statement below) (35). The Pan American Health Organization has developed a strategy to improve environmental health of children in the Americas and launched a regional workshop on children's environmental health in 2003.

The Bangkok Statement
A pledge to promote the protection of Children's Environmental Health

We, the undersigned scientists, doctors and public health professionals, educators, environmental health engineers, community workers and representatives from a number of international organizations, from governmental and non-governmental organizations in South East Asian and Western Pacific countries, have come together with colleagues from different parts of the world from 3 to 7 March 2002 in Bangkok, Thailand, to commit ourselves to work jointly towards the promotion and protection of children's health against environmental threats.

Worldwide, it is estimated that more than one-quarter of the global burden of disease (GBD) can be attributed to environmental risk factors. Over 40% of the environmental disease burden falls on children under 5 years of age, yet these constitute only 10% of the world population. The environmental burden of pediatric disease in Asia and the Pacific countries is not well recognized and needs to be quantified and addressed.

We recognize

That a growing number of diseases in children have been linked to environmental exposures. These range from the traditional waterborne, foodborne and vector-borne diseases and acute respiratory infections to asthma, cancer, injuries, arsenicosis, fluorosis, certain birth defects and developmental disabilities.

That environmental exposures are increasing in many countries in the region; that new emerging risks are being identified; and that more and more children are being exposed to unsafe environments where they are conceived and born, where they live, learn, play, work and grow. Unique and permanent adverse health effects can occur when the embryo, fetus, newborn, child and adolescent (*collectively referred to as "children" from here onwards*) are exposed to environmental threats during early periods of special vulnerability.

That in developing countries the main environmental health problems affecting children are exacerbated by poverty, illiteracy and malnutrition, and include: indoor and outdoor air pollution, lack of access to safe water and sanitation, exposure to hazardous chemicals, accidents and injuries. Furthermore, as countries industrialize, children become exposed to toxicants commonly associated with the developed world, creating an additional environmental burden of disease. This deserves special attention from the industrialized and developing countries alike.

That environmental hazards arise both from anthropogenic and natural sources (e.g. plant toxins, fluoride, arsenic, radiations), which separately and in combination can cause serious harm to children.

That restoring and protecting the integrity of the life-sustaining systems of the earth are integral to ensuring children's environmental health now and in the future. Therefore, addressing global changes such as human population growth, land and energy use patterns, habitat destruction, biodiversity loss and climate change must be part of efforts to promote children's environmental health.

That despite the rising concern of the scientific community and the education and social sectors about environmental threats to children's health and development, progress has been slow and serious challenges still remain.

That the health, environment and education sectors must take concerted action at all levels (local, national, global), together with other sectors, in serious efforts to enable our countries to assess the nature and magnitude of the problem, identify the main environmental risks to children's health and establish culturally appropriate monitoring, mitigation and prevention strategies.

We affirm

That the principle "***children are not little adults***" requires full recognition and a preventive approach. Children are uniquely vulnerable to the effects of many chemical, biological and physical agents. All children should be protected from injury, poisoning and hazards in the different environments where they are born, live, learn, play, develop and grow to become the adults of tomorrow and citizens in their own right.

That all children should have the right to safe, clean and supportive environments that ensure their survival, growth, development, healthy life and well-being. The recognition of this right is especially important as the world moves towards the adoption of sustainable development practices.

That it is the responsibility of community workers, local and national authorities and policy-makers, national and international organizations, and all professionals dealing with health, environment and education issues to ensure that actions are initiated, developed and sustained in all countries to promote the recognition, assessment and mitigation of physical, chemical and biological hazards, and also of social hazards that threaten children's health and quality of life.

We commit ourselves

To developing active and innovative national and international networks with colleagues, in partnership with governmental, nongovernmental and international organizations for the promotion and protection of children's environmental health, and urge WHO to support our efforts in all areas, especially in the following four:

Box continued

1. **Protection and Prevention—To strengthen existing programmes and initiate new mechanisms to provide all children with access to clean water and air, adequate sanitation, safe food and appropriate shelter:**
   - Reduce or eliminate environmental causes and triggers of respiratory diseases and asthma, including exposure to indoor air pollution from the use of biomass fuels and environmental tobacco smoke.
   - Reduce or eliminate exposure to toxic metals such as lead, mercury and arsenic, to fluoride, and to anthropogenic hazards such as toxic wastes, pesticides and persistent organic pollutants.
   - Reduce or eliminate exposure to known and suspected anthropogenic carcinogens, neurotoxicants, developmental and reproductive toxicants, immunotoxicants and naturally occurring toxins.
   - Reduce the incidence of diarrhoeal disease through increased access to safe water and sanitation and promotion of initiatives to improve food safety.
   - Reduce the incidence of accidents, injuries and poisonings, as well as exposure to noise, radiation, microbiological and other factors by improving all environments where children spend time, in particular at home and at school.
   - Commit to international efforts to avert or slow global environmental changes, and also take action to lessen the vulnerability of populations to the impact of such changes.

2. **Health Care and Research—To promote the recognition, assessment and study of environmental factors that have an impact on the health and development of children:**
   - Establish centres to address issues related to children's environmental health.
   - Develop and implement cooperative multidisciplinary research studies in association with centres of excellence, and promote the collection of harmonized data and their dissemination.
   - Incorporate children's environmental health into the training for health care providers and other professionals, and promote the use of the environmental history.
   - Seek financial and institutional support for research, data collection, education, intervention and prevention programmes.
   - Develop risk assessment methods that take account of children as a special risk group.

3. **Empowerment and Education—To promote the education of children and parents about the importance of their physical environment and their participation in decisions that affect their lives, and to inform parents, teachers and caregivers and the community in general on the need and means to provide a safe, healthy and supportive environment to all children:**
   - Provide environmental health education through healthy schools and adult education initiatives.
   - Incorporate lessons on health and the environment into all school curricula.

● Empower children to identify potential risks and solutions.
● Impart environmental health expertise to educators, curriculum designers and school administrators.
● Create and disseminate to families and communities culturally relevant information about the special vulnerability of children to environmental threats and practical steps to protect children.
● Teach families and the community to identify environmental threats to their children, to adopt practices that will reduce risks of exposure and to work with local authorities and the private sector in developing prevention and intervention programmes.

4. **Advocacy—To advocate and take action on the protection and promotion of children's environmental health at all levels, including political, administrative and community levels:**
● Use lessons learned to prevent environmental illness in children, for example by promoting legislation for the removal of lead from all petrol, paints, water pipes and ceramics, and for the provision of smoke-free environments in all public buildings.
● Sensitize decision-makers to the results of research studies and observations of community workers and primary health care providers that need to be accorded high priority to safeguard children's health.
● Promote environmental health policies that protect children.
● Raise the awareness of decision-makers and potential donors about known environmental threats to children's health and work with them and other stakeholders to allocate necessary resources to implement interventions.
● Work with the media to disseminate information on core children's environmental health issues and locally relevant environmental health problems and potential solutions.

For all those concerned about the environmental health of children, the time to translate knowledge into action is now.

Bangkok, 7 March 2002

References

1. US Environmental Protection Agency. *Chemicals-in-commerce information system. Chemical update system database, 1998.* Washington, DC, July 1997.
2. National Academy of Sciences. *Toxicity testing needs and priorities.* Washington, DC, National Academy Press, 1984.
3. US Environmental Protection Agency. Office of Pollution Prevention and Toxic Substances. *Chemical hazard data availability study: What do we really know about the safety of high production volume chemicals?* US EPA, Washington, DC, 1998.
4. National Academy of Sciences. *Pesticides in the diets of infants and children.* Washington, DC, National Academy Press, 1993.

5. World Health Organization. *Healthy environments for children*. World Health Organization, Geneva, 2002 (WHO/SDE/PHE/02.05).

6. Landrigan PJ, Suk WA, Amler RW. Chemical wastes, children's health and the Superfund Basic Research Program. *Environmental Health Perspectives*, 1999, 107:423–427.

7. Landrigan PJ. The toxicity of lead at low dose. *British Journal of Industrial Medicine*, 1989, 46:593–596.

8. Needleman HL, Gunnoe C, Leviton A. Deficits in psychological and classroom performance of children with elevated dentine lead levels. *New England Journal of Medicine*, 1979, 300:689–695.

9. Bellinger D et al. Longitudinal analysis of prenatal and postnatal lead exposure and early cognitive development. *New England Journal of Medicine*, 1987, 316:1037–1043.

10. Jacobson JL, Jacobson SW, Humphrey HEB. Effects of in utero exposure to polychlorinated biphenyls and related contaminants on cognitive functioning in young children. *Journal of Pediatrics*, 1990, 116:38–45.

11. Grandjean P et al. Cognitive deficit in 7-year-old children with prenatal exposure to methylmercury. *Neurotoxicology and Teratology*, 1997, 19:417–428.

12. World Health Organization. *Healthy environments for children. Initiating an alliance for action*. World Health Organization, Geneva, 2002 (WHO/SDE/PHE/02.06).

13. Landrigan PJ, Boffetta P, Apostoli P. The reproductive toxicity and carcinogenicity of lead: a critical review. *American Journal of Industrial Medicine*, 2000, 38:231–243.

14. Nicholson WJ, Perkel G, Selikoff IJ. Occupational exposure to asbestos: population at risk and projected mortality—1980–2030. *American Journal of Industrial Medicine*, 1982, 3:259–311.

15. Mannino DM et al. Surveillance for asthma—United States, 1960–1996. *Morbidity and Mortality Weekly Report*, 1998, 47(SS-1):1–28.

16. Centers for Disease Control and Prevention. Asthma mortality and hospitalization among children and young adults—United States, 1980–1993. *Morbidity and Mortality Weekly Report*, 1996, 45:350–353.

17. Friedman MS et al. Impact of changes in transportation and commuting behaviors during the 1996 summer Olympic Games in Atlanta on air quality and childhood asthma. *Journal of the American Medical Association*, 2001, 285:897–905.

18. Claudio L et al. Socioeconomic factors and asthma hospitalization rates in New York City. *Journal of Asthma*, 1999, 36:343–350.

19. *Children's health and environment: a review of evidence*. Copenhagen, WHO Regional Office for Europe, 2002 (Environmental Issue Report, No. 29).

20. Gurney JG et al. Trends in cancer incidence among children in the U.S. *Cancer*, 1996, 76:532–41.

21. Legler JM et al. Brain and other central nervous system cancers: recent trends in incidence and mortality. *Journal of the National Cancer Institute*, 1999, 91:1382–1390.

22. Ojesina AI, Akang EEU, Ojemakinde KO. Decline in the frequency of Burkitt's lymphoma relative to other childhood malignancies in Ibadan, Nigeria. *Annals of Tropical Paediatrics*, 2002, 22:159–163.

23. Henry SH, Bosch FX, Bowers JC. Aflatoxin, hepatitis and worldwide liver cancer risks. *Advances in Experimental Medicine and Biology*, 2002, 504:229–233.

24. Montesano R, Hainaut P, Wild CP. Hepatocellular carcinoma: from gene to public health. *Journal of the National Cancer Institute*, 1997, 89:1844–1851.

25. Centers for Disease Control and Prevention. Lead poisoning—update. *Morbidity and Mortality Weekly Report*, 1997, 46:141–146.

26. Hernberg S. Lead poisoning in a historical perspective. *American Journal of Industrial Medicine*, 2000, 38:244–254.

27. Bindea V. Blood lead levels in children from Baia Mare, Romania. In: *Proceedings of the International Conference on Lead Exposure, Reproductive Toxicity and Carcinogenicity, Gargagno, Italy, 7–9 June 1999*, Lyon, International Agency for Research on Cancer, 1999.

28. Bulat P et al. Occupational lead intoxication in lead smelter workers. In: *Proceedings of the International Conference on Lead Exposure, Reproductive Toxicity and Carcinogenicity, Gargagno, Italy, 7–9 June 1999*, Lyon, International Agency for Research on Cancer, 1999.

29. Chatterjee A et al. Pollution from a lead smelter in a residential area of Calcutta. In: *Proceedings of the International Conference on Lead Exposure, Reproductive Toxicity and Carcinogenicity, Gargagno, Italy, 7–9 June 1999*, Lyon, International Agency for Research on Cancer, 1999.

30. Koplan J. Hazards of cottage and small industries in developing countries. *American Journal of Industrial Medicine*, 1996, 30:123–124.

31. Weiss B, Landrigan P. The developing brain and the environment: an introduction. *Environmental Health Perspectives*, 2000, 108 (Suppl.):373–374.

32. National Academy of Sciences. *Scientific frontiers in developmental toxicology and risk assessment*. Washington, DC, National Academy Press, 2000.

33. Paulozzi LJ, Erickson JD, Jackson RJ. Hypospadias trends in two US surveillance systems. *Pediatrics*, 1997, 100:831–834.

34. *Declaration of the Environment Leaders of the Eight on Children's Environmental Health.* (http://www.library.utoronto.ca/g7/environment/1997miami/children.html).

35. *International Conference on Environmental Threats to the Health of Children: Hazards and Vulnerability.* Bangkok, 3–7 March 2002 (http://www.who.int/docstore/peh/ceh/Bangkok/bangkokconf.htm).

CHAPTER 2

Windows of susceptibility to environmental exposures in children

S. G. Selevan
National Center for Environmental Assessment/ORD
Environmental Protection Agency, Washington, DC, USA

C. A. Kimmel
National Center for Environmental Assessment/ORD
Environmental Protection Agency, Washington, DC, USA

P. Mendola
National Health and Environmental Effects Research Laboratory/ORD
Environmental Protection Agency, Research Triangle Park, NC, USA

Children have a unique susceptibility to chemical, biological and physical environmental threats. Their tissues and organs grow rapidly, developing and differentiating until maturity. The developmental and growth processes in the fetus, infant, child, and adolescent can define periods of varying vulnerability to environmental toxicants. Furthermore, the exposure patterns and behaviours of children are very different from those of adults, and may result in greater exposures.

A large number of anatomical, biochemical, and physiological changes occur from early intrauterine life through adolescence. These maturational processes may be altered by physical, biological, and chemical environmental factors at various points in time. Furthermore, the changes with maturation may themselves substantially affect the absorption, distribution, metabolism, and elimination of chemicals present in the environment. The younger and less mature the child, the more different its response may be from that of an adult. Additionally, recent evidence suggests that exposure of the embryo, fetus or young child may affect the onset of diseases in adulthood, e.g. cardiovascular and neurodegenerative diseases or cancer.

These susceptible developmental periods, called "windows of susceptibility", are times when a number of systems, including the endocrine, reproductive, immune, respiratory, and nervous systems, may be particularly sensitive to certain chemicals and physical factors. Therefore, a new "child-centred" approach to research, risk assessment and risk management is necessary to identify, understand, control, and prevent childhood or adult diseases of environmental origin.

Timing of exposure

Not only the level of exposure, but also its timing, may ultimately affect the health outcomes observed in children. During the highly susceptible periods of organ formation, timing of exposure is extremely important. For example, in the case of prenatal exposures, the same type of exposure occurring at different times is likely to produce a varied spectrum of malformations with the specific outcomes observed dependent on the organ system(s) most vulnerable at the time of exposure (Figure 2.1) (1).

In addition to highly sensitive windows for morphological abnormalities (birth defects), there are also time windows important for the development of physiological defects and morphological changes at the tissue, cellular and sub-cellular levels (Figure 2.2) (2). An adaptation of the scheme in Figure 2.2 shows the broader range of potential adverse outcomes from exposures during pre-conceptional, prenatal, and postnatal development (Figure 2.3). Many of the existing data are related to preconceptional and prenatal exposures (3). Data on prenatal exposures are based mainly on studies of maternal exposure to pharmaceuticals (e.g. diethylstilbestrol, thalidomide) and parental alcohol use,

Figure 2.1 Syndromes of malformation

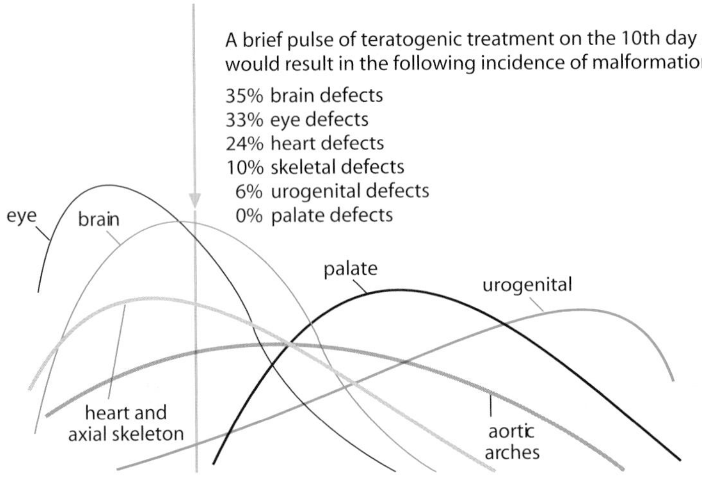

A brief pulse of teratogenic treatment on the 10th day of gestatio
would result in the following incidence of malformations:

35% brain defects
33% eye defects
24% heart defects
10% skeletal defects
 6% urogenital defects
 0% palate defects

eye   brain

palate
urogenital

heart and
axial skeleton

aortic
arches

Hypothetical representation of how the syndrome of malformations produced by a given agent might be expected to change when treatment is given at different times. The percentage of animals affected as well as the incidence ranking of the various types of malformations would be different if treatment were given on day 12 or 14, for example. Reprinted from (1) with permission of University of Chicago Press.

SECTION I: INTRODUCTION

Figure 2.2 Critical periods in human development

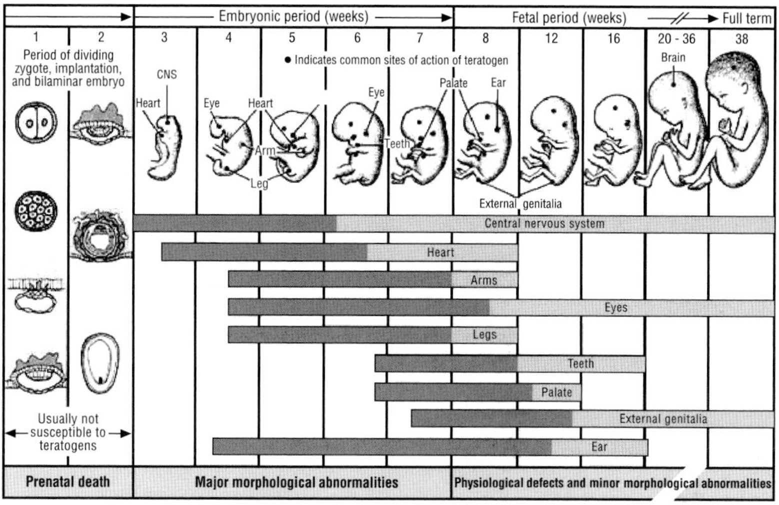

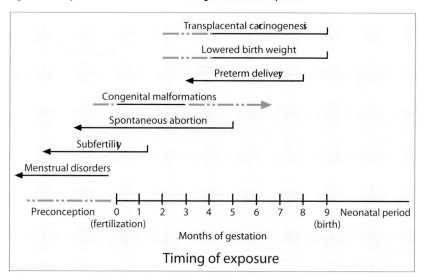

Schematic illustration of the sensitive or critical periods in human development. Dark grey denotes highly sensitive periods; light grey indicates stages that are less sensitive to teratogens. Reprinted from (2) with permission of W.B. Saunders Co.

Figure 2.3 Reproductive outcomes and timing of maternal exposure

Transplacental carcinogenesis

Lowered birth weight

Preterm delivery

Congenital malformations

Spontaneous abortion

Subfertility

Menstrual disorders

Preconception   0   1   2   3   4   5   6   7   8   9   Neonatal period
(fertilization)   (birth)

Months of gestation

Timing of exposure

Solid lines indicate the most probable timing of exposure for a particular outcome; dotted lines indicate less probable but still possible timing of exposure. Arrows suggest that a defined cut-off point for exposure to a specific outcome is not known. Reprinted from (3) with permission of Lippincott, Williams and Wilkins.

smoking, and occupational exposures. Information on critical windows for exposure during the postnatal period is scarce. Postnatal exposures have been examined in detail for only a few environmental agents, including lead, mercury, some pesticides, and radiation.

Developmental exposures may result in health effects observed:

- prenatally and at birth, such as spontaneous abortion, stillbirth, low birth weight, small size for gestational age, infant mortality, and malformation (3–6);
- in childhood, such as asthma, cancer, neurological and behavioural effects (7–10);
- at puberty, such as alterations in normal development and impaired reproductive capacity (11, 12);
- in adults, such as cancer, heart disease, and degenerative neurological and behavioural disorders (13–16).

In 1999, a multidisciplinary group reviewed the data available on preconceptional, prenatal, and postnatal developmental exposures and the subsequent outcomes, looking in detail at the respiratory, immune, reproductive, nervous, cardiovascular and endocrine systems, as well as general growth and cancer. Clear limitations were found in the data available on developmental toxicity (5).[1]

Animal studies done for regulatory testing purposes are well controlled and may include extended periods to simulate long-term human exposure. In humans, the patterns of exposure are much more variable and must be carefully evaluated with systematic studies of environmental exposures and developmental effects. Early evidence of the effects of environmental exposures on parents and children came from data on individuals with atypical exposures (e.g. industrial or environmental accidents, poisoning). These studies of atypical exposures provided information about associations between exposures and outcomes but were not usually sufficient for extrapolation because of limitations in the measurement of exposure and uncertainty as to whether exposure occurred at a biologically plausible time. More recent studies have attempted to better document exposures using environmental and biological sampling as well as measuring the level and timing of exposure.

Exposure issues vary according to the time at which they occur: before conception, prenatally, or postnatally. The preconceptional exposures of concern

---

[1] Developmental toxicity was defined as the occurrence of adverse effects on the developing organism that may result from exposure prior to conception (either parent), during prenatal development, or postnatally to the time of sexual maturation. Adverse developmental effects may be detected at any point in the lifespan of the organism. The major manifestations of developmental toxicity include death of the developing organism, structural abnormality, altered growth, and functional deficiency.

may occur acutely prior to conception or result from an increased body burden in either parent accumulated over a long period of exposure. Prenatally, exposures often change throughout pregnancy, e.g. if a woman reduces her alcohol consumption, quits smoking, or avoids using medicines. In addition to these variations, the altered absorption, distribution, metabolism, and excretion of chemicals during pregnancy result in changes in internal dosing (Table 2.1) (17). For example, pregnant women have an increased cardiac output and pulmonary function (they exchange about 72% more air over 8 hours at rest: 5000 litres in pregnant women versus 2900 litres in nonpregnant women) (18). In practice, studies of prenatal exposures in humans are difficult, as they are typically based upon one or a few measurements of exposure, which are used to estimate exposure for the entire pregnancy.

Difficulties also arise in studies of exposure in children, as these can vary enormously over time. At different developmental stages, the biology, behaviour, settings, and activities of children can result in variable exposures which may also be quite different from those of adults in the same environment (Table 2.2). For example, the ratio of surface area to body mass in infants is approximately 2.7 times that in adults; the respiratory minute ventilation rate is

Table 2.1   Physiological and toxicokinetic changes during pregnancy[a]

PARAMETER	PHYSIOLOGICAL CHANGE	TOXICOKINETIC CHANGE
Absorption		
Gastric emptying time	Increased	Absorption increased
Intestinal motility	Decreased	Absorption increased
Pulmonary function	Increased	Pulmonary exposure increased
Cardiac output	Increased	Absorption increased
Blood flow to skin	Increased	Absorption increased
Dermal hydration	Increased	Absorption +/–
Metabolism		
Hepatic metabolism	+/–	Metabolism +/–
Extrahepatic metabolism	+/–	Metabolism +/–
Plasma proteins	Decreased	Metabolism +/–
Excretion		
Renal blood flow	Increased	Increased renal elimination
Glomerular filtration rate	Increased	Increased renal elimination
Pulmonary function	Increased	Increased pulmonary elimination
Plasma proteins	Decreased	Elimination +/–

[a] Modified from Silvaggio & Mattison (17).

Table 2.2 *Differences between children and adults in certain parameters affecting environmental exposures*

PARAMETER	NEWBORN	YOUNG CHILD	OLDER CHILD	ADULT	REF.
Surface area: body mass (m²/kg)	0.067	0.047	0.033	0.025	(18)
Respiratory ventilation rates	**Infant**			**Adult**	(18)
Respiratory volume (ml/kg per breath)	10			10	
Alveolar surface area (m²)	3			75	
Respiration rate (breaths/min)	40			15	
Respiratory minute ventilation rate[a]	133			2	
	<1 year	**1–10 years**	**11–19 years**	**20–64 years**	
Mean drinking-water intake (ml/kg per day)	43.5	35.5	18.2	19.9	(19)
Fruit consumption (g/kg per day (USA))	**<1 year**	**3–5 years**	**12–19 years**	**40–69 years**	(21)
Citrus fruits	1.9	2.6	1.1	0.9	
Other fruits (including apples)	12.9	5.8	1.1	1.3	
Apples	5.0	3.0	0.4	0.4	
Soil ingestion (mg/day)					(19)
Pica child		500			
		2.5 years	**6 years**	**Adult**	
Outdoors		50	20	20[b]	
Indoors		60	2	0.4	
Differences in absorption of lead	42–53%	30–40%	18–24%	7–15%	(19)

[a] In ml/kg of body weight per m² lung surface area per minute.
[b] Gardening.

SECTION I: INTRODUCTION

more than 65 times greater (17), and consumption of drinking-water more than twice that of adults on a body weight basis (19). Even over the relatively short time span of childhood, exposure levels can vary widely.

Windows of susceptibility

Because of the variety of biological factors mentioned above, there is a greater potential for adverse health effects in children than in adults. Children are still developing in many ways and may be more vulnerable. They may be less able to avoid exposure because of immature detoxification mechanisms. Differences in metabolism, size, and behaviour may mean that they have higher levels of exposure than adults in the same environment.

It is, therefore, crucial to identify and understand the importance of the "windows of susceptibility" in children and the relationships between exposures and developmental outcomes. This requires knowing the key periods of susceptibility for specific outcomes. Information on these critical windows has been compiled in a number of reports (20). However, one of the main constraints in identifying critical windows is the limited information on the exact timing and sensitivity of various developmental stages. This underscores the importance of collecting case-specific information and detailed exposure assessments in children. For cancer, the situation is unique: tumours may be induced in a wide variety of systems at many highly vulnerable developmental stages.

Several issues that are closely related to the windows of susceptibility in children require further attention.

- The consequences of developmental exposures that are manifested in adulthood and old age should be considered: the potential cascade of events that might result in health effects in the adult is poorly understood. For example, if intrauterine growth restriction (IUGR) is associated with exposure to a particular agent, does it have the same later-life effects as nutritionally induced IUGR?
- Limited data are available on gene–environment interactions, an area identified as important for future research. Are those with certain genetic traits more likely to develop cancer or other health conditions associated with developmental exposures? Do these genetic traits impart greater vulnerability during particular developmental stages?
- The peripubertal/adolescent period is under-represented in studies of both exposure and outcomes in the current literature, despite the fact that many organ systems—especially the endocrine system—undergo significant development during this time.

More information is needed on windows of susceptibility in order to improve the risk assessment of potential environmental health threats to children, adolescents and adults. This requires increased interaction across different scientific disciplines. For example, animal laboratory data can help clinicians and epidemiologists identify areas of potential concern in humans. Epidemiological data can raise interest among laboratory researchers for developing mechanistic data and exploring agent–target interactions. Clinicians may contribute case reports that generate hypotheses for follow-up by other scientists. These interactions could help develop more sensitive methods for both clinicians and researchers for validation across species, and for enhancing the value of future studies on children's environmental health.

In summary, increased knowledge and information about children's windows of susceptibility to environmental agents will help to identify the particularly susceptible subgroups/ages and to plan for specific preventive actions. Increased dialogue among scientists from various disciplines will help to fill in the data gaps, improve measurement of exposures, and enhance the use of information to address and prevent the adverse effects of environmental threats on children's health.

References

1. Wilson JG. Embryological considerations in teratology. In: Wilson JG, Warkany J, eds. *Teratology: principles and techniques*. Chicago, The University of Chicago Press, 1965:256.

2. Moore KL, Persaud TVN. *The developing human: clinically oriented embryology*. Philadelphia, W.B. Saunders, 1973:98.

3. Selevan SG, Lemasters GK. The dose-response fallacy in human reproductive studies of toxic exposures. *Journal of Occupational Medicine*, 1987, 29: 451–454.

4. Herbst AL, Scully RE, Robboy SJ. Prenatal diethylstilbestrol exposure and human genital tract abnormalities. *National Cancer Institute Monographs*, 1979, 51:25–35.

5. Horta BL et al. Low birthweight, preterm births and intrauterine growth retardation in relation to maternal smoking. *Paediatric and Perinatal Epidemiology*, 1997, 11:140–151.

6. Gonzalez-Cossio T et al. Decrease in birth weight in relation to maternal bone-lead burden. *Pediatrics*, 1997, 100:856–862.

7. Hu FB et al. Prevalence of asthma and wheezing in public schoolchildren: association with maternal smoking during pregnancy. *Annals of Allergy, Asthma and Immunology*, 1997, 79:80–84.

8. Drews CD et al. The relationship between idiopathic mental retardation and maternal smoking during pregnancy. *Pediatrics*, 1996, 97:547–553.

9. van Duijn CM et al. Risk factors for childhood acute non-lymphocytic leukemia: an association with maternal alcohol consumption during pregnancy? *Cancer Epidemiology, Biomarkers and Prevention*, 1994, 3:457–460.

10. Daniels JL, Olshan AF, Savitz DA. Pesticides and childhood cancers. *Environmental Health Perspectives*, 1997, 105:1068–1077.

11. Blanck HM et al. Age at menarche and tanner stage in girls exposed in utero and postnatally to polybrominated biphenyl. *Epidemiology*, 2000, 11:641–647.

12. Selevan SG et al. Blood lead concentration and delayed puberty in girls. *New England Journal of Medicine*, 2003, 348:1527–1536.

13. Needleman HL et al. The long-term effects of exposure to low doses of lead in childhood. An 11-year follow-up report. *New England Journal of Medicine*, 1990, 322:83–88.

14. Miller RW. Special susceptibility of the child to certain radiation-induced cancers. *Environmental Health Perspectives*, 103(Suppl. 6):41–44.

15. Wadsworth ME, Kuh DJ. Childhood influences on adult health: a review of recent work from the British 1946 national birth cohort study, the MRC National Survey of Health and Development. *Paediatric and Perinatal Epidemiology*, 1997, 11:2–20.

16. Osmond C et al. Early growth and death from cardiovascular disease in women. *British Medical Journal*, 1993, 307:1519–1524.

17. Silvaggio T, Mattison DR. Comparative approach to toxicokinetics. In: Paul M, ed. *Occupational and environmental reproductive hazards: a guide for clinicians.* Baltimore, MD, Williams & Wilkins, 1993:25–36.

18. Snodgrass WR. Physiological and biochemical differences between children and adults as determinants of toxic response to environmental pollutants. In: Guzelian PS, Henry CJ, Olin SS, eds. *Similarities and differences between children and adults: implications for risk assessment.* Washington, DC, ILSI Press, 1992: 35–42.

19. US Environmental Protection Agency. *Exposure factors handbook. Vol 1: General factors.* Washington, DC, 1997:3–7 (EPA/600/P-95/002Fa).

20. Selevan SG, Kimmel CA, Mendola P, eds. Identifying critical windows of exposure for children's health. *Environmental Health Perspectives*, 2000, 108(Suppl 3):449–597.

21. US Environmental Protection Agency. *Exposure factors handbook. Vol. 2: Food ingestion factors.* Washington, DC, 1997:9–13; 9–19 (EPA/600/P-95/002Fa).

CHAPTER 3

Where the child lives and plays

N. Chaudhuri
Environmental Health Professional, Paris, France

L. Fruchtengarten
Paediatrician and Medical Toxicologist,
Poison Control Centre of São Paulo, Brazil

Introduction

Children are more susceptible than adults to the action of environmental toxicants. The environment where children live can cause or prevent illness, disability, and injury. A clean environment is essential for the good health and development of children. There are numerous situations in the home and in schools that may result in exposure to contaminants, such as presence of second-hand smoke (environmental tobacco smoke), spraying of insecticides, and accumulation of different materials in carpets.

The home environment

A healthy physical and psychosocial home environment is essential for the normal development of children, especially during preschool years when they spend much of their time at home. Poor quality housing and hazards found inside the home can affect their health.

In developing countries, housing may be poorly constructed because of a lack of high quality building materials and limited building skills. Housing may be located on contaminated or disaster-prone sites; basic services, such as clean water, sanitation, and waste storage and disposal may be limited; and there may be chronic rodent and insect infestation and other vectors of disease. The use of biomass stoves contributes to poor indoor air quality and overcrowded housing may favour the transmission of disease and adversely affect the mental health of children.

In the developed world, where basic services such as water, sanitation and waste management are usually provided, unhealthy housing is generally a result of poor design, construction, or lighting, or of the use of unhealthy building materials such as lead. Poor heating or ventilation systems may encourage the development of mould and dust mites, triggering chronic diseases such as asthma. Exposure to radon and electromagnetic fields may also occur.

Principles of healthy housing (1)

Protection against communicable diseases:

- safe water supply;
- sanitation;
- disposal of solid wastes;
- drainage of surface water;
- personal and domestic hygiene;
- safe food preparation;
- structural safeguards.

Protection against injuries, poisonings and chronic diseases:

- adequate structural features and furnishing;
- good air quality;
- chemical safety;
- avoidance of use of the home as workplace;

Reduction of psychological and social stress:

- adequate living space, privacy and comfort;
- personal and family security;
- access to recreation and community amenities;
- protection against noise.

Access to supportive living environment:

- security and emergency services;
- health and social services;
- access to cultural and other amenities.

Protection of groups at special risk:

- women and children;
- displaced and mobile population;
- the aged, ill and disabled.

Psychosocial factors

Housing design can influence the ability of people to satisfy their needs in terms of contact with others, privacy, play and development. Restricted opportunities for play and social isolation in high-rise apartments can produce psychological distress in children.

Poor mental health, psychiatric disorders, psychological distress in children, and worry have been found to be related to population density and overcrowding. However, the precise relationship between crowding and mental health depends on many cultural and social factors, and both low and high population densities can be detrimental to health.

Play spaces

Young children like to explore their environment, passing through an intense hand-to-mouth discovery phase, which is necessary to their development; this can place them at risk both inside and outside the home.

Because of their short stature and early crawling activities, they live much closer to the floor than adults. Children are therefore at increased risk from chemicals sprayed on gardens and fields, and during play in polluted industrial sites. An eating disorder, mainly caused by a deficiency of iron, may lead children to ingest soil and any associated toxicants.

SECTION II: HOW AND WHEN EXPOSURE OCCURS

Playgrounds present a potential risk to children and should be made safe and attractive. The majority of injuries are caused by falls. All play equipment should be located on shock-absorbing surfaces, and climbing equipment should have well defined foot and hand grips. All materials used in construction should be non-corroding and maintenance should be carried out regularly. Sand pits should be free of dirt, clay, stones, sticks and other dangerous materials.

Children should be encouraged to learn about water, its pleasures and its dangers. Children can drown in very small amounts of water, and constant supervision is needed. Pools should be covered when not in use. The chemical treatment of swimming-pools can lead to excessive inhalation of chlorine and nitric oxide by young children.

The indoor environment

Indoor air quality is influenced by outdoor air pollution, indoor sources of pollution, the characteristics of the building and the habits of the residents. High levels of indoor air pollution come from the use of open fires and inefficient stoves for cooking or heating, with combustion of biomass fuels, coal and kerosene. Gas stoves or wood-burning units that have been poorly installed and maintained, or that are inadequately ventilated, can increase indoor levels of carbon monoxide, nitrogen dioxide and particles.

There is a risk of pollution by automobile fumes in homes with attached garages. Tobacco smoke is a dangerous combustion product and a major source of fine particulate matter indoors. Pollution from traffic and industry may also influence the quality of indoor air in urban areas.

Other pollutants not associated with fuel combustion may also be of concern, including building materials such as asbestos, cement, and wood preservatives. Volatile organic compounds may be released by various materials including paints, glues, resins, stored petrol, polishing materials, perfumes, spray propellants, building materials, personal care products and cleaning agents. Formaldehyde, a component of some household products, can irritate eyes, nose and airways. The most significant sources of indoor allergens are dust mites, and feathered and furry pets. Mattresses, upholstery and carpets are primary reservoirs for such allergens.

Increased air exchange may dilute indoor airborne pollutants and prevent moisture problems, but can be difficult to achieve in certain countries during winter or with continuous use of air-conditioning in the summer.

Specific chemical contaminants
Lead

Lead is one of the most toxic chemical hazards found in houses. The main source of lead in houses is deteriorating interior and exterior lead-based paint. Lead from petrol or industrial sources may be brought into houses in contaminated dust and soil. Cottage industries that recycle lead batteries, particularly if work is conducted indoors, can be an important source of household lead. Other sources include ceramic pottery glazes, polyvinyl chloride and other plastics, and cosmetics.

Children can be exposed to lead via two pathways—either by directly ingesting paint chips or other lead-containing products (water from lead-based waterpipes) or indirectly by ingesting lead-contaminated house dust or soil through normal hand-to-mouth behaviour. Lead dust may also settle on food, creating another route of exposure.

Asbestos

Another chemical contaminant of significance is asbestos, which is found in ceiling and floor tiles, and as insulation. Exposure to asbestos may affect lung function.

Volatile organic compounds

Volatile organic compounds (VOCs) significantly influence the quality of air in homes. They are found widely in personal care and cleaning products, paints, solvents, adhesives, furnishings, pesticides and building materials, and as a byproduct of chlorinated drinking-water. Acute and chronic effects associated with exposure to VOCs include irritation and sensitization of eyes, nose, lungs and mucous membranes, narcotic effects and depression of the central nervous system.

Particulate matter

Particulate matter is small solid or liquid particles suspended in the air. In the developing world, the greatest source of particulates is the burning of biomass fuels, such as wood, charcoal, crop residues and animal dung. In developed societies, sources include cleaning activities such as vacuuming and dusting; heating, ventilation and air-conditioning systems; consumer products, such as spray disinfectants, cleaners and repellents; unvented clothes dryers; tobacco smoke; particles carried indoors from busy roads, incinerators and industrial sources. Increased rates of respiratory infections in vulnerable groups, such as children and those with pre-existing chronic respiratory disease, have been associated with the presence of high concentrations of particles (3).

Nitrogen dioxide

Nitrogen dioxide is formed at high temperatures in gas appliances, such as stoves, kerosene heaters and wood-burning stoves, as well as in cigarette smoke. Health effects associated with nitrogen dioxide exposure include irritation of the mucous membranes of the lungs; provocation of asthmatic crises either by direct pollutant effect or by inducing an allergic response in the bronchi; increased incidence of respiratory infections, sore throats, and colds.

Carbon monoxide

Carbon monoxide is a colourless, odourless gas, produced by the incomplete combustion of carbon-containing fuels, including coal, natural gas, biomass, and oil. Cigarette smoke can also produce high levels of carbon monoxide. Poorly functioning heating devices (stoves and furnaces), poor ventilation and poor elimination of combustion by-products are the usual sources of carbon monoxide indoors. Carbon monoxide is extremely toxic and exposure can be fatal. In the United Kingdom, for example, more children die from carbon monoxide poisoning than from any other poisoning (4). Acute effects include headache, fatigue and impaired exercise tolerance. Higher concentrations produce a wide range of symptoms that resemble those of gastroenteritis, influenza, cerebrovascular disease and drunkenness. Chronic exposure can produce headache, fatigue, confusion, dizziness, chest pain, visual disturbances, nausea, diarrhoea, and abdominal pain.

Pesticides

Residual insecticides have played an important role in vector control activities. Concerns exist, however, over the prolonged use of pesticides, including the development of resistance in pest species, and exposure of children to residues. Pesticides may also be found in breast milk.

Commonly used insecticides include pyrethroids, chlorpyrifos, diazinon, propoxur, dichlorvos, malathion and piperonyl butoxide. Children are at increased risk of exposure to pesticides used in residential areas because of higher concentrations near the floor and the persistence of some insecticides on carpets, furniture and soft toys. Activities of young children, such as crawling, playing on the floor, playing outdoors and hand-to-mouth behaviour, contribute to higher exposure. Ingestion and inhalation of, and contact with, house dust can be primary routes of exposure for small children. Accidental exposures may also occur when pesticides spill, leak or are improperly used, because label

Radiation

Radiation is carcinogenic to humans, and children and fetuses are especially sensitive to its effects. This is probably due to the higher rate of cell division during growth and development. While some exposure comes from natural radiation, most people are also exposed to man-made radiation. The biggest source of this is medical radiation, from diagnostic X-rays and imaging techniques, cancer treatments, etc., though these procedures do provide benefits to patients. Children may be exposed to radiation in their homes and communities, from television sets, nuclear weapons tests, waste generated from the production of nuclear power, and radon from soil and stone. High levels of radiation exposure have been linked to cancer: childhood exposure, in particular, increases the risk of leukaemia, and breast and thyroid cancer. Health risks are higher for children than for adults. Whenever possible, medical X-ray examinations of children should be avoided; in any case, the radiation doses should be kept to a minimum.

instructions are not followed or pesticides are placed in unmarked containers or in unsafe places.

In some countries, the pesticide chlorpyrifos is frequently used indoors, where it can accumulate on soft toys, furniture and carpets and later volatilize in the air. Under these conditions children may be exposed to high levels. Pesticides used to treat head lice, such as lindane, are considered as possibly carcinogenic (5). Few studies have examined the potential health effects of chronic exposure to insecticides used to control Chagas disease or malaria.

Health effects associated with pesticide use may include endocrine disruption, behavioural abnormalities, cancers and damage to the immune system. Integrated pest management (IPM) techniques, which use the least possible amount of pesticide, are recommended to avoid unnecessary exposure.

Second-hand tobacco smoke

Tobacco smoke is a mixture of gases and particles. Second-hand tobacco smoke includes sidestream smoke, the smoke emitted from a burning cigarette, cigar, or pipe, and mainstream smoke from the smoker. Health effects in infants have been correlated with close contact with smoking mothers (6). Acute health effects include eye, nose and throat irritation. Other effects include cancer, lower respiratory tract infections, respiratory symptoms (cough, phlegm and wheezing), childhood asthma, retarded lung growth and development, and middle ear disease. Some evidence exists that second-hand smoke is related to sudden infant death syndrome.

Specific biological contaminants
Dampness and mould

Dampness in a dwelling can promote the growth of several agents, such as viruses, bacteria, dust mites and mould. Damp conditions are related to prevailing climatic conditions, poor housing design and construction, and poor ventilation.

Condensation, in combination with organic materials found on walls (such as wallpaper paste), ceilings and floors, provides a good medium for mould growth. Kitchens and bathrooms are particularly prone to mould growth because of the moist conditions. The health effects of moulds include respiratory allergies, such as asthma, rhinitis, bronchitis, alveolitis, fever, chills, hoarseness, fatigue, coughing, and wheezing.

Dust mites

Dust mites are microscopic organisms, which tend to breed at a constant temperature of around 25 °C and a relative humidity of between 70% and 80%. They do not survive in cool and dry conditions. Furnishing, flooring materials, heating systems and type of house also influence the concentration of mites, which are mostly found on soft furnishings, such as sofas, fabrics, carpets, sheets, duvets, pillows and mattresses. Health effects associated with dust mite exposure include allergic reactions, bronchial asthma, allergic rhinitis and atopic dermatitis.

Pets and livestock

In many developing countries, people share their home with domestic animals, including sheep, pigs, cattle and poultry. Animal diseases may be transmitted to children through contact or via soil and dust. These diseases include anthrax, tetanus, brucellosis, tuberculosis, listeriosis, salmonellosis, rabies, psittacosis, larva migrans, histoplasmosis and mycotic dermatophytosis.

In industrialized countries, approximately 50% of households have some type of animal living in the home. Dogs, cats and other companion animals have been shown to produce health benefits. However, up to 60% of asthmatic patients show an IgE mediated hypersensitivity to cat or dog allergen. Many allergic individuals are not willing to give up a family pet for psychological reasons. In this case, pets should be kept out of the bedroom, and should preferably stay outdoors or in a well ventilated area. Soft furnishings, such as carpets or sofas, should be removed or cleaned regularly.

Water and sanitation

The availability of water of good quality is essential for children's health. Unsanitary conditions and practices in households, such as unsafe waste disposal and unhygienic behaviour in child care and food preparation, account for a large number of diseases that are transmitted via water, food and contact between individuals. Diseases such as diarrhoea, intestinal parasitic infection and resulting malnutrition, anaemia and retarded growth, blindness from trachoma, and arsenic poisoning have all been attributed to an unsafe water supply and inadequate sanitation.

Chemical contaminants may be introduced into drinking-water by various means. Naturally occurring chemicals, such as arsenic and radon, may dissolve in groundwater. Industrial and human wastewater may be discharged into surface water or groundwater. Pesticides and fertilizers applied to land and crops may wash into water sources. Lead may leach from pipes during water distribution. As far as possible, water sources should be protected to prevent chemical or microbiological contamination. Water treatment plants should be designed and operated to take all these factors into consideration to avoid health hazards.

Health benefits accrue from the provision of sufficient quantities of water through good quality community facilities, and even more so from household connections. As regards sanitation, health benefits are achieved through facilities ranging from hygienic on-site sanitation to flushing toilets to sewerage systems with effective wastewater treatment. The full health benefits of water supply and sanitation facilities can only be achieved in combination with hygiene education.

Accidents

Environmental hazards associated with home accidents may be related to bad design, poor quality of housing materials, poor maintenance, or use of defective and improperly installed equipment and appliances. Injuries, falls, burns and poisonings may result from inadequate storage of poisonous substances and dangerous items such as medicines and cleaning products; poorly placed or maintained heat sources such as open fires, and wood, oil, gas or kerosene burners; inadequate floor coverings and surfaces; poorly designed stairways and storage areas; and improperly designed or installed windows.

Crowding and density

There are several hypotheses about the health effects of crowding and population density. Crowding is a perceived condition (lack of privacy, social demands) whereas density refers to the amount of space available. High population density may increase the risk of early and repeated disease transmission in children. In addition, it increases the risk of repeated exposure to toxins. Intensive exposure at home (secondary cases) increases the severity of infection and the case–fatality ratio for infectious diseases, such as measles, chickenpox, pertussis and poliomyelitis. However, high population density may have some positive effects, e.g. children may get mild forms of viral infections which stimulate the immune system and protect against more severe infection.

Outdoor air

Outdoor air pollution can influence the quality of air found in the household. The effect is dependent on various factors, including the concentration of outdoor pollutants, the rate of infiltration, the reactivity of the contaminant, the efficiency of any mechanical filtration system and, for solids, particle size and shape. Some pollutants that have been identified as particularly hazardous include total suspended particulates ($>$10 μg) and fine particulates ($<$10 μg) from diesel exhaust, sulfur dioxide, sulfuric acid, polycyclic aromatic hydrocarbons, nitrous oxides, ozone, carbon monoxide and heavy metals such as lead.

Vector-borne diseases

Several vector-borne diseases, such as malaria, Chagas disease and dengue fever are related to housing construction and design. Malaria risk has been shown to be greater for people living in poorly constructed houses (e.g. with incomplete thatched roofs) than for those living in houses with complete brick and plaster walls and tiled roofs. Malaria risk also increases if housing is located near a body of water where mosquitoes can breed. Similar results have been found for dengue fever, where people living in houses that are fully screened are at lowest risk.

Chagas disease, which is caused by a protozoan parasite, *Trypanosoma cruzi*, is transmitted to humans by triatomine bugs. Triatomine bugs proliferate in houses made of earth, wood, and roughly plastered wattle daub, in thatch and palm roofs on a timber structure, and in walls of split and flattened bamboo.

Replacement of uneven, cracked, earth floors by cement or ceramic tiles has reduced infestation rates of *Triatoma dimidiata*. Replacement of palm-thatched roofs by corrugated tin sheets or ceramic tiles also decreases the number of infestations.

Cockroaches can be vectors of disease, such as dysentery, salmonellosis, hepatitis A, poliomyelitis, and legionnaire disease (7); cockroach antigens are also important provokers of asthma. Housing conditions and housekeeping practices influence the severity of cockroach infestations, which are fostered by the presence of food through improper storage or disposal, water from leaky pipes and taps, and points of entry such as cracks, crevices and holes in plasterwork and flooring.

Four key vector-borne diseases

A considerable proportion of the disease burden for four key vector-borne diseases—malaria, schistosomiasis, Japanese encephalitis and dengue/dengue haemorrhagic fever—falls on children under 5 years of age. Because of the vastness of this topic, readers are referred to WHO manuals and guidelines on such diseases (see www.who.int/tdr and www.who.int/ceh/risks). The particular concerns for children in relation to vector-borne diseases are summarized here.

In sub-Saharan Africa and in many countries in Asia and Latin America, children under 5 years suffer high mortality and morbidity due to **malaria**. In older children malaria remains an important cause of mortality and morbidity and significantly contributes to low educational achievement. **Schistosomiasis** is a waterborne disease that affects children and adolescents mainly because of lack of hygiene and specific behaviour, such as playing and swimming in contaminated water. High infection rates and individual worm loads produce a debilitating infection which may cause severe damage to liver and kidneys over many years, and can result in premature death. The occurrence of **Japanese encephalitis** is restricted to south and south-east Asia, where it is associated with irrigated rice production ecosystems. The annual number of clinical cases is estimated at between 30 000 and 50 000, some 90% of which are in children in rural areas. **Dengue** affects mainly urban populations (the *Aedes* species that transmit dengue are adapted to the man-made environment), and the infection can develop into dengue haemorrhagic fever or dengue shock syndrome with high levels of mortality. Annually, mortality due to dengue fever is estimated at around 13 000; more than 80% of these deaths occur in children.

Several methods are available for controlling these diseases. A combination of four interventions in different settings is proposed for the mosquito-borne diseases: the use of insecticide-impregnated mosquito nets; the screening of windows, doors and eaves of houses; the application of zooprophylaxis in places where mosquitoes are distinctly zoophilic; and the use of insect repellents. For the control of schistosomiasis, a combination of case detection and drug treatment is most cost-effective in the short term, but as prevalence drops it becomes increasingly expensive. Environmental management and community health education are then needed to make the achievement of drug treatment sustainable.

Specific physical factors
Electric and magnetic fields

Extremely low frequency (ELF) electric and magnetic fields are produced by the movement of charged particles, such as the transmission of electricity through power lines. Electric fields arise from electric charges. Common materials such as wood and metal can shield against them. The motion of electric fields gives rise to magnetic fields, which are not easily shielded and are therefore of most concern for health.

Electric and magnetic field strength in homes depends on many factors, including the distance from local power lines, the number and type of electrical appliances used in the home, and the configuration and position of household electrical wiring. Both fields decrease rapidly with distance.

The International Agency for Research on Cancer (IARC) has concluded that ELF magnetic fields above 0.4 microtesla are possibly carcinogenic to humans (8), based on consistent statistical associations of high-level magnetic fields in residential areas with increased risk of childhood leukaemia.

Noise

Noise pollution is an often overlooked environmental risk that can be detrimental to human health. As with many other environmental health concerns, children are more vulnerable than adults to noise pollution. This is because of behavioural factors, such as a child's inability to move away from a noisy situation, or a teenager's tendency to listen to loud music. Children and teenagers can have problems with learning, language development, and concentration, as well as hearing damage and tinnitus, from overexposure to noise. Exposure to excessive noise in the womb can cause babies to be born with high-frequency hearing loss. Exposure to noise above 70 decibels (dB) can cause physiological changes, such as an increase in heart rate and blood pressure. It is likely that children are routinely exposed to levels of noise even higher than this (2).

Noise pollution is not always as obvious as air or water pollution, but it is important to protect children from its harmful effects. Parents should discourage children from playing with loud toys and listening to loud music. Hearing protection should be used in cases where noise cannot be avoided, such as in work situations.

Radon

Radon is an inert radioactive gas that arises from the decay of radium 226 contained in various minerals found in soil and rock. The main source of radon gas is soil, so that highest concentrations are found in basements. Some evidence exists to suggest that 5–15% of lung cancer deaths may be associated with residential radon exposure.

References

1. *Health principles of housing.* Geneva, World Health Organization, 1989.
2. Roche AF et al. Longitudinal study of hearing in children: baseline data concerning auditory thresholds, noise exposure, and biologic factors. *Journal of the Acoustic Society of America*, 1978, 64:1593–1616.
3. Goren A et al. Respiratory problems associated with exposure to airborne particles in the community. *Archives of Environmental Health*, 1999, 54:165–171.
4. Flanagan RJ, Rooney C. Recording acute poisoning deaths. *Forensic Science International*, 2002, 128:3–19.
5. *Overall evaluations of carcinogenicity to humans.* Lyon, International Agency for Research on Cancer (www.iarc.fr).
6. Prietsch SO et al. [Acute disease of the lower airways in children under five years of age: role of domestic environment and maternal cigarette smoking.] *Journal of Pediatrics (Rio de Janeiro)*, 2002, 78:415–422 [in Portuguese].
7. Baumholtz MA et al. The medical importance of cockroaches. *International Journal of Dermatology*, 1997, 36:90–96.
8. Non-ionizing radiation, Part 1: static and extremely low-frequency (ELF) electric and magnetic fields. Lyon, International Agency for Research on Cancer, 2002 (IARC Monographs on the Evaluation of Carcinogenic Risks to Humans, No. 80).

CHAPTER 4

Where the child learns

J. Pronczuk

Department for the Protection of the Human Environment,
World Health Organization, Geneva, Switzerland

A healthy school environment is crucial for protecting children's health and promoting effective learning. Throughout the world, most children attend primary school, spending up to eight hours a day for nine months a year within classrooms and laboratories or in playgrounds and the surrounding school areas. Myriad physical, chemical and biological threats to children's health and development may be present inside or near the school (1).

A contaminated school environment can cause or exacerbate health problems such as infectious diseases or asthma, which can reduce school attendance and adversely affect learning ability. Pollutants in the school environment may also be associated with chronic health effects, such as cancer or neurological diseases, that may appear much later in life.

Environmental threats vary considerably among schools in urban and rural areas, within communities, countries and regions. The health and pollution problems are generally related to levels of prosperity, and some may exist only in certain climates or geographical areas, but many problems are global. Contaminated water or food can result in diarrhoeal disease, which is more common in poor countries, but may also affect schoolchildren in industrialized countries. Air pollution around a school may result from industries or heavy traffic, and this happens both in developed and developing countries. Exposure to lead in paint is a risk in the old urban schools of some industrialized countries. Exposure of schoolchildren to pesticides may occur following their application to combat vectors of disease or may result from drift after field application in agricultural areas (2).

Infectious diseases carried by water and physical risks associated with poor construction and maintenance are examples of risks children face in schools throughout the world.

What is the physical school environment?

The physical school environment includes the school building and all its contents (physical structure, furniture, chemicals and biological agents in use or storage), the site on which the school is located, and the surrounding environment (air, water, materials that children use or touch, nearby land uses and roadways) (3).

What are the main threats in the school environment?

Potential environmental threats present in the school and surroundings include indoor and outdoor air pollution, contaminated drinking- and recreational water, lack of sanitation, contaminated food, vector-borne diseases, unsafe buildings, and ultraviolet radiation. Other conditions that can adversely affect children are extreme temperatures (very cold or hot buildings), lack of light and ventilation, and overcrowding.

Lack of adequate sanitation facilities not only represents a health threat to children but also leads to absenteeism, especially among girls (who in some countries leave school once they reach adolescence, because of the lack of adequate toilets).

In urban areas, children are exposed to outdoor air pollution from industry and traffic exhaust on their way to school, and these pollutants may enter the classrooms. Many children spend much of their school day indoors. The air they breathe inside their school may be more polluted than outdoor air. For example, in many rural schools, biomass fuels are used for heating and for the preparation of school meals, potentially exposing children to high levels of indoor air pollution. Carbon monoxide, resulting from inadequate combustion in heating devices, poses a very severe risk to the health and life of children. Indoor air pollution results also from deficient heating systems, as well as mould, cockroach and rat detritus, and lack of ventilation. Poor indoor air quality may increase the incidence of asthma, allergies, and infectious and respiratory diseases, and also affect the performance of intellectual tasks involving concentration, calculation, and memory (1).

In some parts of the world, rural areas are polluted by the smoke from burning forests ("haze"). Drinking- and recreational water in schools may be contaminated with metals (e.g. lead and arsenic), fluorides, organic solvents, viruses and bacteria. Vector-borne diseases, such as malaria, yellow fever, and dengue fever, may also affect children at school. Unsafe building structures increase the risk of falls, trauma and lesions. This may be the case especially in schools that are installed in old houses, which are totally unfit for educational purposes. Old buildings may have lead in paint, asbestos insulation, and mould in the walls.

New schools may be constructed on undesirable land, on sites that pose health hazards. A famous example in the USA is the Love Canal dumpsite in Niagara Falls, New York, where schools constructed on a former industrial landfill were closed after testing showed excessive levels of contamination (4).

Exposure to ultraviolet radiation occurs when children play and do sports in non-shaded areas around the school.

Children's behaviour may increase the risks of exposure (e.g. exploring dangerous areas, touching objects and placing fingers in the mouth, not washing the hands, rubbing the eyes). Adolescents often tend to act on impulse and take risks (e.g. climbing and jumping or experimenting with drugs) and may lack the experience to judge the risks associated with their behaviour.

What health effects can result from an adverse school environment?

Acute respiratory infections (ARI). They are the most common disease in children throughout the world, and pneumonia is the biggest cause of childhood mortality. ARI are linked to indoor and outdoor air pollution and other environmental factors (5).

Asthma. Asthma and chronic respiratory illnesses such as bronchitis are growing problems, especially in industrialized countries. Both indoor and outdoor air pollution may increase the severity of the disease. Wood smoke, moulds, and many volatile chemicals found in indoor environments can affect the respiratory function in schoolchildren. School absenteeism associated with these respiratory diseases can adversely affect both intellectual and emotional development (6).

Diarrhoeal diseases. The second most common global illness affecting young children and a major cause of death in low-income countries, diarrhoeal diseases are closely associated with poor sanitation, poor hygiene, and lack of access to clean water and food. Although diarrhoeal diseases are most deadly in the developing world, they are also a significant health threat in developed countries (7).

Vector-borne diseases. Mosquitoes, ticks, rodents, and flies may be present in the school and are significant disease vectors. Mosquitoes can transmit malaria, dengue fever, yellow fever, filariasis, and Japanese encephalitis. Ticks can transmit Lyme disease, tick-borne encephalitis, and different fevers. Rodents are capable of spreading plague (transmitted from rats to humans by fleas), leptospirosis, and various viral and rickettsial diseases. In sub-Saharan Africa, tsetse flies can cause trypanosomiasis (8).

Foodborne disease. In developing countries, a polluted environment, lack of safe water supply and poor sanitation increase the likelihood of food becoming contaminated. However, in all countries outbreaks of foodborne illness may result from improper food handling, such as use of contaminated equipment, contamination by infected persons, use of contaminated raw ingredients, cross-contamination, and addition of toxic chemicals or use of food containing natural toxins (9).

Accidents and injuries. In high-income countries road traffic accidents are the most common cause of death among school-age children (5 out of every 100 000 deaths) and in low- and middle-income countries they are the third leading cause of death along with drowning (nearly 15 out of every 100 000 deaths). Children attending schools located near busy roads or water bodies are at increased risk of these types of accidents. Falls and other accidents within the school grounds can occur as a result of poor construction and poor maintenance (10).

Poisoning. Children can be poisoned at school as a result of the improper storage or application of pesticides, or from exposure to lead in paint chips and air, or chemicals in cleaning products. The effects of long-term exposure to lead, pesticides and other pollutants on children's health and development are likely to outweigh the effects of acute poisonings (10).

Cancer. Some environmental childhood exposures, such as to ionizing and ultraviolet radiation, environmental tobacco smoke, some pesticides, solvents, radon and arsenic, may contribute to the cancers that develop in adulthood (2).

Developmental disabilities. Environmental factors are suspected to play a role in the "epidemic" of learning and behavioural disabilities observed in some parts of the world. Developmental disabilities are believed to be a significant and frequently undetected health problem in developing countries, where malnutrition and parasitosis (especially helminth infections) may contribute to these illnesses (11). For example, in India, undernourished rural children 10–12 years of age had learning deficiencies when compared with normally nourished children. Schools could play an important role in ensuring that students have nutritious food to eat every day.

Exposure to toxic substances such as lead and mercury may induce developmental disorders. Children may suffer permanent brain damage from exposure to lead, causing learning disabilities, hearing loss, reduced attention span, and behavioural abnormalities.

What is a healthy physical school environment?

WHO defines a health promoting school as "one that constantly strengthens its capacity as a healthy setting for living, learning and working". A healthful school environment protects students and staff against immediate injury or disease, promotes prevention activities, and teaches about risk factors that might lead to disease or disability.

Access to safe water and sanitation and shelter from the elements are the basic necessities for a healthy physical learning environment. Equally important is protection from biological, physical, and chemical risks that can threaten children's health (see box below).

Why do children need a safe school environment?

Children require safe schools, with clean water to drink, adequate sanitation facilities for boys and girls, clean air to breathe, safe and nutri-

Components of a healthy school environment

Provision of basic necessities
Shelter
Warmth
Water
Food
Light
Ventilation
Sanitary facilities
Emergency medical care

Protection from biological threats
Moulds
Waterborne pathogens
Foodborne pathogens
Vector-borne diseases
Venomous animals
Rodents
Hazardous insects

Protection from physical threats
Traffic and transport
Violence and crime
Accidents
Radiation

Protection from chemical threats
Air pollution
Water pollution
Pesticides
Hazardous waste
Hazardous materials and finishes
Cleaning agents

tious food, and a clean and quiet place to learn and play. This allows them to grow and develop normally, and enhances their learning capacity.

Furthermore, schools represent an example for the community. As people become aware of how environmental risks are dealt with at school they will recognize ways to make other environments (home, playground, workplace) safer. In addition, students who learn about the link between the environment and health will be able to recognize and remedy health threats in their own homes when they become adults.

It is therefore important to provide the information that will help people understand the relationship between the environment and health, identify key hazards in the places where children live, play, learn and work, in particular in the school environment, and recognize children's special vulnerability and exposure to environmental health threats. The health care provider should be able to detect and prevent those childhood diseases and effects that may be linked to the environment where the child learns.

References

1. *The physical school environment. An essential component of a health-promoting school*. Geneva, World Health Organization, 2003.

2. Sanborn M et al. *Pesticides literature review*. Toronto, Ontario College of Family Physicians, 2004 (www.ocfp.on.ca).

3. *School health and youth health promotion*. Geneva, World Health Organization (www.who.int/hpr/gshi/index.htm).

4. Brown P, Clapp R. Looking back on Love Canal. *Public Health Reports*, 2002, 117:95–98.

5. *Health and environment in sustainable development. Five years after the Earth Summit*. Geneva, World Health Organization, 1997.

6. Aubier M. Air pollution and allergic asthma. *Revue des Maladies Respiratoires*, 2000, 17:159–165.

7. Martines J et al. Diarrhoeal diseases. In: Jamison DT et al., eds. *Disease control priorities in developing countries*. Oxford, Oxford Medical Publications, 1993.

8. Vectors of diseases, hazards and risks for travelers. Part 1. *Weekly Epidemiological Record*, 2001, 76:189–196.

9. International Life Sciences Institute. Global approach to prevent, detect, and treat food-borne disease. *ILSI News*, 1997, 159.

10. *Healthy environments for children: initiating an alliance for action*. Geneva, World Health Organization, 2002.

11. Oberhelman RA et al. Correlations between intestinal parasitosis, physical growth, and psychomotor development among infants and children from rural Nicaragua. *American Journal of Tropical Medicine and Hygiene*, 1998, 58:470–475.

CHAPTER 5

Where the child works[1]

M. Tennassee
Division of Health and Environment, Pan American Health
Organization, Washington, DC, USA

Introduction

Every day, around the world, millions of children go to work instead of school. The main reason for this is poverty, especially in developing countries. But poverty is not the only reason for the existence of child labour; other factors play a role, including inefficiency in educational systems and in enforcement of relevant legislation, and lack of public awareness (1).

Children are different from adults in anatomy, physiology and psychology. They are more vulnerable to hazards, such as long hours at work, exposure to chemicals and physical risk factors, and psychological conditions. Many children work in dangerous occupations and industries, and are exposed to extremely dangerous situations and exploitative and abusive conditions. Dangerous occupations are included in Convention No. 182 of the International Labour Organization (ILO) on the worst forms of child labour. Governments, employers, workers' organizations, universities, nongovernmental organizations (NGOs), occupational health professionals and other interested parties need to work together to establish programmes to eliminate these dangerous forms of child labour and to protect children at work.

Characteristics and trends in child labour

In 2002, ILO estimated the number of working children aged between 5 and 14 years to be about 211 million worldwide. Of these, 127.3 million are in the Asia–Pacific region, 48 million in sub-Saharan Africa, 17.4 million in Latin America and the Caribbean, and 13.4 million in the Eastern Mediterranean and North Africa (2). Developed and transition economies have the lowest numbers of child labourers, with 2.5 million and 2.4 million, respectively.

According to the World Bank (1), in general, child labour participation rates in the workforce are much higher in rural than in urban areas, and three-quarters of working children work in a family enterprise. In rural areas, 90% of working children are engaged in agricultural or similar activities, while their urban counterparts are found mainly in trade and services, with fewer in manufacturing and construction. The same report of the World Bank found relatively

---

[1]Reviewed by **Dr Gerry Eijkemans**, Occupational and Environmental Health, WHO, Geneva, Switzerland.

few child workers in export industries (such as textile, clothing, carpets, and footwear) compared with the numbers involved in activities geared to domestic consumption.

In the United States, more than 5 million adolescents under 18 years are legally employed, and a further 1–2 million are believed to be employed in violation of wage, hours, or safety regulations (3). According to household surveys (4), there are 11.6 million children between 10 and 14 years old working in Latin America and the Caribbean. If children under 10 years working in domestic service are included, the total child workers in Latin America and the Caribbean reach almost 18 million. The ILO estimates that one in five children in Latin America is economically active (Table 5.1).

Table 5.1 Economically active child population in Latin America

COUNTRY	TOTAL POPULATION AGED 10–14 YEARS	ECONOMICALLY ACTIVE POPULATION 10–14 YEARS	
		NO.	%
Argentina	3 197 582	214 238	6.70
Bolivia	386 222	54 549	14.10
Brazil	16 664 591	1 935 269	11.61
Chile*	755 227	14 914	2.00
Colombia*	2 327 823	367 796	15.80
Costa Rica*	203 893	26 009	12.80
Ecuador	1 391 433	420 663	30.20
El Salvador	661 176	85 516	12.90
Guatemala	1 325 725	316 061	23.80
Haití	847 706	158 182	18.66
Honduras	778 714	88 264	11.30
Mexico	10 934 134	1 233 353	11.30
Nicaragua	575 137	42 310	7.35
Panama	278 631	12 603	4.50
Paraguay	602 417	49 097	8.15
Peru**	4 928 899	801 033	16.20
Dominican Republic	871 144	42 302	4.80
Uruguay	253 846	5 278	2.08
Venezuela	3 205 592	80 781	2.52
TOTAL	**50 189 892**	**5 948 720**	**11.85**

*Figures refer to population aged 12 to 14 years.
**Figures refer to population aged 6 to 14 years.
Source: ref. 5.

Working conditions

There are some conditions that increase the risk to child workers. As noted in an earlier chapter, children are not "little adults". Most biological systems in the human body do not mature until about the age of 18. Many differences in anatomy, physiology, and psychology distinguish children from adults. These differences may translate into unique risk factors for occupational injuries and illnesses (6), stemming from the nature of the work or from poor working conditions. Because they are physically immature, children are more vulnerable to the effects of arduous work and exposure to dangerous chemical substances. Children are not physically suited to long hours of strenuous and monotonous work and they suffer the effects of fatigue more than adults. Such labour can have an effect on their intellectual development and physical health. Although most working children combine work and school, often child labourers lack educational opportunities (2, 7).

What is particularly important is not so much the fact that the child works, but the conditions in which he or she works. There is a huge difference between a child who does 2 hours of light work a day, after going to school, and one who works long hours in hazardous conditions. It is fundamental to make this distinction in order to prioritize action at national and local level.

Risk factors related to the physical environment

Most information about the health outcomes of child workers relates to injuries, but illness may also result when children and adolescents are exposed to hazardous materials, processes or tasks, or working conditions. Child workers may be exposed to pesticides during farm work, benzene during work at petrol stations, lead during vehicle repair, asbestos and silica during construction and maintenance work, and loud noise during manufacturing, construction, and farm work, to name a few. Exposures to hazardous materials and working conditions may result in immediate illness or illness that is not detected for months or years after exposure. In both cases, the association with work exposure may or may not be recognized (Table 5.2) (6).

According to ILO (9), a large number of working children are affected by various physical, chemical and biological hazards; more than two-thirds (69%) of them are found in the same countries. Many children suffer injuries or illness, including punctures, burns and skin diseases, eye and hearing impairment, respiratory and gastrointestinal illnesses, fever, and headache from excessive heat. The surveys carried out so far have assisted in identifying the specific industries and occupations that are harmful to children. According to ILO (4), hazardous workplaces for children include brick mould factories, mines, quarries, marketplaces, rocketry manufacturing sites, domestic service, and agriculture. Although more than two-thirds (70.4%) of all working children are in the agricultural sector, where a large proportion of injuries occur, injuries also occur in the construction, mining and transport sectors (10).

Table 5.2 **Some examples of hazardous agents to which working children may be exposed**

HAZARDOUS AGENT	SOURCES OF EXPOSURE	HEALTH EFFECTS
Biological agents		
Contact with bacteria or viruses, through contact with domestic and wild animals	Abattoirs, agricultural animals, bone and meat processing, butcher's shops, ivory and horn processing, poultry, stock, tanneries	Anthrax, asthma, brucellosis, catarrh, dermatitis, herpes, Q fever, leptospirosis, rabies, rat bite fever, ringworm, salmonellosis, toxoplasmosis, tuberculosis
Cotton, flax, linen	Mixing and carding rooms, rope-making, textiles, twine-making, ball-pressing plants, cotton ginneries	Byssinosis
Physical agents		
Compressed air	Deep-sea diving	Decompression sickness
Noise	Textile engineering works, boilers, explosives, compressors	Hearing impairments
Chemical agents (including metals)		
Organophosphorus compounds	Use of pesticides in agriculture	Severe poisoning, neurological impairment, death
Chromium and its compounds	Production or use of chromium salts, chromium plating, leather tanning, metallurgy, refractory bricks	Asthmatic bronchitis, impaired lung function, lung cancer, ulcerations and perforation of nasal septum
Coal dust (associated with silica) coal tar derivatives	Coal mines	Anthracosilicosis (pulmonary fibrosis), lung cancer
Asbestos dust	Brake linings, cement filter for plastics, fire smothering blankets, mining of asbestos, safety garments, thermal and electrical insulation	Asbestosis (pulmonary fibrosis), lung cancer

Source: Modified from ref. 8.

Factors related to work organization (amount of safety training and supervision) may increase the risk of injuries and illnesses among children and adolescents. In a telephone survey, cited by the US National Institute for Occupational Safety and Health (NIOSH) (6), 54% of workers aged 14 to 16 years with work injuries reported receiving no training in methods to prevent their injuries. According to NIOSH, in the United States, every year at least 70 children under 18 years die at work, and more than 77 000 are injured severely enough to seek care in emergency departments (6).

The usual routes of exposure of children at work are:

- dermal—especially to chemicals such as pesticides (in lawn care and agriculture), nicotine (while harvesting tobacco) and solvents (in vehicle bodywork repair);
- inhalation—from metal fumes (such as lead), ammonia, isocyanates and shellac;
- ingestion—of dangerous agents such as lead and other heavy metals (10).

Child labour is more common in rural areas and concentrated in the informal sector of the economy. In some countries, a significant percentage of working children are under the age of 10. Children not only work long hours and may be exposed to physical, psychological, and social hazards that prevent their normal development; they may also suffer intolerable exploitation such as slavery, servitude, forced labour, and sexual abuse.

In urban areas, children can be found working in trade, domestic service, construction and manufacturing sectors, as well as begging and performing different tasks on the street.

In manufacturing, they may suffer serious cuts, fractures, burns, skin diseases, and respiratory illnesses. Table 5.3 shows some potential job-related exposures of child workers.

Psychosocial risk factors

"Child labour damages children's physical and mental health . . . Working children are more vulnerable than adult workers not only for physiological reasons, but also because of a combination of psychological and social reasons. Some children at work are under psychological stress. The motivation for them to start working and to retain the job is to contribute to the financial support of the family, which is a heavy responsibility at an early age. . . . [they] may prefer to face a challenge rather than be considered weak by the other playmates and therefore may attempt the riskiest tasks" (8).

The psychosocial risk factors are extremely important in children who work under the unconditional worst forms of child labour, such as defined in ILO convention C182 (1999). In slavery and forced labour systems, the most common of which is debt bondage, children work to pay off a debt or other obligations incurred by the family. There are also less "formal" types of child slavery and forced labour, in which rural children are lured to the city with false promises of work, only to be forced into domestic service or sweatshops. Children are

Table 5.3 Potential job-related exposures of child workers

Bloodborne pathogens—in nursing homes and hospitals

Cleaning agents—in restaurants, nursing homes, schools

Pesticides—in lawn care, farm work, and when buildings are sprayed

Isocyanates—during vehicle bodywork repair or roofing with newer forms of roofing materials

Benzene—when pumping petrol

Lead—from radiators in vehicle repair and home renovation

Asbestos—in vehicle brake repair, renovation/demolition of old buildings

Solvents—in T-shirt screening

Second-hand smoke—in restaurants and bars

Heat—in washing dishes, in working outdoors in hot weather

Cold—in outdoor jobs in cold weather

Wood dusts—in furniture making

Fumes and eye damage—in welding

Chemicals and dyes—in cosmetic manufacture

Biological/infectious hazards—in farming, work with animals

Noise-induced hearing loss—in farms and factories

Nicotine—in harvesting of tobacco

Source: adapted from ref. 11.

also being used in drug trafficking in many cities of Latin America, and are themselves victims of drug trafficking organized by criminal networks.

As they grow, children experience profound psychological changes as well as physical and physiological ones. The psychological transition is often less visible than the physical one, requires more time to complete, and typically lags behind physical maturation. Thus psychological immaturity may be obscured by a relatively mature physical appearance in an adolescent. As a result, a child worker may be assigned to a task for which he or she is emotionally or cognitively unprepared. In addition, young workers often do not have adequate experience to judge their ability to complete an assignment safely. There is no easy way of characterizing the complex psychological development that takes place during adolescence and the potential consequences for working adolescents. A general lack of work experience, coupled with normal adolescent psychological development, places adolescents at high risk of injury at work.

It is important to mention the situation of live-in child domestic workers, i.e. children who work full-time in other people's households, doing domestic chores, caring for children, running errands, etc., in exchange for room, board, care, and some remuneration (12). The number of children in this position is literally uncountable at present because of the "hidden" nature of the work, which lies largely beyond the scope of conventional labour market mechanisms. However, improved statistical survey methods being pioneered by the ILO indicate that the practice, especially in the case of girls, is extensive. In Brazil, for example, 22% of working children are employed in domestic service. The majority of child domestic workers are between 12 and 17 years old, but some surveys have identified children as young as 5 or 6 years. Their hours of work are usually long—15 or 16 hours a day is not uncommon. There is also alarming evidence of physical, mental and sexual abuse (12).

Child domestic workers usually come from poor families and the majority will probably remain poor throughout their lives. Work as a child domestic worker perpetuates poverty, as it usually does not allow for an education. In addition, it is rare for the child to receive payment directly, if at all; wages may be paid directly to the parents, if contact is maintained, but often the employer provides food, shelter and clothing instead of payment. Regardless of the type of employment, the assigned duties often go beyond the children's ability.

Children may often work 15 or more hours a day, seven days a week. In studies that have examined their physical wellbeing, children complain of fatigue, headaches and other health problems. Accidents are a risk, in particular when the child is exhausted. There are hazards associated with cooking, boiling water, chopping vegetables, using cleaning fluids and carrying heavy items. Burns are relatively common among child domestic workers. The Innocenti Digest on Child Domestic Work, issued in May 1999, states that the possibility of sexual abuse or exploitation presents risks of sexually transmitted diseases and early pregnancy in these girls. Usually pregnancy leads to dismissal and in some countries rejection by the girl's own family. In addition, the isolation and ill-treatment that child domestic workers endure may lead to low self-esteem. Health care providers should be alert to any signs, symptoms, or indications that may suggest that there is child labour. In this case, they should explain and discuss the problem with parents and care-givers and involve the relevant social actors who could take appropriate action.

References

1. Fallon PR. *Child labour: issues and directions for the World Bank*. Washington, DC, World Bank, 1998.
2. *Every child counts: new global estimates on child labour*. Geneva, International Labour Office, 2002 (www.ilo.org).
3. American Academy of Pediatrics, Committee on Environmental Health. The hazards of child labour. *Pediatrics*, 1995, 95:311–313.
4. *Action against child labour 1999–2001. Progress and future priorities*. Geneva, International Programme on the Elimination of Child Labour, International Labour Office, 2001.
5. International Programme on the Elimination of Child Labour. *Working Document*, San José, International Labour Office, 2002 (Brochure).

6. National Institute for Occupational Safety and Health. *Child labour research needs. Recommendations from the NIOSH Child Labour Working Team.* Washington, DC, US Department of Health and Human Services. Public Health Service. Centers for Disease Control and Prevention, 1997.

7. *Action against child labour: lessons and strategic priorities for the future. A synthesis report.* Geneva, International Labour Office, 1997.

8. Forastieri V. *Children at work. Health and safety risks.* 2nd ed. Geneva, International Labour Office, 2002, 169 pages.

9. International Programme on the Elimination of Child Labour. *Action against child labour. Achievements, lessons learned and indicators for the future (1998–1999).* Geneva, International Labour Office, 1999.

10. Fassa AG. *Health benefits of eliminating child labour.* Geneva, International Labour Organization, 2003.

11. Workplaces. In: *Handbook of pediatric environmental health.* Elk Grove Village, IL, American Academy of Pediatrics, 1999:295–304.

12. *Child domestic work. Innocenti Digest.* New York, United Nations Children's Fund, 1999.

CHAPTER 6

Where the child is under extreme stress[1]

R. Bu-Hakah
Department of Emergency and Humanitarian Action, World Health Organization, Geneva, Switzerland

How and when does exposure happen?

Too many children throughout the world are confronted with extreme stress from a variety of sources, including war and conflict, environmental disasters, physical and emotional abuse, loss of parents and being forced to abandon their homes. In such situations, survival becomes the child's instinctive and primary concern.

Mechanisms of exposure

Under extreme circumstances, such as floods, droughts, environmental and technological disasters, and wars and conflict situations, and the consequent displacement and refugee movement, the whole spectrum of threats to children's health changes. Extreme situations can be described in terms of four characteristics:

- speed of onset (sudden or gradual);
- duration;
- type (natural, technological, conflict);
- impact.

Children's exposure to these threats can be (1) sudden or slow, (2) acute or chronic, (3) direct or indirect, (4) purposeful or unintentional. Exposure may occur in the familiar environment, with minimal change in its physical characteristics. Alternatively, exposure can take place in a completely new environment, as in the case of refugee children. Table 6.1 summarizes the various situations, their characteristics, effects and consequences.

Despite the characterizations mentioned above, there is tremendous complexity surrounding each extreme situation. For example, an earthquake can occur in a known physical environment but it causes the destruction of familiar landmarks, such as homes, schools and churches. An unfamiliar and

---

[1] Reviewed by **C. Corvalan**, Department for the Protection of the Human Environment, World Health Organization, Geneva, Switzerland; **A. Loretti**, Department of Emergency and Humanitarian Action, World Health Organization, Geneva, Switzerland; **D. Rasmussen**, Department of Emergency and Humanitarian Action, World Health Organization, Geneva, Switzerland.

Table 6.1 Summary of various types of traumatic situations, their characteristics, initial effects and consequences

SITUATION	ONSET	INCREASED EXPOSURE TO ENVIRONMENTAL THREATS	NEW RISKS	CHANGE IN SURROUNDINGS	BREAKDOWN OF SOCIETY/COMMUNITY STRUCTURE	VIOLENCE	INCREASED POVERTY
Drought	slow	+	−	+	−	−	+
Flood	sudden	++	++	+ or ++	−	−	+
Earthquake	sudden	+++	++	+++	−	−	+
Volcano	sudden	+++	++	+++	−	−	+
War	sudden	+	+++	+++	++	+++	+
	chronic	+	++	+++	+++	+++	+
Refugee/displacement	chronic	+	++	+++	+++	+++	+
Technological	slow	++	++	+++	−	−	++
	sudden	+++	+++	++	−	−	+

+, slight; ++, moderate; +++, significant; −, no change.

6. WHERE THE CHILD IS UNDER EXTREME STRESS

unsettled environment surrounds the child when he or she is on the move, displaced or seeking refuge in another province or in another country as a result of a natural disaster or conflict. Alternatively, in conflicts and ongoing wars, the physical environment may be only mildly damaged but the normal life activities, and even the societal structure, change.

Under these extreme circumstances, the risk of exposure to environmental threats is typically increased. There may be greater potential for water- and food-borne diseases, poisoning, air pollution, electrocution, traffic accidents and other injuries. Other risks may be rare, unforeseen or unconventional, including injury by landmines and unexploded ordnance, exposure to nuclear radiation or depleted uranium, or spewing of hot ashes and burning lava from a volcanic eruption. Sadly, in some countries these formerly unanticipated threats are becoming commonplace. In Angola, for example, which is plagued with an extraordinary number of landmines, the probability of stumbling on a landmine is higher than that for any other trauma (1, 2).

Health consequences

The consequences of extreme stress can be severe in both physical and psychological terms. Lack of adequate nutrition, unavailability of water, spread of communicable disease, exposure to toxic chemicals, loss of housing and increased violence are just some of the physical threats that confront children in such situations. Children living in war zones or areas of conflict are subject to violence, which they either witness or experience directly. Environmental threats may provoke respiratory illnesses, enteric infections, and vector-borne diseases. Many children die in infancy, and maternal mortality and incidence of miscarriage and stillbirth often rise significantly. During flight from an acute threat, such as war or natural disaster, children often become separated from their families and their communities and ethnic groups. Many are orphaned. In some countries, large numbers of children have been kidnapped to serve as "military slaves" or recruited as child soldiers in prolonged situations of conflict.

Emotional trauma, depression, grief and fear are some of the psychological effects manifested in children under extreme stress. In a war situation, children may become accustomed to violence, losing the ability to empathize, and may become aggressive. In one study, emotional and stress disorders were observed in children in situations of extreme stress, in the form of sleep disorders and nightmares. Children become fearful, their personalities may change, they become withdrawn, and are unable to play (3).

What to do for a child who is extremely stressed

The United Nations Children's Fund (UNICEF) publication, *Facts for life* (4), serves as an excellent resource on assisting children who are especially stressed. This publication offers key messages on addressing the challenges that children confront in such situations. Providing access to basic nutrition, water and sanitation are the first challenges. Consideration of psychological stability, stress management and emotional health is important for children, both during and after the crisis. Other important steps for alleviating stressful situations are summarized in the box opposite.

Remedial action, prevention and education

Disasters can kill large numbers of people at one time. The number will depend on the vulnerability or susceptibility of a community to hazards and its resilience. Emergency preparedness at the individual, community and national level can alleviate the physical and emotional effects on all citizens. Children largely depend on families, communities and other sources of aid to prepare for disasters. Information resources are available that provide guidelines and recommendations for emergency preparedness for different types of situations (5). These are summarized in Table 6.2.

Key messages on action in emergency situations

What every family and community has a right to know about disasters and emergencies

1. In disaster or emergency situations, children should receive essential health care, including measles vaccination, adequate food and micronutrient supplements.
2. Breastfeeding is particularly important in emergency situations.
3. It is always preferable for children to be cared for by their parents or other familiar adults, especially during conflict situations, because it makes children feel more secure.
4. Violence in the home, war and other disasters can frighten and anger children. When such events occur, children need special attention, extra affection and the opportunity to express their feelings and to describe their experiences in ways that are appropriate for their age.
5. Landmines and unexploded ammunition are extremely dangerous. They should never be touched or stepped over. Establish safe play areas for children and warn them not to play with unknown objects.

Source: ref. 4.

Table 6.2 Summary of emergency preparedness and mitigation

DISASTER	NATIONAL LEVEL	COMMUNITY LEVEL	FAMILY LEVEL	HEALTH PROFESSIONAL
Natural disasters Earthquake Floods Drought Landslide Volcanic eruption Bush fires Cyclones	National disaster plan Disaster committee National drills Organization of training and re-certification for health, search and rescue teams, police, army Early warning system Communication networks and alternatives Laws Hazard mapping Insurance Disaster funds Public information campaigns (media, schools, health facility) for public education, warning and for support during response Emergency stocks (food, water purification, drugs and medical supplies) Health facilities assessments and reduction of vulnerability Evacuation plans and responsibilities Development of provincial/ district and sector-specific disaster plans	Community disaster committee Participation of sector/ societies representatives from health, water, engineering, police, fire fighters, civil defence, education, local media, clerics and social workers Community disaster plan, education campaign targeting schools, health facilities and industrial plants Hazard identification at the level of community Drills and simulation Identification of possible shelter facilities Emergency stocks Early warning system based on communication facilities and networks Evacuation routes, responsibilities and plans First aid courses and volunteer training and identification Coordination with other neighbouring communities	Family disaster plan: knowing what disasters are most likely to happen, learning about community warning signals, knowing location of emergency shelters, knowing where family members are likely to be and ensure numbers/contacts, explaining danger of fire, severe weather, floods, and earthquakes to children, having a place to meet outside house in case of a disaster, stocks for at least 3 days, supplies, change of clothes, blankets, sanitation supplies, first-aid kit and prescriptions, learning how to turn off water, electric fuse box and gas, keeping radio and batteries, taking first-aid course.	Participation or identifying community disaster committee Training in disasters and emergencies Participating in drills Maintain updated knowledge and information about hazards Ensuring that health facility/workplace has a disaster plan and reducing its vulnerability to disasters Participating in public education and information campaigns, distributing information material Educating families and children about disaster risks and protection Preparing with social workers for support in case of a disaster Ensuring stocks of essential drugs and supplies Disease surveillance networks and alternatives

| Epidemics | In addition to above and especially for the Ministry of Health:

Procedures for obtaining funds and other resources such as transportation, drugs, vaccines, health workers

Intersectoral collaboration

Coordination with private sector and with NGOs, implementation of key environmental measures

Surveillance systems activated and level of alert heightened

Training of health care staff, and a core of epidemiologists

Ensuring communication systems at health facility and timely reporting

Establishing network of laboratories and procedures for collection and testing samples

Case management protocols

Public health mapping | In addition to the above (disaster committee):

Updated lists of health providers, laboratories, pharmacists and facilities

Identification of alternatives for health facilities and isolation wards

Public health community disaster plan

Public education and information campaign (media and special events) and community health education programmes

First aid/volunteers training

Dissemination of simplified protocols and flowcharts to teachers, social workers

Early warning and reporting procedures

Health education in school curricula/youth clubs

Ensuring regular and adequate implementation of environmental measures for controlling infections such as spraying, sanitization of food preparation areas, solid waste disposal, disinfecting and protecting water sources | Health education on basic hygiene and disease transmission, protective measures, signs of some epidemic diseases

Training on home-based care

Immunization and regular visits to health facilities

List of emergency contacts (doctor, nurse, health worker) | Training and keeping updated knowledge

Simulations and drills

Delivering health education messages

Participating in community activities with health focus

Distributing information booklets and brochures about epidemic diseases

Documenting cases and reporting cases of epidemic prone diseases

Ensuring and advocating environmental protection measures such as sanitization of food preparation areas, spraying, solid waste disposal, disinfecting and protecting water sources |

Table 6.2 *continued*

DISASTER	NATIONAL LEVEL	COMMUNITY LEVEL	FAMILY LEVEL	HEALTH PROFESSIONAL
Armed conflicts	In addition to the above:	In addition to the above:	Ensure access to information	Training in first aid/trauma care
	Focus on advocacy for peace and negotiation for preventing conflict	Develop community contingency plan	Evacuation routes	Participate in community activities
	Preparing in case negotiations fail	Train community health workers on counselling and psychological support	Access to shelter	Training in counselling and psychological support
	Coordinating mechanisms of health-related interventions	Strengthen community participation and consultation mechanisms	Information to children and logical explanation provided	Network with other health professionals
	Vulnerability assessment	Identify possible reception sites in case of displaced population	First-aid kit and essential supplies stock	Advocate for peace
	Information collection, analysis and management systems	Conduct vulnerability assessments	Contacts lists, addresses of relatives	Ensure that health facilities have disaster plan and stocks in place
	Develop contingency plans, security issues	Prepare stocks of emergency supplies, identify supply routes	Maps	Identify vulnerable areas in health facilities
	Training on war surgery	Evacuation routes and procedures		
	Identification of safe facilities	Security issues		
	Blood transfusion campaigns			
	Special arrangements and agreements for wounded/deaths			
	Mass casualty management			
	Identification of intensive care facilities and development of referral protocols			

SECTION II: HOW AND WHEN EXPOSURE OCCURS

Technological accidents	In addition to the above:	In addition to the above:	In addition to the above:
	Implement local awareness and preparedness plans for emergencies at local level	Coordinate with local industry emergency plans	Participate in emergency planning
	Engaging industries and communities	Raise public awareness and mobilize support for emergency plan	Training on identification and management of toxic spillages
	Enforce implementation of labelling, sites planning, storage facilities monitoring and regulation	Improve fire fighting capacities at plants and in surrounding areas	Procedures and protocols disseminated
	Requirements of insurance for industries handling hazardous chemicals	Evaluate risk and hazards of storage sites and map them, review plans regularly	Identification of possible decontamination areas
		Regular inspection of chemical plants and storage facilities	Drills and simulation exercise
		Land use planning and zoning	Stock of protective equipment and supplies
		Maintain monitoring and database about transportation hazards	
		Conduct drills, evacuation exercises	
		Monitor pollution level and report incidents	

(additional column)

In addition to the above:

Be familiar with hazards around them, alarm signals, evacuation plans

Ensuring that doors and windows are equipped with tight fastenings

Table 6.2 *continued*

DISASTER	NATIONAL LEVEL	COMMUNITY LEVEL	FAMILY LEVEL	HEALTH PROFESSIONAL
Terrorist attacks	In addition to the above:	In addition to the above:	In addition to the above:	In addition to the above:
	Mass casualty plans	Maintaining databases of specialists, laboratories and essential supplies providers	Family kit	Preparing and training health care staff to deal with stress and anxiety and to provide counselling and advice
	Ensure surveillance systems are able to detect unusual pattern of diseases or injuries	Participation of health providers in preparedness activities	Water (for at least 3 days)	Training/refresher course in trauma care, triage
	Coordination and intersectoral collaboration	Report suspicious incidents and coordinate with national levels	Food: canned meats, fruits, vegetables, sugar, high-energy food, food for infants	Training and awareness of signs and symptoms of diseases, exposure to chemical agents, decontamination, personal protective equipment, support and therapy
	Evaluation of health facilities preparedness	Mobilization plans for volunteers and community members	First aid supplies: bandages, gauze, scissors, tape, safety pins, soap, antiseptic, thermometer, pain reliever	Simulation exercises, drills
	Disaster plans, practice drills	Emergency plans to ensure alternatives to main utilities such as electricity and water sources	Clothing and bedding	Stocks of antidotes, drugs and protective equipment maintained
	Stockpile appropriate drugs, antidotes and vaccines	Mass communication systems	Tools and supplies (paper cups, plates, battery-operated radio, batteries, flashlight, can opener or knife, fire extinguisher, compass, paper, pencil, whistle, map, toilet paper, chlorine	Documenting and reporting
	Prepare educational materials that will inform and reassure the public during and after biological or chemical attack	Mechanisms for informing health providers on possible threats	Special items for specific needs of infants, the elderly and family documents	Health facilities plans
	Disseminate public health guidelines to local level	Expertise of epidemiologists enhanced and resources available		
	Collection, analysis and information sharing	Drills and exercises		
		Prepare adaptation of educational material to be distributed in case of an attack		

References

1. Chaloner EJ. The incidence of landmine injuries in Kuito, Angola. *Journal of the Royal College of Surgeons of Edinburgh*, 1996, 41:398–400.

2. Landmine-related injuries, 1993–1996. *Morbidity and Mortality Weekly Report*, 1997, 46:724.

3. McDermott BM, Palmer LJ. Post disaster emotional distress, depression and event-related variables: findings across child and adolescent developmental stages. *Australian and New Zealand Journal of Psychiatry*, 2002, 36:754.

4. *Facts for life*, 3rd ed. New York, United Nations Children's Fund, 2002.

5. *Health action in crises: reducing the impact of crises on people's health*. Geneva, World Health Organization, 2003.

CHAPTER 7

When the child uses alcohol and other drugs[1]

M. Monteiro
Department of Mental Health and Substance Dependence,
World Health Organization, Geneva, Switzerland

Introduction

There has been a considerable increase worldwide in the production and consumption of psychoactive drugs, including new drugs such as ecstasy, amfetamines, and other synthetic substances. Five of the ten leading causes of disability worldwide are mental disorders, including alcohol dependence (1). In 2000, alcohol, tobacco and illicit drug use ranked among the top twenty risks to health worldwide, with tobacco and alcohol among the top five (2).

Psychoactive drugs are substances that, when taken into a living organism, may modify its perception, mood, cognition or behaviour. They include alcohol, tobacco, volatile solvents, illicit drugs and psychotropic medications (prescribed or taken illicitly or not as prescribed). There has been an increase in the availability and use of alcohol, tobacco and other drugs among children and young people, marked by a change in the social context in which drugs are taken and in patterns of drug use.

Routes of exposure: how do children gain access to alcohol and drugs?

Globalized marketing and trade in many consumer goods, improvements in transportation networks, increases in disposable incomes, and rapid social changes are some of the factors related to the increase in the availability of alcohol and other drugs worldwide. Populations have been brought into contact with each other's customs and behaviour through tourism, migration, and internal displacements, particularly from rural to urban areas, bringing new cultural norms and attitudes towards alcohol and other drug use. Rapid urbanization leads to overcrowding, adverse living conditions, poor sanitation, and lack of access to recreational activities, placing an increased burden on the lives of children and their parents. Changes in work opportunities, and social isolation and disintegration are also related to an increase in the consumption of alcohol, tobacco and other drugs.

---

[1]Reviewed by **V. Poznyak**, Department of Mental Health and Substance Dependence, World Health Organization, Geneva, Switzerland.

In some parts of the world, the majority of the population remains in poverty, and destitution has increased. In some places particularly affected by famine and warfare, government functions have essentially ceased and illicit drug production has flourished. In others, the economic power of the illicit drug market has become a threat to the stability of the government and its ability to function (3).

Substance use and health in children and adolescents

Alcohol and other substance use is related to key determinants of population health, such as poor education, low income and social status, lack of social support networks, unemployment and adverse working conditions, unhealthy physical environments, and lack of or inadequate access to health services (4). It is also an independent determinant of population health linked to overall mortality and hospitalizations. Risky patterns of alcohol consumption are more prevalent among young males, and unemployed or poorly educated individuals; consumption is increasing in developing societies where drinking is not part of the tradition and culture, and where alcohol is very cheap (5). Poor health and living conditions can also lead to alcohol and other substance use problems, and drug use can serve as a paradigm for understanding and analysing inequalities and inequities in health (4, 6).

Alcohol and other drug use needs to be seen as multidimensional and complex behaviour, which cannot simply be said to be the result of a "free choice". It often occurs in the context of difficult social, environmental and economic conditions, in which the freedom to choose whether or not to take a substance is seriously compromised by several individual and environmental factors. Alcohol and other drug use may serve as coping strategies in dealing with difficult life circumstances, including physical, emotional and sexual abuse at home (7).

The role of psychoactive substances in the lives of children and adolescents is related to the environmental conditions in which they live. They can serve to solve temporary problems including hunger, boredom, fear, feelings of shame, depression, hopelessness, lack of medicine and medical care, difficulty falling asleep because of noise or overcrowding, cold or heat, tiredness, risk of attack and abuse, lack of recreational facilities or after-school activities, social isolation, lack of proper parenting, loneliness and physical pain.

Under difficult economic and social conditions young people may resort to drug dealing in order to make enough money to provide basic needs and a better quality of life for themselves and their families. Trafficking of small amounts of illicit drugs provides an appealing opportunity for young people, who are often naïve about the legal consequences of their acts, may feel protected by gangs or see no other opportunity to obtain goods and services advertised widely in the media.

Alcohol and other substance use problems are growing faster in societies undergoing rapid social change and as a result of the globalization of markets and increases in the availability of these substances (both legal and illegal), particularly in countries without strong policies to counteract these problems. For example, alcohol consumption is increasing rapidly in eastern Europe and Asia (8). Intravenous drug use is the major factor in the spread of human immunodeficiency virus in eastern Europe and Asia (9), where new trafficking routes have been established, and rapid socioeconomic changes are taking place (10). The age at which people start to use drugs and tobacco is decreasing.

Patterns of drug use depend on the living conditions of children and young people. For example, studies have found that between 25% and 90% of street children use psychoactive substances of some kind. Other marginalized and vulnerable groups, such as gypsies, indigenous populations, sex workers, homeless people and prisoners, also have relatively high rates of use and related problems. These behaviours often begin in early adolescence and can interfere with development, affect school performance, and be linked with other behavioural problems that can have an impact later in life (11, 12).

Schoolchildren also use alcohol, tobacco and other drugs. Marketing and promotion of alcohol and tobacco create a permissive environment that glamorizes the use of these substances, and links their use with particular lifestyles which are often very appealing to young people but are unaffordable or unrealistic. Experimentation with other drugs, often illicit, is related not only to access and street price, but also to youth culture.

Profiles of problems can vary dramatically from region to region, even for the same drug. Health consequences are strongly related to the characteristics of the drug itself, the mode of administration and the pattern of use. Social consequences of drug use are determined not only by the behaviour of the user but also by the reaction of those in the social environment. These include the levels of tolerance towards alcohol and other drug use, existing laws and their enforcement, and cultural norms regarding drug use and consequences.

Remedial action, prevention and education

The environment can also offer a range of protective factors that decrease the chances of a child or young person using alcohol and other drugs. These include limited availability of drugs and alcohol, restricted access, opportunities for education and leisure activities, support for parents and youth groups, a culture that is not permissive towards alcohol and other drug use, an environment that promotes dialogue and offers opportunities for young people to express their views, and opportunities for confidential counselling and information on substance use and related topics. Positive and strong attachments or close relationships with other people, either parents, relatives or friends, can have a positive influence on the behaviour of young people. Negative attachments are connections to people or institutions associated with substance use, abuse or exploitation, such as drug syndicates or peers who use drugs: such attachments make substance use more likely. Finally, young people need to develop physical, psychological, social, moral and vocational competencies as a part of their healthy development, in order to be less likely to harm themselves with psychoactive drugs.

In conclusion, the environment in which children and adolescents live can have both risk and protective factors that strongly influence the decision to experiment with a psychoactive substance or to continue to use it, as well as the health and social consequences. Rather than just trying to convince individual users to avoid any contact with drugs, environmental responses need to be promoted to strengthen protective factors and weaken the risk factors that contribute to substance use among young people.

References

1. *The World Health Report 1999: making a difference*. Geneva, World Health Organization, 1999.
2. *The World Health Report 2002: reducing risks, promoting healthy life*. Geneva, World Health Organization, 2002:
3. *WHO Expert Committee on Drug Dependence: twenty-eighth report*. Geneva, World Health Organization, 1993 (WHO Technical Report Series, No. 836).
4. Single E. Substance abuse and population health. *Paper presented at the Workshop on Addiction and Population Health, Edmonton, June 1999* (http://www.ccsa.ca/ADH/single.htm).
5. Room R et al. *Alcohol in a changing world: drinking patterns and problems in developing societies*. Helsinki, Finnish Foundation of Alcohol Studies, 2002.
6. Leon DA, Walt G, Gilson L. International perspectives on health inequalities and policy. *British Medical Journal*, 2001, 322:591–594.
7. Radford J, King A, Warren W. *Street youth and AIDS*. Kingston, Health and Welfare Canada, 1989.
8. *Global status report alcohol*. Geneva, World Health Organization, 1999.
9. *AIDS epidemic update: December 2000*. Geneva, Joint United Nations Programme on AIDS, World Health Organization, 2000 (UNAIDS/00.44E; WHO/CDS/CSR/EDC/2000.9).
10. *Global illicit drug trends, 2000*. Vienna, United Nations International Drug Control Programme, 2000 (ODCCP Studies on Drugs and Crime).
11. Brown SA et al. Conduct disorder among adolescent alcohol and drug misusers. *Journal of Studies on Alcohol*, 1996, 57:314–324.
12. Linskey M, Hall W. The effects of adolescent cannabis use on educational attainment: a review. *Addiction*, 2000, 95:1621–1630.

Specific environmental threats: sources of exposure and health effects

CHAPTER 8

Water quality[1]

T. Boonyakarnkul
Sanitation and Health Impact Assessment Division,
Department of Health, Ministry of Public Health, Bangkok,
Thailand

P. A. Kingston
Queensland Environmental Protection Agency, Brisbane,
Australia

K. M. Shea
Division of Occupational and Environmental Medicine,
Department of Community and Family Medicine, Duke
University Medical Center, Raleigh, USA

Overview

Viewed from space the earth appears to be mostly water; but only 2.5% of that water is fresh, and most of that lies frozen and inaccessible. As a result, less than 1% of fresh water is accessible in lakes, river channels and underground. Geography, environment, and pollution from human activities reduce this by a further two-thirds, and what remains is unequally distributed around the world (1).

It is estimated that between 1990 and 2000, the global population increased from 5.25 billion to over 6 billion, an increase of over 15%. Within that total, there was a 25% increase in the urban population, and an 8% increase in the rural sector. This population increase meant that an additional 800 million people required access to safe water supplies, just to maintain coverage at a constant level. During this period an additional 900 million people gained access to an improved source of water, resulting in an increase in coverage from 77% to 82%. Despite these gains, there are still more than 1.1 billion people, or 1/6 of the world's population, without access to adequate sources of drinking-water (2).

The decade also saw a marked shift in the urban–rural population ratio; by 2000, the proportion of urban dwellers had risen from 43.5% to 47%, and the growth showed no signs of slowing. The rate of urbanization is greater in the developing world, particularly in Africa and Asia, and this, together with lower

[1] Reviewed by **J. Bartram** and **J. Hueb,** Department for the Protection of the Human Environment, Water, Sanitation and Health, World Health Organization, Geneva, Switzerland.

levels of safe water supply, make these locations particularly vulnerable to the risk of water-related diseases. By 2000, 81% of Asians and only 64% of Africans had access to safe sources of drinking-water, despite worldwide efforts.

Even with the modest increases in water supply coverage, there is evidence that, because of the rural to urban shift, urban water supply coverage has decreased, and the total number of people who lack access to water supply has remained constant. With urban populations in the developing world expected to double over the next 25 years, the water supply sector faces enormous challenges. In rural areas, considerable work and investment will be needed to narrow the existing gap in coverage.

It should be noted that access to safe water, provision of sufficient supplies of water, and access to sanitation are three factors that together can contribute to the health and safety of the world's population. A lack of adequate water supplies of good quality, together with poor sanitation, exacts a high health toll, particularly in rural areas, hindering both social and economic development. This makes the promotion of hygienic behaviour a high priority.

Diarrhoea is the major public health problem caused by unsafe water and lack of sanitation. To give an indication of the scale of health problems caused by lack of safe water, there are approximately 4 billion cases of diarrhoea each year, causing 1.8 million deaths. These deaths occur mostly among children under the age of five and represent 15% of all deaths in this age group in developing countries. Waterborne intestinal worms infect nearly 10% of the population of the developing world, leading to malnutrition, anaemia, and retarded growth. Some 6 million people are blind from trachoma, while research suggests that provision of safe water could reduce infections by 25%. Some 200 million people are infected with schistosomiasis, while the provision of safe water and sanitation could reduce infections by as much as 77% (2). Contamination of drinking-water by chemicals, particularly arsenic and fluoride, has been increasingly recognized as a major health problem in some parts of the world (3).

Interventions in water supply and sanitation and the promotion of hygienic practices have been shown to lower dramatically the incidence of waterborne

Household water treatment: a success story

Diarrhoeal diseases are a leading cause of illness and death among children under 5 years old in developing countries; they are associated with approximately 1.6 million deaths in these children every year. Provision and use of microbiologically safe drinking-water are key to decreasing diarrhoeal disease in children. Discover how the *Safe Water System*, led by the Pan American Health Organization and World Health Organization, with support from the United States Centers for Disease Control and Prevention, has improved household management of clean and disinfected drinking-water in poor areas of South and Central America (Case study 7, page 299).

SECTION III: SPECIFIC ENVIRONMENTAL THREATS

diseases, particularly in infants and children, who—because of their physiological immaturity—are at higher risk (4). These health risks vary by climate, geography, economic development, education, and by urban/rural status, and are particularly acute among the rural poor of developing countries.

Major contaminants of water

The primary public health concern regarding water contamination is microbiological contamination of drinking-water. Water-related infections can be classified in four categories: waterborne diseases (directly acquired from drinking-water), water-washed (indirectly acquired) diseases, water-based diseases, and diseases transmitted by water-related insect vectors (see Table 8.1).

Water contains many trace elements and minerals which, depending on their concentration, may be inert, beneficial, or toxic. Some minerals can be beneficial at low concentrations but toxic at higher levels. These minerals may occur naturally, arising from the surrounding geological features, particularly in groundwater. Chemicals may also be introduced into water from human activities, particularly into surface waters. Contamination may be from agricultural chemicals, such as pesticides and fertilizers, human activity, such as waste disposal, urban run-off from human settlements, industrial chemicals, or the process of water treatment itself.

Many of these substances are not harmful to humans, or are present in concentrations so low as to cause no health effects. However, some are known to cause serious health effects at low concentrations, and treatment is needed to remove or reduce their concentration in drinking-water.

Guideline values for a number of contaminants of drinking-water are given in Appendix 8.1.

Mechanisms of exposure

Contamination of water can be conveniently divided into two categories—biological and chemical. Exposure to biologically contami-

Table 8.1 Examples of water-related infections

Waterborne diseases
• Cholera
• Poliomyelitis
• Diarrhoeal diseases
• Roundworm
• Enteric fevers: typhoid
• Whipworm
• Hepatitis A

Water-washed diseases
• Scabies
• Typhus
• Trachoma
• Louse infestation
• Leishmaniasis

Water-based diseases
• Schistosomiasis
• Dracunculiasis (guinea-worm disease)

Diseases transmitted by water-related insect vectors
• Malaria
• Onchocerciasis
• African trypanosomiasis
• Yellow fever
• Dengue
• Filariasis

Source: ref. 5.

nated materials often results in acute health effects, such as outbreaks of gastroenteritis and diarrhoea, allowing the source of contamination to be quickly traced. Exposure of the skin during bathing and recreational water use can also be important, particularly with infectious diseases such as schistosomiasis and amoebic meningoencephalitis.

While there are many clear instances of directly acquired (waterborne) disease, such as outbreaks of cholera and typhoid, a large number of less dramatic diseases, resulting from infections or from chronic exposure to toxic chemicals, can reduce work capacity and quality of life. Major outbreaks, which occur in both developed and developing countries, are usually transmitted by the faecal–oral route and may not be effectively detected. Diseases that are either very common or localized are even more difficult to address, as often only the sufferer and local health care workers are aware of their extent. Disease may also result from the consumption of foods that have been grown on land irrigated with contaminated water, or from fish or fish products gathered from contaminated water sources.

Indirectly acquired (water-washed) disease occurs when the quantity of safe water is insufficient, resulting in low levels of personal and domestic hygiene, and allowing the spread of diseases, such as scabies, trachoma, and louse infestation.

Adequate quantities of safe water are required for consumption and to promote hygienic behaviour. The quantity of water used often depends on the ease of access: greater quantities of water will be used if it is readily available, while if it is in short supply, people will use less or will turn to unsafe water sources.

Water quality and sanitation are directly linked, and it is of the greatest importance to protect water supplies from contamination by human faeces. Nevertheless, improvements in sanitation alone are less effective than an improved water supply in preventing disease. Children are the main victims of diarrhoea and other faecal-oral disease, and are also the most likely source of infection, so both the safe disposal of their faeces and hygiene education are of critical importance.

Chemical contamination, though less easy to determine, is often self-limiting, as high levels of contamination usually result in water becoming undrinkable because of its taste, smell, or colour. However, some chemical contaminants produce long-term health effects at concentrations undetectable by the consumer; these include inorganic chemicals such as arsenic, fluoride, lead, nitrates, and selenium.

The major pollutants found in drinking-water are listed in Table 8.2.

Microbial contamination
Occurrence

Microbial contamination usually results from the contamination of water with human or animal faeces. If drinking-water is contaminated with faeces,

Table 8.2 Selected water pollutants, their common sources and major adverse health outcomes

CONTAMINANT	WHO guideline value (mg/litre)	COMMON SOURCES	MAJOR ADVERSE HEALTH OUTCOMES
Inorganic chemicals			
Arsenic	0.01	Natural erosion, pesticide run-off, coal burning, smelting, glass and electronic production waste	Skin damage, circulatory damage, increased risk of cancer
Fluoride	1.5	Natural erosion, discharge from fertilizer and aluminium factories	Bone disease, mottled teeth
Lead	0.01	Natural erosion, plumbing, solder, lead-glazed ceramics, old paint, deposits from leaded petrol	Impaired growth and development, behavioural problems, kidney damage
Mercury (inorganic)	0.001	Natural erosion, discharge from refineries and factories, run-off from landfills and croplands	Kidney damage
Nitrite/nitrate	3/50	Run-off from fertilized land, septic tanks, sewers, erosion from natural deposits	Methaemoglobinaemia in young infants
Selenium	0.01	Natural erosion, occupational exposure	Nail deformities, gastrointestinal problems, dermatitis, dizziness
Organic chemicals			
Disinfection by-products		Drinking-water disinfection	Increased risk of cancer
Dioxins		Combustion by-products, discharge from chemical plants	Reproductive problems, increased risk of cancer
Methylmercury		Contaminated fish	Impaired neurological development
Pesticides		Urban and rural run-off	Multiple, including endocrine and neurological damage
Polychlorinated biphenyls		Transformers, industry, run-off from landfills	Impaired neurological development, increased risk of cancer, skin changes

Table 8.2   continued

CONTAMINANT	COMMON SOURCES	MAJOR ADVERSE HEALTH OUTCOMES
Radionuclides		
Radium	Natural erosion	Increased risk of cancer
Bacteria		
Campylobacter	Human and animal faeces	Gastroenteritis, Guillain-Barré syndrome
Escherichia coli	Human and animal faeces	Gastroenteritis
Escherichia coli O157:H7	Human and animal faeces	Bloody diarrhoea, haemolytic uraemic syndrome
Salmonellae	Human and animal faeces	Enteric fever, gastroenteritis
Shigellae	Human faeces	Dysentery
Vibrio cholerae	Human and animal faeces	Dysentery
Viruses		
Enterovirus	Human faeces	Gastroenteritis
Poliovirus	Human faeces	Poliomyelitis
Hepatitis A virus	Human faeces	Hepatitis A
Rotavirus	Human faeces	Gastroenteritis
Parasites		
Cryptosporidium	Human and animal faeces	Gastroenteritis
Entamoeba	Human faeces	Gastroenteritis
Giardia	Human and animal faeces	Gastroenteritis, anaemia
Schistosoma	Human faeces/infected snails	Schistosomiasis
Natural toxins		
Microcystins	Cyanobacteria in nutrient-rich surface waters	Gastrointestinal, neurological effects

Source: compiled from data in ref. 6.

pathogens are likely to be widely and rapidly dispersed. If the contamination is recent, and if the faeces are from carriers of communicable enteric diseases, the microorganisms (bacteria, viruses, or protozoa) that cause these diseases may be present in the water. The diseases range from mild gastroenteritis to severe and sometimes fatal diarrhoea, dysentery, hepatitis, cholera, or typhoid. Helminths and amoebae may also be transmitted in water and are common in poor quality water supplies. There are also some organisms of environmental origin that may cause disease in humans in certain circumstances, e.g. *Legionella* may be transmitted through aerosols. Some toxins occur naturally, particularly in nutrient-rich surface waters where there is high algal growth.

Health considerations

Adverse health effects arise primarily from the ingestion of pathogenic bacteria. People with low immunity, including infants, young children, the sick and the elderly are particularly vulnerable to microbial contamination even from ordinarily mild pathogens. Outbreaks of waterborne disease can lead to infection across a wide community.

Chemical contamination
Arsenic
Occurrence

Arsenic is a naturally occurring element, which can be introduced into water through the dissolution of minerals, from industrial effluent (drainage from goldmines) and from atmospheric deposition (burning of fossil fuels and wastes). These sources make significant contributions to arsenic concentrations in drinking-water and may be harmful to health (7). The body rapidly excretes organic forms of arsenic, and it is the inorganic trivalent form that is of most concern.

While concentrations in natural water are generally less than 0.005 mg/litre, some countries have reported very high concentrations particularly in groundwater supplies. In Bangladesh, for example, over 25 000 wells are contaminated with arsenic at levels above 0.05 mg/litre. Food is also a significant source of arsenic, but usually in highly complex forms that are biologically unavailable and essentially non-toxic.

Health considerations

Although studies indicate that arsenic may be essential for some animal species, there is no indication that it is essential for humans. Arsenic compounds are readily

Arsenic exposure and child health

In an effort to reduce the occurrence of diarrhoeal disease in Bangladesh, tube wells were installed in the 1970s and 1980s. Unfortunately, many of these wells were contaminated with arsenic and resulted in serious health effects. Read about the case, actions taken and lessons learned in Case study 6, page 294.

absorbed by the gastrointestinal tract, and then bind to haemoglobin and are deposited in the liver, kidneys, lungs, spleen, and skin. Inorganic arsenic does not appear to cross the blood–brain barrier, but can cross the placenta (8). Approximately 45–85% of ingested arsenic is excreted in the urine within 1–3 days. The major health effects are caused by low-level chronic exposure from the consumption of arsenic-contaminated water. A number of studies in Bangladesh and West Bengal have documented the effects of consuming water containing elevated concentrations of arsenic (>0.3 mg/litre). Consumption over periods of 5 to 25 years was reported to produce skin lesions, skin cancer, vascular disease, effects on the nervous system, and possibly cancer of other organs (9). The only available treatment for chronic arsenic poisoning is to remove the patient from the source of exposure and provide supportive care.

Fluoride
Occurrence
Fluoride occurs naturally in soil and water, and is a by-product of industrial activities such as the aluminium and fertilizer industries. It is also added to drinking-water to help prevent dental caries. Concentrations in surface water are usually relatively low (<0.5 mg/litre) while deeper groundwater wells in areas high in fluoride minerals may have concentrations as high as 10 mg/litre.

A fluorotic village

An estimated 100 million people suffer health effects from overexposure to fluoride. A wide strip from North to South Africa, and including the Syrian Arab Republic, Jordan, Egypt, Sudan, Ethiopia, Kenya, the United Republic of Tanzania and South Africa, is known to have high concentrations of fluoride in groundwater as a result of the natural weathering of volcanic and sedimentary rocks. In one village of 2000 people, 95% of children are affected by dental fluorosis. Other effects, such as skeletal fluorosis and crippling fluorosis, are also present in this village, as in other parts of the so-called "African fluoride belt". Read about the effects suffered by children and learn how reducing exposure to fluoride can help (Case study 9, page 306).

Health considerations
Fluoride may be an essential trace element for humans, but this has yet to be established. It is widely dispersed in the environment, and all living organisms tolerate modest amounts. Fluoride is absorbed quickly following ingestion, but is not metabolized, and diffuses throughout the body. About 40% is excreted in urine within 9 hours, and 50% over 24 hours.

Fluoride has an affinity for mineralizing tissues of the body—in young people the bones and teeth, and in older people the bones. As the excretion rate is greater in adults, mineralization is proportionally less than in children. The most readily identifiable health effects of consuming water with elevated levels of fluoride are a mottling of the teeth, known as fluorosis, and sclerosis of the bones. Children are particularly affected by fluorosis, because teeth take up fluoride during their formation (10).

Fluoride has been shown to be effective in preventing dental caries, from the observed association of low dental caries with naturally occurring fluoride in drinking-water (at about 1 mg/litre). As a result, many health authorities around the world, including the World Health Organization, recommend fluoridation of public water supplies as an important public health measure. However, at concentrations above 1.5 mg/litre fluoride may affect tooth mineralization in children leading to a mottling of the teeth, which can in some cases be unsightly. Where exposure to high fluoride concentrations in drinking-water has occurred over prolonged periods (several years), skeletal fluorosis may appear. If the exposure is removed, some of the effects may be reversible, and the fluoride levels in bone gradually decline. The regular consumption of water with fluoride concentrations above 4 mg/litre, however, can cause progressively increasing skeletal fluorosis. This is the maximum acceptable level in drinking-water. People with kidney impairment may retain fluoride to a greater degree, thus lowering their margin of safety for fluoride intake (11). Patients with evidence of exposure to fluoride should avoid the contaminating source.

Lead
Occurrence
Lead may be found in drinking-water at high levels. This is most commonly a result of human activities, particularly where lead piping is still being used, or water supply fittings use leaded solders. Concentrations are affected by factors such as water acidity, water hardness, and contact time with water. Urban run-off, particularly where leaded fuels are common, is a source of lead contamination, particularly of surface waters (11).

Health considerations
Lead is a neurodevelopmental toxicant. It interferes with haem synthesis, and can damage the peripheral nervous system, the kidneys, and the reproductive system. It can be absorbed by the body through inhalation, ingestion, or placental transfer. In adults, approximately 10% of ingested lead is absorbed, but in children this figure can be 4–5 times higher. After absorption, the lead is distributed in soft tissues such as the kidneys, liver, and bone marrow, where it has a biological half-life in adults of less than 40 days. In skeletal bone lead may persist for 20 to 30 years. Lead is a cumulative poison, and can severely affect the central nervous system. Infants and fetuses are the most susceptible. Placental transfer of lead occurs in humans as early as the 12th week of gestation and continues throughout development.

Many epidemiological studies have been carried out on the effects of lead exposure on the intellectual development of children. Although there are some conflicting results, on balance the studies demonstrate that exposure to lead adversely affects intelligence.

Other adverse effects associated with exposure to high amounts of lead include kidney damage, and interference with the production of red blood cells and the metabolism of calcium needed for bone formation (11).

Nitrates and nitrites
Occurrence
Nitrates and nitrites occur primarily as a result of run-off from the agricultural use of fertilizers and bacterial action on animal wastes. The intensification of farming practices and sewage effluent disposal to streams have led to increasing amounts of nitrate in some waters, particularly groundwater. Nitrite is formed by the reduction of nitrate in poorly oxygenated waters and is relatively unstable. It is rapidly oxidized to nitrate and is rarely present in well oxygenated or chlorinated supplies. Other processes reduce it to other compounds such as ammonia. While food is the major source of nitrate intake for adults, bottle-fed infants may be exposed to nitrates if contaminated water is used for mixing formula.

Health considerations
The toxicity of nitrate in humans is thought to be solely due to its reduction to nitrite. The major biological effect of nitrite in humans is its involvement in the oxidation of normal haemoglobin to methaemoglobin, which is unable to transport oxygen to the tissues, a condition known as methaemoglobinaemia or more commonly, "blue baby syndrome". Young infants and pregnant women are most susceptible to methaemoglobin formation. Laboratory experiments with animals suggest that neither nitrite nor nitrate acts directly as a carcinogen, but there is concern that nitrite may react with foods rich in secondary amines to form N-nitroso compounds in the stomach, many of which are known to be carcinogenic in animals. Some epidemiological evidence suggests a relationship between nitrate and gastric cancer in humans, but this has yet to be confirmed (11).

Selenium
Occurrence
Selenium, although widespread in the environment, is generally found in very low concentrations. There are some regions where elevated levels have resulted in health effects, and groundwater

Contaminated water distribution
In an area of Uzbekistan, a study was undertaken to determine the causes of increased diarrhoeal disease during certain seasons. It was found that agricultural irrigation reduced water supply during certain months, and as a result an overhaul of the water supply and quality management were carried out. Case study 8 (page 303) illustrates the usefulness of field epidemiology as an analytical tool to address a problem and guide policy and decision-making.

SECTION III: SPECIFIC ENVIRONMENTAL THREATS

concentrations as high as 6 mg/litre have been reported in the United States, for example.

Health considerations

Selenium is an essential element for many species, including humans. Selenium deficiency in humans is not well established but may include a chronic disorder of the heart muscle and cancer. The gastrointestinal tract effectively absorbs most water-soluble selenium compounds, which are then distributed to most organs, with the highest concentrations found in the kidneys, liver, and spleen. The toxicity of selenium varies considerably depending on the compound, with selenite and selenate being more toxic than the sulfide. There have been a number of reports of ill-effects attributed to short-term and long-term exposure to selenium, most of which have been linked to occupational exposure or accidental poisoning. Acute or chronic nutritional toxicity is comparatively rare. Intakes above about 1 mg/day over prolonged periods may produce nail deformities characteristic of selenosis. Other features of excess selenium intake include non-specific symptoms, such as gastrointestinal disturbances, dermatitis, dizziness, lassitude, and a garlic odour on the breath (11).

Mercury
Occurrence

Mercury occurs naturally in drinking-water at extremely low levels, but contamination can result from industrial emissions or spills. Inorganic mercury compounds are generally insoluble in water and the major concern is the organic methylmercury, formed from inorganic mercury by bacteriological action. Methylmercury is known to accumulate in fish and fish products, and the consumption of these foods may cause human illness (12).

Health considerations

A developmental neurotoxicant, when exposure occurs *in utero* methylmercury interferes with neuronal migration, organization of brain nuclei and layering of the cortex. These experimental findings are consistent with the severe cerebral palsy, seizure disorders, blindness, deafness and mental retardation that have been documented in children whose mothers ate heavily contaminated fish during pregnancy (13). More subtle neurodevelopmental deficits have been observed in some children who received much lower exposures *in utero* (14). Methylmercury can also damage the brain after birth. Long-term exposures outside the developmentally vulnerable periods also cause central nervous system damage. Progressive signs include paraesthesia, ataxia, tremor, and muscle spasticity, leading to coma and death.

Studies of workers occupationally exposed to mercury have reported health effects including tremors, mental disturbances, and gingivitis. Methylmercury compounds are almost completely absorbed by the gastrointestinal tract and can cross biological membranes, especially in the brain, spinal cord, and peripheral nerves. The main effects of methylmercury poisoning are severe, irreversible, neurological disorders and mental disability. In Minamata Bay, Japan, two major epidemics of methylmercury poisoning were caused by the release of methylmercury and other mercury compounds from industrial processes. These compounds accumulated in fish, which were subsequently eaten by humans. Other countries have reported cases of poisoning caused by mercury contamination of bread and cereals (11).

Less than 15% of inorganic mercury in drinking-water is absorbed by the gastrointestinal tract. Inorganic mercury compounds have a long biological half-life, accumulating in the kidneys where the toxic effects may lead to kidney failure.

Pesticides
Occurrence
Pesticides are of increasing concern due to their widespread and often indiscriminate use. In both urban and rural settings, pesticides may reach water supplies from agricultural run-off. While not specifically removed by conventional water treatment processes, natural filtration and biodegradation prior to and during treatment means that these substances are rarely detected in treated water. However, elevated levels are often found in rural areas where intensive agricultural practices can result in direct contamination of the water source.

Health considerations
Public health concerns regarding pesticides arise from their potential to cause poisoning and to accumulate in the body. These chemicals can be absorbed by the oral, inhalation, and dermal routes; health effects depend on the specific type of pesticide. For instance, organophosphorus compounds produce an anticholinergic syndrome (salivation, vomiting, diarrhoea, etc.), while organochlorine compounds induce neurological signs and symptoms.

Disinfection by-products
Occurrence
Disinfection by-products (DBPs) occur when treatment chemicals such as chlorine are added to water to control microbial contamination, where they combine with organic materials (15).

Health considerations
A variety of halogenated DBPs found in treated drinking-water have been linked to cancer in laboratory animals at high doses (15, 16). There are few data on the effects of low doses on humans, particularly infants and children. While there is some concern that these chemicals may pose a health risk, the potential risks arising from not treating drinking-water are considerably greater, and the disinfection of water should never be compromised as a result (11, 17).

Radionuclides
Occurrence
Radionuclides occur naturally in the environment from deposits of radioactive minerals, and from the disposal and storage of radioactive materials. Concentrations in surface waters are likely to be extremely low, and groundwater concentrations vary according to the type of aquifer minerals and dissolved anions.

Health considerations
Radioactive materials cause changes in the DNA of cells, with an increased risk of cancer being the most serious outcome. The most common exposure route is via the respiratory system by inhalation of aerosolized droplets (11). The US Environmental Protection Agency estimates that 168 cancer deaths per year in the USA are related to radon in water, of which 89% are lung cancers, and 11% stomach cancers (18).

Diagnosis
Diagnosis of illnesses suspected to be caused by contaminated water supplies requires a thorough knowledge of the history of exposure, a complete physical examination of the patient and, where possible, confirmatory laboratory tests. Standard stool cultures, tests for ova and parasites, and measurement of antibody titres may be feasible for patients who present at hospitals or health care centres. Laboratory tests are more likely to be useful for microbial exposures and acute effects from chemical exposures than for chronic low-dose chemical exposures. Testing for low concentrations of chemicals requires sophisticated analytical techniques unlikely to be found outside research settings. Measuring methaemoglobin in the blood will confirm acute nitrate poisoning. Testing blood lead levels can indicate lead exposure. Urinary arsenic levels are of limited value as arsenic is rapidly excreted from the body. None of these tests however, will identify the source of exposure, which is important for case management and prevention of further exposure. If elevated levels of chemical contaminants are known to exist then exposure can be inferred, and confirmed by detailed patient and environmental histories and by chemical and microbiological analyses.

Treatment guidelines
Diarrhoeal illness is treated by controlling the infection and by aggressive fluid management. Antimicrobial drugs are used only in cases of severe cholera and bloody diarrhoea (dysentery). In young children, the most common cause of death is from dehydration. Correct management may prevent up to 90% of deaths (19). Dehydration can usually be treated using oral rehydration fluids. Intravenous rehydration may be needed in cases of severe dehydration, or where the patient cannot drink or absorb water. The rehydration treatment of diarrhoeal disease is summarized in the box below.

Guidelines for treating children and adults with some dehydration
Approximate amount of ORS^a solution to give in the first 4 hours

Age[b]	Less than 4 months	4–11 months	12–23 months	2–4 years	5–14 years	15 years or older
Weight	Less than 5 kg	5–7.9 kg	8–10.9 kg	11–15.9 kg	16–29.9 kg	30 kg or more
In ml	200–400	400–600	600–800	800–1200	1200–2200	2200–4000
In local measure						

[a] Oral rehydration salts.
[b] Use the patient's age only when you do not know the weight. The approximate amount of ORS required (in ml) can also be calculated by multiplying the patient's weight in kg by 75.

- If the patient wants more ORS than shown, give more.
- Encourage the mother to continue breastfeeding her child.
- For infants under 6 months who are not breastfed, if using the old so-called standard WHO ORS solution containing 90 mmol/L of sodium, also give 100–200 ml clean water during this period. However, if using the new reduced (low) osmolarity ORS solution containing 75 mmol/L of sodium, this is not necessary.

NOTE: During the initial stages of therapy, while still dehydrated, adults can consume up to 750 ml per hour, if necessary, and children up to 20 ml per kg body weight per hour.

Sources of infection should be identified and made safe. If the infected person is potentially contagious, isolation, strict hand-washing by staff, and the safe disposal of faeces are the recommended control measures. For non-infectious diseases resulting from contaminated water supplies, treatment involves removing the patient from the source of exposure and providing supportive care. In some cases the use of a specific pharmaceutical or antidote may be indicated (e.g. succimer for lead, atropine for organophosphorus pesticides, methylene blue for reversal of methaemoglobinaemia).

Registration, recording and reporting of data
It is critical that information is registered and recorded after diagnosis. Some diseases are notifiable by law.

A systematic approach to recording this information is vital in building up a knowledge base. It provides a basis for effective communication both within the health care system and with the community, and ensures that the relevant authorities receive the information they need to make informed decisions and respond appropriately to the sources of contamination and disease. The harmonized recording of clinical case data will show trends over time and seasonal occurrence.

Prevention, remedial action, and education

Prevention of contamination is an essential feature of effective water quality management. A comprehensive assessment of the water supply system enables effective risk management strategies to be identified from the source to the consumer. When a situation that can give rise to water contamination is recognized, preventive strategies can be identified to minimize the exposure (17).

Surface and groundwater sources should be protected from contamination. Possible sources of contamination include animal and human waste, agriculture, industry, mining and quarrying run-off, and the disposal of hazardous wastes. These and other polluting activities should be identified and controlled, or where feasible, excluded from the water catchment area.

Groundwater in deep or confined aquifers is usually protected from local sources of contamination and microbiological quality is generally high. However, groundwater supplies may contain high concentrations of naturally occurring elements with health or aesthetic effects.

Groundwater with a high salinity may be unpalatable, while high levels of nitrates, arsenic, boron, fluoride and radionuclides may make water unfit for use. Groundwater may also be polluted by some practices, such as drilling of wells.

Even in areas without safe drinking-water systems, home treatment is possible. Filtration can remove some microbial contamination and parasites, as can disinfection and boiling. While it is possible to remove some chemical contaminants, methods tend to be expensive and the costs must be weighed against the risks involved in drinking water with potentially high levels of chemical contaminants. Water treatment carried out in the home requires scrupulous and continuous maintenance to ensure a safe and effective supply (7, 17).

Education is vitally important to ensure that consumers of water understand the routes by which contaminants may enter the system. Health promotion activities are needed to show the importance of correct hygiene regarding both sanitation and water supply, particularly for those most at risk. Communities should be involved to ensure that everyone understands the importance of clean water to health, and that the protection of safe water sources is essential in reducing health risks.

APPENDIX 8.1

Guideline values for drinking-water contaminants[1]

Inorganic constituents

	GUIDELINE VALUE (mg/litre)	REMARKS
Antimony	0.005 (P)[a]	
Arsenic	0.01[b] (P)	For excess skin cancer risk of 6×10^{-4}
Barium	0.7	
Beryllium		NAD[c]
Boron	0.5 (P)	
Cadmium	0.003	
Chromium	0.05 (P)	
Copper	2 (P)	Based on acute gastrointestinal effects
Cyanide	0.07	
Fluoride	1.5	Climatic conditions, volume of water consumed, and intake from other sources should be considered when setting national standards
Lead	0.01	It is recognized that not all water will meet the guideline value immediately; meanwhile, all other recommended measures to reduce the total exposure to lead should be implemented
Manganese	0.5 (P)	ATO[d]
Mercury (total)	0.001	
Molybdenum	0.07	
Nickel	0.02 (P)	
Nitrate (as NO_3^-)	50 (acute)	
Nitrite (as NO_2^-)	3 (acute) 0.2 (P)(chronic)	
Selenium	0.01	
Uranium	0.002 (P)	

[1] Based on ref. 17.

SECTION III: SPECIFIC ENVIRONMENTAL THREATS

Organic constituents

	GUIDELINE VALUE (µg/litre)	REMARKS
Chlorinated alkanes		
Carbon tetrachloride	2	
Dichloromethane	20	
1,1-dichloroethane		NAD
1,2-dichloroethane	30[b]	For excess risk of 10^{-5}
1,1,1-trichloroethane	2000 (P)	
Chlorinated ethenes		
Vinyl chloride	5[b]	For excess risk of 10^{-5}
1,1-dichloroethene	30	
1,2-dichloroethene	50	
Trichloroethene	70 (P)	
Tetrachloroethene	40	
Aromatic hydrocarbons		
Benzene	10[b]	For excess risk of 10^{-5}
Toluene	700	ATO
Xylenes	500	ATO
Ethylbenzene	300	ATO
Styrene	20	ATO
Benzo [*a*] pyrene	0.7[b]	For excess risk of 10^{-5}
Chlorinated benzenes		
Monochlorobenzene	300	ATO
1,2-dichlorobenzene	1000	ATO
1,3-dichlorobenzene		NAD
1,4-dichlorobenzene	300	ATO
Trichlorobenzenes (total)	20	ATO
Miscellaneous		
Di(2-ethylhexyl)adipate	80	
Di(2-ethylhexyl)phthalate	8	
Acrylamide	0.5[b]	For excess risk of 10^{-5}
Epichlorohydrin	0.4 (P)	
Hexachlorobutadiene	0.6	
Edetic acid (EDTA)	600	Applies to the free acid
Nitrilotriacetic acid	200	
Dialkyltins		NAD
Tributyltin oxide	2	
Microcystin-LR	1 (P)	Applies to total microcystin-LR (free plus cell-bound)

Pesticides

	GUIDELINE VALUE (µg/litre)	REMARKS
Alachlor	20[b]	For excess risk of 10^{-5}
Aldicarb	10	
Aldrin/dieldrin	0.03	
Atrazine	2	
Bentazone	300	
Carbofuran	7	
Chlordane	0.2	
Chlorotoluron	30	
Cyanazine	0.6	
DDT	2	
1,2-dibromo-3-chloropropane	1[b]	For excess risk of 10^{-5}
1,2-dibromoethane	0.4–15[b] (P)	For excess risk of 10^{-5}
2,4-dichlorophenoxyacetic acid (2,4-D)	30	
1,2-dichloropropane (1,2-DCP)	40 (P)	
1,3-dichloropropane		NAD
1,3-dichloropropene	20[b]	For excess risk of 10^{-5}
Diquat	10 (P)	
Heptachlor and heptachlor epoxide	0.03	
Hexachlorobenzene	1[b]	For excess risk of 10^{-5}
Isoproturon	9	
Lindane	2	
(4-chloro-2-methylphenoxy)acetic acid (MCPA)	2	
Methoxychlor	20	
Metolachlor	10	
Molinate	6	
Pendimethalin	20	
Pentachlorophenol	9[b] (P)	For excess risk of 10^{-5}
Permethrin	20	
Propanil	20	
Pyridate	100	
Simazine	2	
Terbuthylazine (TBA)	7	
Trifluralin	20	

Chlorophenoxy herbicides other than 2,4-D and MCPA		
2,4-DB	90	
Dichlorprop	100	
Fenoprop	9	
4-(4-chloro-2-methylphenoxy)butanoic acid (MCPB)		NAD
Mecoprop	10	
2,4,5-T	9	

SECTION III: SPECIFIC ENVIRONMENTAL THREATS

Disinfectants and disinfectant by-products

DISINFECTANTS	GUIDELINE VALUE (mg/litre)	REMARKS
Monochloramine	3	
Di- and trichloramine		NAD
Chlorine	5	ATO. For effective disinfection there should be a residual concentration of free chlorine of 0.5 mg/litre after at least 30 minutes contact time at pH < 8.0
Chlorine dioxide		A guideline value has not been established because of the rapid breakdown of chlorine dioxide and because the chlorite guideline value is adequately protective for potential toxicity from chlorine dioxide
Iodine		NAD

DISINFECTANT BY-PRODUCTS	GUIDELINE VALUE (μg/litre)	REMARKS
Bromate	10[b] (P)	For 7×10^{-5} excess risk
Chlorate		NAD
Chlorite	700 (P)	
Chlorophenols		
2-chlorophenol		NAD
2,4-dichlorophenol		NAD
2,4,6-trichlorophenol	200[b]	For excess risk of 10^{-5}, ATO
Formaldehyde	900	
3-chloro-4-dichloromethyl-5-hydroxy-2(5H)-furanone (MX)		NAD
Trihalomethanes		The sum of the ratio of the concentration of each to its respective guideline value should not exceed 1
Bromoform	100	
Dibromochloromethane	100	
Bromodichloromethane	60[b]	For excess risk of 10^{-5}
Chloroform	200	
Chlorinated acetic acids		
Monochloroacetic acid		NAD
Dichloroacetic acid	50 (P)	
Trichloroacetic acid	100 (P)	
Chloral hydrate (trichloroacetaldehyde)	10 (P)	
Chloroacetone		NAD

DISINFECTANTS	GUIDELINE VALUE (µg/litre)	REMARKS
Halogenated acetonitriles		
Dichloroacetonitrile	20 (P)	
Dibromoacetonitrile	70 (P)	
Bromochloroacetonitrile		NAD
Trichloroacetonitrile		NAD
Cyanogen chloride (as CN)	70	
Chloropicrin		NAD

[a] (P)—Provisional guideline value. This term is used for constituents for which there is some evidence of a potential hazard but where the available information on health effects is limited; or where an uncertainty factor greater than 1000 has been used in the derivation of the tolerable daily intake (TDI). Provisional guideline values are also recommended: (1) for substances for which the calculated guideline value would be below the practical quantification level, or below the level that can be achieved through practical treatment methods; or (2) where disinfection is likely to result in the guideline value being exceeded.

[b] For substances that are considered to be carcinogenic, the guideline value is the concentration in drinking-water associated with an excess lifetime cancer risk of 10^{-5} (one additional cancer per 100 000 of the population ingesting drinking-water containing the substance at the guideline value for 70 years). Concentrations associated with estimated excess lifetime cancer risks of 10^{-4} and 10^{-6} can be calculated by multiplying and dividing, respectively, the guideline value by 10.

In cases in which the concentration associated with an excess lifetime cancer risk of 10^{-5} is not feasible as a result of inadequate analytical or treatment technology, a provisional guideline value is recommended at a practicable level and the estimated associated excess lifetime cancer risk presented.

It should be emphasized that the guideline values for carcinogenic substances have been computed from hypothetical mathematical models that cannot be verified experimentally and that the values should be interpreted differently from TDI-based values because of the lack of precision of the models. At best, these values must be regarded as rough estimates of cancer risk. However, the models used are conservative and probably err on the side of caution. Moderate short-term exposure to levels exceeding the guideline value for carcinogens does not significantly affect the risk.

[c] NAD—No adequate data to permit recommendation of a health-based guideline value.

[d] ATO—Concentrations of the substance at or below the health-based guideline value may affect the appearance, taste, or odour of the water.

Chemicals not of health significance at concentrations normally found in drinking-water

CHEMICAL	REMARKS
Asbestos	U
Fluoranthene	U
Glyphosate	U
Silver	U
Tin	U

U—It is unnecessary to recommend a health-based guideline value for these compounds because they are not hazardous to human health at concentrations normally found in drinking-water.

Bacteriological quality of drinking-water[a]

ORGANISMS	GUIDELINE VALUE
All water intended for drinking	
E. coli or thermotolerant coliform bacteria[b,c]	Must not be detectable in any 100-ml sample
Treated water entering the distribution system	
E. coli or thermotolerant coliform bacteria[b]	Must not be detectable in any 100-ml sample
Total coliform bacteria	Must not be detectable in any 100-ml sample
Treated water in the distribution system	
E. coli or thermotolerant coliform bacteria[b]	Must not be detectable in any 100-ml sample
Total coliform bacteria	Must not be detectable in any 100-ml sample. In the case of large supplies, where sufficient samples are examined, must not be present in 95% of samples taken throughout any 12-month period

[a] Immediate investigative action must be taken if either *E. coli* or total coliform bacteria are detected. The minimal action in the case of total coliform bacteria is repeat sampling; if these bacteria are detected in the repeat sample, the cause must be determined by immediate further investigation.

[b] Although *E. coli* is the more precise indicator of faecal pollution, the count of thermotolerant coliform bacteria is an acceptable alternative. If necessary, proper confirmatory tests must be carried out. Total coliform bacteria are not acceptable indicators of the sanitary quality of rural water supplies, particularly in tropical areas where many bacteria of no sanitary significance occur in almost all untreated supplies.

[c] It is recognized that in the great majority of rural water supplies in developing countries faecal contamination is widespread. Under these conditions, the national surveillance agency should set medium-term targets for the progressive improvement of water supplies, as recommended in the Guidelines for drinking-water quality, released by WHO (www.who.int/water_sanitation_health/dwq)

Radioactive constituents of drinking water

	SCREENING VALUE (Bq/litre)
Gross alpha activity	0.1
Gross beta activity	1

Substances and parameters in drinking-water that may give rise to complaints from consumers

	LEVELS LIKELY TO GIVE RISE TO CONSUMER COMPLAINTS[a]	REASONS FOR CONSUMER COMPLAINTS
Physical parameters		
Colour	15 TCU[b]	Appearance
Taste and odour	—	Should be acceptable
Temperature	—	Should be acceptable
Turbidity	5 NTU[c]	Appearance; for effective terminal disinfection, median turbidity = 1 NTU, single sample = 5 NTU
Inorganic constituents		
Aluminium	0.2 mg/litre	Depositions, discoloration
Ammonia	1.5 mg/litre	Odour and taste
Chloride	250 mg/litre	Taste, corrosion
Copper	1 mg/litre	Staining of laundry and sanitary ware (health-based provisional guideline value 2 mg/litre)
Hardness	—	High hardness: scale deposition, scum formation
Low hardness: possible corrosion		
Hydrogen sulfide	0.05 mg/litre	Odour and taste
Iron	0.3 mg/litre	Staining of laundry and sanitary ware
Manganese	0.1 mg/litre	Staining of laundry and sanitary ware (health-based guideline value 0.5 mg/litre)
Dissolved oxygen	—	Indirect effects
pH	—	Low pH: corrosion / High pH: taste, soapy feel
	Preferably <8.0 for effective disinfection with chlorine	
Sodium	200 mg/litre	Taste
Sulfate	250 mg/litre	Taste, corrosion
Total dissolved solids	1000 mg/litre	Taste
Zinc	3 mg/litre	Appearance, taste
Organic constituents		
Toluene	24–170 µg/litre	Odour, taste (health-based guideline value 700 µg/l)
Xylene	20–1800 µg/litre	Odour, taste (health-based guideline value 500 µg/l)
Ethylbenzene	2–200 µg/litre	Odour, taste (health-based guideline value 300 µg/l)

SECTION III: SPECIFIC ENVIRONMENTAL THREATS

	LEVELS LIKELY TO GIVE RISE TO CONSUMER COMPLAINTS[a]	REASONS FOR CONSUMER COMPLAINTS
Styrene	4–2600 µg/litre	Odour, taste (health-based guideline value 20 µg/l)
Monochlorobenzene	10–120 µg/litre	Odour, taste (health-based guideline value 300 µg/l)
1,2-dichlorobenzene	1–10 µg/litre	Odour, taste (health-based guideline value 1000 µg/l)
1,4-dichlorobenzene	0.3–30 µg/litre	Odour, taste (health-based guideline value 300 µg/l)
Trichlorobenzenes (total)	5–50 µg/litre	Odour, taste (health-based guideline value 20 µg/l)
Synthetic detergents	—	Foaming, taste, odour
Disinfectants and disinfectant by-products		
Chlorine	600–1000 µg/litre	Taste and odour (health-based guideline value 5 µg/l)
Chlorophenols		
2-chlorophenol	0.1–10 µg/litre	Taste, odour
2,4-dichlorophenol	0.3–40 µg/litre	Taste, odour
2,4,6-trichlorophenol	2–300 µg/litre	Taste, odour (health-based guideline value 200 µg/l)

[a] The levels indicated are not precise numbers. Problems may occur at lower or higher values according to local circumstances. A range of taste and odour threshold concentrations is given for organic constituents.
[b] TCU, true colour unit.
[c] NTU, nephelometric turbidity unit.

References

1. *Water for health—taking charge.* Geneva, World Health Organization, 2001.

2. WHO/UNICEF Joint Monitoring Programme for Water Supply and Sanitation. *Global water supply and sanitation assessment 2000 report.* Geneva, World Health Organization, United Nations Children's Fund, 2000 (http://www. who.int/water_sanitation_health/Globassessment/Global1.htm#Top).

3. Smith AH, Lingas EO, Rahman M. Contamination of drinking-water by arsenic in Bangladesh: a public health emergency. *Bulletin of the World Health Organization,* 2000, 78:1093–1103 (http://www.who.int/bulletin/pdf/2000/issue9/bu0751.pdf).

4. Special considerations based on age and developmental stage. In: Etzel RA, Balk SJ. *Handbook of pediatric environmental health.* Elk Grove Village, American Academy of Pediatrics, 1999:9–19.

5. Satterthwaite D et al. *The environment for children.* New York, United Nations Children's Fund & Earthscan, 1996.

6. Environmental Protection Agency. *Drinking water contaminant candidate list.* 1998 (www.epa.gov/safewater/ccl/cclfs.html).

7. *United Nations Synthesis Report on Arsenic in Drinking Water* (http://www.who.int/water_sanitation_health/dwq/arsenic3/en/print.html).

8. Kreiss K. *Arsenic toxicity*. Atlanta, GA, US Department of Health and Human Services, Agency of Toxic Substances and Disease Registry, 1990 (Case Studies in Environmental Medicine, No. 5).

9. International Programme on Chemical Safety. *Arsenic*. Geneva, World Health Organization, 1981 (Environmental Health Criteria No. 18).

10. Marcus R. Agents affecting calcification and bone turnover. In: Hardman JG, Limbird LE. *Goodman & Gillman's the pharmacological basis of therapeutics*, 9th ed. New York, McGraw-Hill, 1996:1538–1539.

11. National Health and Medical Research Council. *Australian drinking water guidelines and framework for management of drinking water quality* (http://www.health.gov.au/nhmrc/publications/synopses/eh19syn.htm).

12. Wheeler M. Measuring mercury. *Environmental Health Perspectives*, 1996, 104:826–831 (http://ehpnet1.niehs.nih.gov/docs/1996/104-8/focus.html).

13. Goyer RA. Toxic effects of metals. In: Klaassen CD. *Casarett & Doull's toxicology: the basic science of poisons*, 5th ed. New York, McGraw-Hill, 1996:691–736.

14. Grandjean P et al. Cognitive deficit in 7-year-old children with prenatal exposures to methylmercury. *Neurotoxicology and Teratology*, 1997, 6:417–428.

15. International Programme on Chemical Safety. *Disinfectants and disinfectant by-products*. Geneva, World Health Organization, 1999 (WHO Environmental Health Criteria No. 216) (www.inchem.org/documents/ehc/ehc/ehc216.htm).

16. Booker SM. TNP taps disinfection by-products for study. *Environmental Health Perspectives*, 2000, 108:A64–A66.

17. *Guidelines for drinking-water quality, 3rd ed.* Geneva, World Health Organization, 2004 (www.who.int/docstore/water_sanitation_health/GDWQ/Updating/draftguidel/draftchap1.htm).

18. US Environmental Protection Agency. Proposed radon in drinking water rule. EPA 815-F-99-009, 2000 (http://www.epa.gov/safewater/radon/proposal.html).

19. *The treatment of diarrhoea. A manual for physicians and other senior health workers.* Geneva, World Health Organization, 2003 (WHO/FCH/CAH/03.7).

CHAPTER 9

Sanitation and hygiene

J. Hueb

*Water, Sanitation and Health, Department for the
Protection of the Human Environment, World Health
Organization, Geneva, Switzerland*

Introduction

Global sanitation needs are enormous. An estimated 42% of the world's population has no access to sanitation facilities. In sub-Saharan Africa and South Asia, the situation is critical, with 64% and 63% of the respective populations without adequate sanitation facilities. Of the 2.6 billion people without access to sanitation services, 75% live in Asia (Figure 9.1) (1).

Although major improvements have been made over the past decade (Figure 9.2), the world population not served with adequate sanitation has hardly decreased (see Appendix 9.1), primarily because of rapid population growth among the poorest sectors of society, particularly in isolated rural communities and periurban slums. Sanitation has been given a low priority compared with other development issues. One assessment found that only 20% of the total investment in water supply and sanitation infrastructure over the 1990s was dedicated to sanitation (1, 2).

In developed countries, nearly all human excreta are collected safely in sewerage systems or septic tanks; however, not all wastewater is treated before being discharged to the environment. In developing countries, the percentage of treated wastewater is discouragingly low: 14% in Latin America and the Caribbean; 34% in Asia; and practically no treatment at all in Africa (1).

Lack of access to sanitation services aggravates and in turn is aggravated by poverty, inequity and poor health. Without access to these basic services, people, especially children, miss out on opportunities to improve their own lives with dignity and good health. As long as the human right of access to adequate sanitation and safe water supply is denied to the poor, the health status of millions of children around the world will not improve in a sustainable manner.

Health aspects of sanitation

Lack of sanitation is a critical determinant in the contamination of drinking-water by microbes. Faecal pollution of drinking-water can lead to a number of diseases, including cholera, typhoid fever, paratyphoid fever, salmonellosis, shigellosis, giardiasis, hepatitis and poliomyelitis. Of particular concern is the evidence that the burden of disease associated with the lack of sanitation services falls disproportionately upon children. In 2000, for example,

Figure 9.1 Global population without access to improved sanitation (unserved population in 2002: 2.6 billions)

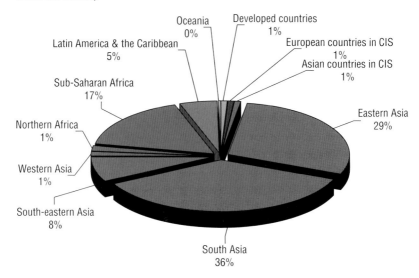

Source: ref. 1.
CIS, Commonwealth of Independent States (countries of the former Union of Soviet Socialist Republics).

Figure 9.2 Global access to improved sanitation, 1990, 2002

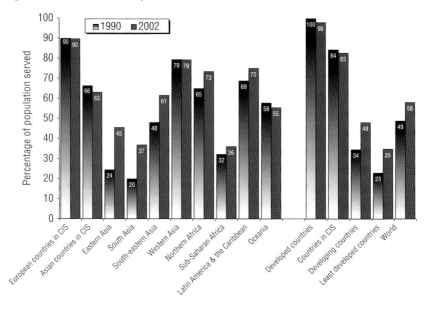

[a] Source: ref. 1.
CIS, Commonwealth of Independent States (countries of the former Union of Soviet Socialist Republics).

SECTION III: SPECIFIC ENVIRONMENTAL THREATS

Table 9.1   Main diseases related to poor sanitation

DISEASE	ANNUAL NO. OF CASES (THOUSANDS)	ANNUAL NO. OF DEATHS (THOUSANDS)	CAUSAL RELATIONSHIP TO POOR SANITATION
Diarrhoeal diseases	4 000 000	1800	Unsafe excreta disposal; poor personal and domestic hygiene; unsafe drinking-water
Ascariasis and other diseases caused by intestinal helminths	1 500 000	100	Unsafe excreta disposal; poor personal and domestic hygiene
Schistosomiasis	200 000	200	Unsafe excreta disposal; poor personal and domestic hygiene
Trachoma	150 000	—	Poor personal and domestic hygiene
Poliomyelitis	114	—	Unsafe excreta disposal
Bancroftian filariasis	72 800	—	Unsafe disposal of excreta; poor domestic hygiene; wastewater disposal and drainage

approximately 60% of the 2.1 million deaths from diarrhoeal diseases were among children under five years of age (2). The data clearly show that children cannot be healthy without access to adequate sanitation and a safe water supply. Providing access to sanitation and hygiene interrupts the disease transmission cycle and reduces the incidence of infectious diseases.

Water-borne diseases (see Chapter 8) are transmitted by contaminated drinking-water. Contaminated water is a direct result of a lack of adequate sanitation facilities, poor wastewater treatment, and unhygienic behaviour.

Water-washed diseases, which produce skin and eye infections, are caused by a lack of soap and insufficient water for washing hands and clothes and for personal hygiene. Again, children are particularly vulnerable to these diseases. The main water-washed diseases are scabies, trachoma, leishmaniasis, typhus, and louse infestation. Trachoma, for example, is an infectious disease that can lead to blindness (3). Children are often a reservoir for the bacteria that cause trachoma.

Water-based diseases are transmitted to aquatic hosts, such as freshwater crustaceans, which may then be ingested by people. The main water-based diseases are schistosomiasis and dracunculiasis (guinea-worm disease).

Water-related vector-borne diseases are caused by bacteria, viruses and parasites (protozoa and helminths) that are transmitted by water-related agents (vectors or intermediate hosts). Often, the vector is an insect that transmits infectious agents from one infected person to another, or from infected animals to people (4). The main water-related vector-borne diseases are malaria, African trypanosomiasis, dengue, onchocerciasis, yellow fever and filariasis.

Inadequate water supply, sanitation and hygiene are estimated to be responsible for 4.0% of all deaths and 5.7% of the total disease burden in disability-adjusted life years (DALYs).[1] Most of this burden could be prevented with interventions to improve sanitation. Other diseases related to water supply, sanitation and hygiene remain to be evaluated (5). Also, the burden of hygiene-related diseases needs to be analysed separately for water-, sanitation- and hygiene-related risk factors. Estimates of morbidity and mortality related to poor sanitation are shown in Table 9.1 for selected main diseases.

Barriers to progress in sanitation

The barriers to improving sanitation are complex and interrelated. The main problems are listed below (6):

- A lack of political will: governments have little interest in dealing with sanitation issues.
- Low prestige and recognition: promoting low-cost sanitation and hygiene education has never been popular with politicians and technical staff because such projects carry little prestige.
- Poor policy on sanitation at global and country level.
- Poor institutional framework: responsibilities for sanitation are fragmented and poorly coordinated among country agencies.
- Inadequate and poorly used resources: scarce financial resources are frequently used inefficiently, such as for improving existing services.
- Inappropriate approaches: frequently, the approach used to provide sanitation services is not in line with local culture, technical limitations or affordability criteria.
- Failure to recognize the disadvantages of conventional excreta management systems. Although water-borne sanitation systems have been used successfully in many parts of the world, often the wastewater is not treated before being discharged to rivers, lakes or the ocean. In many situations, on-site alternatives are more appropriate in terms of both cost and their low impact on the environment.
- Neglect of user preferences: sanitation programmes should consider user preferences for affordability, cultural aspects, etc.
- Ineffective promotion and low public awareness: often both the potential users of sanitation services and those responsible for policy and decision-making are not aware or convinced of the importance of good sanitation for health.
- The low importance given to women and children: women are potential agents of change in hygiene education, and children are the most vulnerable to poor sanitation.

---

[1]DALY = the sum of years of potential life lost due to premature mortality and years of productive life lost due to disability.

Lessons learned

- Sanitation development should not be based on a supply-driven approach, which frequently runs into problems (7). With such an approach, for the same type of service, the investment per capita is normally higher, since the population does not participate. Users may not be willing to pay for the recurrent costs of facilities that were selected without their participation. This also leads to insufficient cost-recovery, making it impossible to operate and maintain the facilities effectively. Also, such investments are generally focused on improving services for those already served, and the unserved or underserved poor are not considered a priority. Supply-driven approaches may also not consider the environmental impact of a programme, such as when flushing toilets are connected to a sewerage system with no wastewater treatment.

- An adequate institutional framework is a major factor facilitating sector development. Centrally managed sanitation services, especially in urban areas, tend to be hampered by ineffective financial performance and a rigid bureaucracy, and to have little budget autonomy. Decentralization of services appears to be an effective alternative. However, in moving from a centralized to an effective decentralized management system, the central agencies have a vital role to play in organizing the decentralized agencies, mobilizing resources for investment and recurrent costs, and providing strong technical and financial support, during at least the transition process. As the decentralization process progresses, the central agencies should act as facilitators of services, rather than as providers.

- The operation and maintenance of sanitation systems have been traditionally neglected. This is true both of large sewerage systems and of small-scale family-owned sanitation facilities. Many small systems fall into disrepair as early as a few weeks after their installation. A number of large wastewater treatment plants that use sophisticated instrumentation and equipment are operated manually because of a lack of knowledge about the system, a lack of spare parts, or simply a lack of interest in making the most of the facility. Operation and maintenance should therefore not be viewed as purely technical issues, since they have connections with many institutional and management issues.

- Hygiene behaviour has often been the missing link between sanitation, water supply and health. While past efforts have built new water supply and sanitation systems, little has been done to maximize the health benefits from these efforts by changing the behaviour of people. Neglected school sanitation is a typical indicator that hygiene education is not a priority in schools, especially in poor urban agglomerations and in rural areas. According to a 1995 pilot survey conducted in 14 developing countries, the average number of children per toilet in urban schools was often more than 50. None of the 14 countries had increased the number of school toilets by more than 8% since 1990, suggesting that they were barely managing to keep up with the rise in student populations (8).

Future perspectives

Even though sanitation coverage increased from 45% to 58% globally during the 1990s, it is still far below the water supply coverage (82% in 2000). The Asian region, which had a sanitation coverage of only 27% in 1990, made great progress and coverage increased to 47% by 2000. Coverage in Africa, by contrast, was essentially unchanged (59% in 1990; 60% in 2000). If these trends continue, Asia is more likely than Africa to achieve the target set at the World Summit on Sustainable Development in Johannesburg, South Africa, in August 2002 of halving the proportion of people unserved by 2015. Coverage in Latin America and the Caribbean increased from 72% in 1990 to 78% in 2000.

Currently, 2.4 billion people globally do not have access to any type of sanitation facility and are thus heavily exposed to health risks. To achieve the target set in Johannesburg, an additional 1870 million people will need to be provided with sanitation facilities between 2000 and 2015 (taking 1990 as the baseline year). Even if the target is achieved, more than 2 billion people (28% of the 2015 population) will remain unserved.

The task will involve the mobilization of significant financial and human resources, and will require (6):

- a change in political attitude;
- the formulation and implementation of policies at all levels;
- a better organization of the sanitation subsector at country level;
- the use of affordable approaches and technologies that can be operated and maintained by households, communities or agencies in charge;
- that user preferences be considered;
- that people, especially women and children, become a central concern.

Three principles are fundamental for introducing sanitation systems that are sustainable socially, economically and ecologically (1):

- *Equity*. All segments of society should have access to safe, appropriate sanitation systems, adapted to their needs and means.
- *Health promotion and protection from disease*. Sanitation systems should prevent users and others from contracting excreta-related diseases, and should interrupt the cycle of disease transmission.
- *Protection of the environment*. Sanitation systems should neither pollute ecosystems nor deplete scarce resources.

The construction and maintenance of sanitation facilities in rural or poor periurban areas are often carried out by the users themselves. In urbanized areas, public or private organizations generally manage the sewerage system and raise service charges. Increasingly, people in rural and many periurban areas are adopting on-site sanitation (e.g. pit latrines). A marketing approach is needed, with a focus on developing and distributing products that match consumer needs in both quality and price. In turn, this requires understanding the reasons why people want sanitation (1).

Hygiene education, especially in primary schools, should be a fundamental component of sanitation and water-supply programmes. Much of the health benefit of water supply and sanitation is realized through changes in behaviour and improved hygiene. To obtain the full health benefits of sanitation programmes, key issues will need to be addressed, including: how to change habits and long-held beliefs about hygiene; how to discuss sanitation issues in societies where the topic is unmentionable; and how to achieve the necessary commitment of effort and time. Involving children in the process would offer hope for sustainability, because as the children grow, they will continue to implement better sanitation practices and influence their own children and community to do the same (6).

Regional and global use of improved drinking water and sanitation in 1990 and 2002

		1990 POPULATION (THOUSANDS)				2002 POPULATION (THOUSANDS)			
		TOTAL POPULATION	POPULATION SERVED	POPULATION UNSERVED	% SERVED	TOTAL POPULATION	POPULATION SERVED	POPULATION UNSERVED	% SERVED
Worldwide	Urban water	2 273 241	2 165 476	107 765	95	2 980 995	2 820 494	160 501	95
	Rural water	2 990 351	1 893 020	1 097 331	63	3 243 990	2 328 654	915 336	72
	Total water	5 263 592	4 058 496	1 205 096	77	6 224 985	5 149 148	1 075 837	83
	Urban sanitation	2 273 241	1 804 813	468 428	79	2 980 995	2 413 465	567 530	81
	Rural sanitation	2 990 351	752 651	2 237 700	25	3 243 990	1 192 692	2 051 298	37
	Total sanitation	5 263 592	2 557 464	2 706 128	49	6 224 985	3 606 157	2 618 828	58
Developed countries	Urban water	672 945	672 945	0	100	744 438	744 438	0	100
	Rural water	261 158	258 846	2 612	99	248 708	233 786	14 922	94
	Total water	934 103	931 491	2 612	100	993 146	978 224	14 922	98
	Urban sanitation	672 945	672 945	0	100	744 438	744 438	0	100
	Rural sanitation	261 158	258 546	2 612	99	248 708	228 811	19 897	92
	Total sanitation	934 103	931 491	2 612	100	993 146	973 249	19 897	98
Countries in CIS	Urban water	184 339	179 371	4 968	97	179 798	177 029	2 769	98
	Rural water	97 360	80 522	16 838	83	101 172	82 775	18 397	82
	Total water	281 699	259 892	21 807	92	280 970	259 804	21 166	92
	Urban sanitation	184 339	171 598	12 741	93	179 798	166 276	13 522	92
	Rural sanitation	97 360	66 184	31 176	68	101 172	66 310	34 862	66
	Total sanitation	281 699	237 781	43 918	84	280 970	232 586	48 384	83

SECTION III: SPECIFIC ENVIRONMENTAL THREATS

Region	Indicator							
Developing countries	Urban water	1 415 957	1 313 161	102 796	93	2 056 759	1 899 027	157 732	92
	Rural water	2 631 833	1 553 952	1 077 881	59	2 894 110	2 012 094	882 016	70
	Total water	4 047 790	2 867 113	1 180 677	71	4 950 869	3 911 121	1 039 748	79
	Urban sanitation	1 415 957	960 270	455 687	68	2 056 759	1 502 751	554 008	73
	Rural sanitation	2 631 833	427 921	2 203 912	16	2 894 110	897 571	1 996 539	31
	Total sanitation	4 047 790	1 388 191	2 659 599	34	4 950 869	2 400 322	2 550 547	48
European countries in CIS	Urban water	152 300	149 254	3 046	98	147 422	145 948	1 474	99
	Rural water	62 513	54 386	8 127	87	59 772	53 795	5 977	90
	Total water	214 813	203 640	11 173	95	207 194	199 743	7 451	97
	Urban sanitation	152 300	144 685	7 615	95	147 422	140 051	7 371	95
	Rural sanitation	62 513	48 760	13 753	78	59 772	46 024	13 748	77
	Total sanitation	214 813	193 445	21 368	90	207 194	186 075	21 119	90
Asian countries in CIS	Urban water	32 039	30 117	1 922	94	32 376	31 081	1 295	96
	Rural water	34 847	26 135	8 712	75	41 400	28 980	12 420	70
	Total water	66 886	56 252	10 634	84	73 776	60 061	13 715	82
	Urban sanitation	32 039	26 913	5 126	84	32 376	26 225	6 151	81
	Rural sanitation	34 847	17 424	17 424	50	41 400	20 286	21 114	49
	Total sanitation	66 886	44 336	22 550	66	73 776	46 511	27 265	63
Northern Africa	Urban water	57 349	54 482	2 867	95	76 101	73 057	3 044	96
	Rural water	60 719	49 790	10 929	82	71 217	59 822	11 395	84
	Total water	118 068	104 271	13 797	88	147 318	132 879	14 439	90
	Urban sanitation	57 349	48 173	9 176	84	76 101	67 730	8 371	89
	Rural sanitation	60 719	28 538	32 181	47	71 217	40 594	30 623	57
	Total sanitation	118 068	76 711	41 357	65	147 318	108 324	38 994	73
Sub-Saharan Africa	Urban water	141 445	115 985	25 460	82	241 439	197 980	43 459	82
	Rural water	362 929	130 654	232 275	36	443 334	199 500	243 834	45
	Total water	504 374	246 639	257 735	49	684 773	397 480	287 293	58
	Urban sanitation	141 445	76 380	65 065	54	241 439	132 791	108 648	55
	Rural sanitation	362 929	87 103	275 826	24	443 334	115 267	328 067	26
	Total sanitation	504 374	163 483	340 891	32	684 773	248 058	436 715	36

		1990 POPULATION (THOUSANDS)				2002 POPULATION (THOUSANDS)			
		TOTAL POPULATION	POPULATION SERVED	POPULATION UNSERVED	% SERVED	TOTAL POPULATION	POPULATION SERVED	POPULATION UNSERVED	% SERVED
Latin America & the Caribbean	Urban water	313 879	291 907	21 972	93	409 168	388 710	20 458	95
	Rural water	127 647	74 035	53 612	58	126 458	87 256	39 202	69
	Total water	441 526	365 943	75 583	83	535 626	475 966	59 660	89
	Urban sanitation	313 879	257 381	56 498	82	409 168	343 701	65 467	84
	Rural sanitation	127 647	44 676	82 971	35	126 458	55 642	70 816	44
	Total sanitation	441 526	302 057	139 469	69	535 626	399 343	136 283	75
Eastern Asia	Urban water	367 169	363 497	3 672	99	548 285	509 905	38 380	93
	Rural water	859 254	515 552	343 702	60	826 553	562 056	264 497	68
	Total water	1 226 423	879 050	347 373	72	1 374 838	1 071 961	302 877	78
	Urban sanitation	367 169	234 988	132 181	64	548 285	378 317	169 968	69
	Rural sanitation	859 254	60 148	799 106	7	826 553	247 966	578 587	30
	Total sanitation	1 226 423	295 136	931 287	24	1 374 838	626 283	748 555	45
South Asia	Urban water	311 514	280 363	31 151	90	437 431	411 185	26 246	94
	Rural water	863 076	552 369	310 707	64	1 042 856	834 285	208 571	80
	Total water	1 174 590	832 731	341 859	71	1 480 287	1 245 470	234 817	84
	Urban sanitation	311 514	168 218	143 296	54	437 431	288 704	148 727	66
	Rural sanitation	863 076	60 415	802 661	7	1 042 856	250 285	792 571	24
	Total sanitation	1 174 590	228 633	945 957	20	1 480 287	538 989	941 298	37

SECTION III: SPECIFIC ENVIRONMENTAL THREATS

South-eastern Asia	Urban water	138 937	126 433	12 504	91	221 161	201 257	19 904	91
	Rural water	300 989	195 643	105 346	65	314 451	220 116	94 335	70
	Total water	439 926	322 076	117 850	73	535 612	421 372	114 240	79
	Urban sanitation	138 937	93 088	45 849	67	221 161	174 717	46 444	79
	Rural sanitation	300 989	117 386	183 603	39	314 451	154 081	160 370	49
	Total sanitation	439 926	210 474	229 453	48	535 612	328 798	206 814	61
Western Asia	Urban water	84 161	79 111	5 050	94	121 130	115 074	6 057	95
	Rural water	52 283	33 984	18 299	65	62 831	46 495	16 336	74
	Total water	136 444	113 095	23 349	83	183 961	161 568	22 393	88
	Urban sanitation	84 161	80 795	3 366	96	121 130	115 074	6 056	95
	Rural sanitation	52 283	27 187	25 096	52	62 831	30 787	32 044	49
	Total sanitation	136 444	107 982	28 462	79	183 961	145 861	38 100	79
Oceania	Urban water	1 503	1 383	120	92	2 044	1 860	184	91
	Rural water	4 936	1 925	3 011	39	6 410	2 564	3 846	40
	Total water	6 439	3 308	3 131	51	8 454	4 424	4 030	52
	Urban sanitation	1 503	1 247	256	83	2 044	1 717	327	84
	Rural sanitation	4 936	2 468	2 468	50	6 410	2 949	3 461	46
	Total sanitation	6 439	3 715	2 724	58	8 454	4 666	3 788	55

Source: ref. 1.
CIS, Commonwealth of Independent States (countries of the former Union of Soviet Socialist Republics).

References

1. WHO/UNICEF *Meeting the MDG drinking Water and Sanitation target.* Geneva, World Health Organization, United Nations Children's Fund, 2004.

2. *The World Health Report 2000. Health systems: improving performance.* Geneva, World Health Organization, 2000.

3. *Children in the new millennium—environmental impact on health.* Geneva, World Health Organization, 2002.

4. Cairncross S, Feachem RG. *Environmental health engineering in the tropics: an introductory text.* Chichester, John Wiley and Sons, Ltd, 1983.

5. Pruess A et al. Estimating the burden of disease from water, sanitation and hygiene at a global level. *Environmental Health Perspectives*, 2002, 110:537–542.

6. *Sanitation promotion.* Geneva, World Health Organization, 1998.

7. Wright A. *Toward a strategic sanitation approach: improving the sustainability of urban sanitation in developing countries.* Washington, DC, UNDP/World Bank Water and Sanitation Programme, 1997.

8. *The progress of nations.* New York, United Nations Children's Fund, 1997.

CHAPTER 10

Air[1]

R. A. Etzel
Department of Environmental and Occupational Health,
School of Public Health and Health Services, George
Washington University, Washington, DC, USA

K. Balakrishnan
College of Allied Health Sciences, Sri Ramachandra
Medical College and Research Institute, Porur, India

INDOOR AIR
Overview

Indoor air pollutants are now recognized to pose potential health risks to exposed children throughout the world (*1, 2*). Indoor air pollutants have various sources and hazard profiles. Some key indoor air pollutants and their sources are listed in Table 10.1.

Indoor air quality problems are strikingly different between developed and developing nations. The most significant factor affecting indoor air quality in rural areas of developing countries is emissions from combustion of biomass fuels (wood, dung and crop residues) and coal used for cooking and heating. Use of open fires for cooking and heating in poorly ventilated homes exposes an estimated 2.4 billion people to concentrations of particulate matter and gases up to 60 times higher than ambient concentrations (*3, 4*).

Women who cook with these fuels and children, who often stay close to their mothers, are usually the most exposed groups (*5–8*). Although solid fuels make up only 10–15% of total fuel use, indoor exposures are likely to exceed outdoor exposures globally since nearly half the world's population cooks and heats their homes with biomass fuels.

Indoor air quality has also become a health concern in developed countries in recent years as rising energy costs have led to building designs that reduce air exchange. In addition, new synthetic materials are now widely used in home furnishings. As a result, there are a range of airborne pollutants in indoor environments, including particulate matter, gases, vapours, biological materials, and fibres (*9, 10*). In homes, common sources of air pollutants include tobacco smoke, gas and wood stoves, and furnishings and construction materials that release organic gases and vapours. Allergens and biological

[1]Reviewed by **D. Schwela**, Physical and Chemical Exposure Unit, Institute for Health and
Consumer Protection, Joint Research Centre, Ispra, Italy.

Table 10.1   Principal pollutants and sources of indoor air pollution, grouped by origin

PRINCIPAL POLLUTANTS	SOURCES
Predominantly outdoor sources	
Sulfur dioxide, suspended particulate matter, respirable suspended particles	Fuel combustion, smelters
Ozone	Photochemical reactions
Pollens	Trees, grass, weeds, plants
Lead, manganese	Automobiles
Lead, cadmium	Industrial emissions
Volatile organic compounds, polycyclic aromatic hydrocarbons	Petrochemical solvents, vaporization of unburned fuels
Indoor and outdoor sources	
Oxides of nitrogen, carbon monoxide	Fuel burning
Carbon dioxide	Fuel burning, metabolic activity
Suspended particulate matter, respirable suspended particles	Environmental tobacco smoke, resuspension of dust, condensation of vapours and combustion products
Water vapour	Biological activity, combustion, evaporation
Volatile organic compounds	Volatilization, fuel burning, paint, metabolic activity, pesticides, insecticides, fungicides
Spores	Fungi, moulds
Predominantly indoor sources	
Radon	Soil, building construction materials, water
Formaldehyde	Insulation, furnishing, environmental tobacco smoke
Asbestos	Fire-retardant, insulation
Ammonia	Cleaning products, metabolic activity
Polycyclic aromatic hydrocarbons, arsenic, nicotine, acrolein	Environmental tobacco smoke
Volatile organic compounds	Adhesives, solvents, cooking, cosmetics
Mercury	Fungicides, paints, spills or breakage of mercury-containing products, Santeria (traditional medicine in some Latin American countries)
Aerosols	Consumer products, house dust
Allergens	House dust, animal dander

Source: ref. 3.

SECTION III: SPECIFIC ENVIRONMENTAL THREATS

materials include animal dander, faecal material from house dust mites and other insects, fungal spores, and bacteria.

Main indoor air pollutants
Solid fuel smoke

Air pollutants emitted from combustion of biomass fuels, such as wood, woodchips, agricultural produce and cow dung, are the result of incomplete combustion and are practically the same for any type of biomass. However, the amount and characteristics of the pollutants produced depend on several factors including composition of the fuel, combustion conditions (temperature and air flow), mode of burning, and even shape of the fireplace (11). Hundreds of different chemical substances are emitted during the burning of biomass fuels, in the form of liquids (suspended droplets), solids (suspended particles), and gases such as nitrogen dioxide (NO_2) and sulfur dioxide (SO_2) (12). The aerosol mixture of very fine solid and liquid particles, or "smoke", contains particles in the inhalable range, i.e. less than 10 μm in diameter.

The aerosol produced from burning solid fuel is made up of organic and inorganic matter. In addition to particulates, it contains many toxic and carcinogenic compounds, including polycyclic aromatic hydrocarbons (PAHs), benzene, and formaldehyde. The inorganic matter is mostly ash and is produced in very small amounts during regular combustion in stoves. Smoke from burning coal has all of the above in addition to high levels of sulfur and toxic elements such as heavy metals and fluorine, depending on the geographical location.

Combustion pollutants are also emitted from gas ranges, particularly when they function incorrectly or are used as space heaters. Combustion of natural gas results in the emission of nitrogen dioxide (NO_2) and carbon monoxide (CO). Levels of NO_2 in the home generally increase during the winter, when ventilation is reduced to conserve energy. During the winter, average indoor concentrations of NO_2 in homes with gas cooking stoves may be twice as high as outdoor levels. Some of the highest indoor NO_2 levels have been measured in homes where ovens were used as space heaters (12).

Routes of exposure

Exposure to the products of solid fuel combustion is essentially an everyday occurrence in homes that use these fuels. Recent large-scale assessments of household level concentrations and exposures have shown that concentrations of respirable particulate matter (used as an indicator pollutant for overall levels of biomass smoke) in kitchens and living areas during the cooking period can be several thousand μg per m³, while 24-hour average concentrations are around several hundred μg per m³. Households that have indoor kitchens that are not partitioned from the living area have the highest concentrations (13, 14). Young children who spend a considerable time with their mother indoors are at high risk of high exposure.

In homes where coal is burned, concentrations of particulate matter, sulfur dioxide and fluorine have been found to reach 10–100 times the standards set for outdoor air. In cold regions, the use of coal for heating further compounds the situation as these stoves are often kept burning all day long. Release of certain pollutants, such as lead, arsenic and fluorine, where food grains are stored creates the potential for secondary routes of exposure through contaminated food (15).

Health effects in children

While exposure to solid fuel smoke has been associated with several health effects in women who cook with these fuels, including chronic bronchitis in biomass users and lung cancer in coal users, there is strong evidence that high levels of indoor smoke are an important risk factor for acute lower respiratory illnesses in children (16, 17). Acute lower respiratory illnesses in children are a leading contributor to infant mortality. In certain situations, e.g. where coal contains high amounts of arsenic or fluorine, the potential for secondary toxicity exists. Arsenic-induced skin lesions and skeletal fluorosis have been documented in children in communities using so-called "dirty coal".

Exposure to high levels of NO_2 and SO_2 may result in acute mucocutaneous irritation and respiratory effects. The relatively low water solubility of NO_2 results in minimal irritation of the mucous membranes of the upper airway; the principal site of toxicity is the lower respiratory tract (18). In contrast, the high water solubility of SO_2 makes it extremely irritating to the eyes and upper respiratory tract. Whether exposure to the relatively low levels of these gases in houses is associated with any health effects remains to be determined. Exposure to inhalable particles in wood smoke may result in irritation and inflammation of the upper and lower respiratory tract, resulting in rhinitis, cough, wheezing, and worsening of asthma (19).

Diagnosis

The specific etiology of a respiratory illness may be difficult to establish because most respiratory signs and symptoms are nonspecific and may occur only in association with significant exposure. The effects of low exposures may be mild. Multiple pollutants may be involved in a given situation. Establishing an environmental cause for a respiratory illness is further complicated by the similarity of effects to those of allergies and respiratory infections. Diagnosis of an environmentally related disease requires a high index of suspicion and a thorough environmental history. While health workers cannot always assess the causal association between indoor air and health effects, they should consider a possible environmental cause when a child's illness does not follow usual patterns. Exposure reduction should be recommended whenever possible.

Registering the data

Health or environmental databases for registering data on childhood acute respiratory infections and household fuel use are unlikely to be available in developing country settings where such exposures predominate. In this case, an entry may be made on the patient's health chart to indicate the main type of fuel such as natural gas or renewables (e.g. solar heat or biomass fuel used in the home for cooking or heating).

Remedial action, prevention, and education

Recognition that indoor air pollution from solid fuel use is a potential source of significant health risks to children is relatively new. Existing community health and education programmes may not therefore be specifically focused on raising awareness of the threats from indoor air pollution. While interventions to reduce exposure to solid fuel smoke are difficult to implement and often involve substantial cost (such as switching to clean fuels or installing better ventilation systems), health workers can recommend simple behavioural interventions, such as keeping children away from the stove during cooking, using lids on pots during cooking, using dry wood, and cooking outdoors, whenever possible. This may be difficult in some areas, yet the need to reduce exposure of children remains. This information could be disseminated through community health or social workers.

Second-hand tobacco smoke

Environmental tobacco smoke (ETS) or second-hand smoke is exhaled smoke or smoke released from the smouldering end of cigarettes, cigars, and pipes. Environmental tobacco smoke is composed of more than 3800 chemical compounds.

Routes of exposure

Around 700 million, or almost half, of the world's children breathe air polluted by tobacco smoke, particularly at home (20). Because many young children spend a large proportion of their time indoors, they may have significant exposure to second-hand smoke. This exposure may occur in a variety of environments, such as in homes, child care settings, and motor vehicles (21).

> **Children deserve a smoke-free world**
> Smoking tobacco is dangerous, both for users and for those nearby. Growing evidence points to second-hand smoke as an important factor in health problems such as sudden infant death syndrome, asthma, and pulmonary and middle ear infections. The tobacco industry has successfully lobbied worldwide to open doors for tobacco crops, cigarette manufacture, and sales. However, some countries are learning to fight back. Read how the Philippines established a Clean Air Act in 1999, which included the right for children to learn in a smoke-free setting (Case study 11, page 313).

Mechanism of action and clinical effects in children

Infants whose mothers smoke are 38% more likely to be hospitalized for pneumonia than those whose mothers do not smoke. The number of hospitalizations increases with the number of cigarettes the mother smokes each day (22, 23). Infants with two smoking parents are more than twice as likely to have had pneumonia than infants whose parents do not smoke (24, 25).

Children whose parents smoke are about 60% more likely to develop middle ear effusion, as measured by tympanometry; overall, between 8% and 15% of middle ear effusions are attributable to passive smoking (26). In one study, at least one-third of cases of middle ear effusion among children were attributable to passive smoking (27).

Children whose mothers smoke may be more likely to develop asthma. Children with asthma whose parents smoke may have more frequent exacerbation and more severe symptoms (28–30). Conversely, if asthmatic children's exposure to cigarette smoke is reduced, their asthmatic symptoms will be less severe (31).

There is substantial evidence linking exposure to ETS to sudden infant death syndrome (32). This association appears to be independent of birth weight and gestational age (33). Most reviewers consider the association to be causal (34).

Registering the data

It may be difficult to determine the extent of a child's exposure to ETS. At each clinic visit, the child's parents should be asked about their smoking behaviour. Every child's medical chart should include in a prominent place information about smoking and passive smoking.

Remedial action, prevention, and education

Discussions related to ETS exposure and parental smoking are appropriate in the context of paediatric visits. Most parents do not want to damage the health of their children. Messages about risks to children from ETS may become an important factor in their decision to quit smoking. When a child has a medical condition exacerbated by ETS exposure (e.g. asthma or recurrent otitis media), parent education is an important element of the child's medical care. The health worker should advise the parents to reduce their child's exposure to ETS and to attempt to quit smoking. Smoking cessation counselling by physicians has been found to almost double smoking cessation rates. In the United States, approximately 10% of smokers who received smoking cessation counselling from a physician stopped smoking (35). Although this may not seem significant within the context of an individual practice, it reflects a tremendous public health impact at the population level. Over time, advice from physicians may also influence other family members to stop smoking.

Smoking cessation by parents is the most effective means of reducing their children's exposure to ETS. Even if the parents and other family members do not quit, efforts to reduce their children's exposure to ETS may reduce their risk of disease and may also motivate those who smoke to quit.

Carbon monoxide

Carbon monoxide (CO) is a colourless, odourless, tasteless toxic gas that is produced by the incomplete combustion of carbon-based fuels.

Routes of exposure

Unintentional exposure to CO can be largely attributed to smoke from fires, automobile exhaust, faulty or improperly vented combustion appliances, and tobacco smoke. Confined, poorly ventilated spaces such as garages, caravans, tents, and boats are particularly liable to have elevated levels of CO. Common sources of CO exposure are wood and coal fires, gas furnaces and heaters, gas ranges and ovens, gas clothes dryers, other fuel-powered equipment and appliances, fireplaces, and charcoal grills. Exposure to CO may occur in and around automobiles when there is inadequate combustion resulting from substandard vehicle maintenance and poor ventilation.

Carbon monoxide poisoning in children in France

An unusually high incidence of carbon monoxide poisoning was noted in the north of France in the 1980s, associated with the use of kerosene lamps. Public health authorities responded by implementing monitoring, reporting of cases and strict regulations requiring the lamps to have carbon monoxide detection devices. These measures resulted in a noticeable decrease in poisonings the following year. Learn how ongoing surveillance is necessary to protect public health and why carbon monoxide is particularly hazardous to children in Case study 10, page 309.

Mechanism of action and clinical effects in children

Intoxication from exposure to CO and the resultant tissue hypoxia affect multiple organ systems. Systems with high metabolic rates and high oxygen demand are preferentially affected. Carbon monoxide is inhaled, diffuses across the alveolar-capillary membrane, and is measurable in the bloodstream as carboxyhaemoglobin. CO has approximately 240 times greater affinity for haemoglobin than oxygen, and decreases the oxygen-carrying capacity of the blood. Carbon monoxide in the bloodstream also causes a leftward shift of the oxyhaemoglobin dissociation curve, causing decreased delivery of oxygen to the tissues.

The clinical presentation of CO intoxication is highly variable and the severity of the symptoms may not correlate to carboxyhaemoglobin levels in the blood. Low levels of carboxyhaemoglobin may be present in cases of severe poisoning. Symptoms of CO intoxication include: headache, dizziness, fatigue, weakness, drowsiness, nausea, vomiting, loss of consciousness, skin pallor, dyspnoea on exertion, palpitations, confusion, irritability, and irrational behaviour. The prevalence of unintentional nonfatal CO poisonings is difficult to estimate because early symptoms of intoxication are often nonspecific (36, 37).

Infants and children are particularly susceptible to CO toxicity because of their higher metabolic rates (38). The fetus is especially vulnerable to maternal CO intoxication. The risk of complications increases with the severity of the maternal poisoning, as the amount of oxygen available to the fetus decreases.

Diagnosis

A thorough history and physical examination, as well as a high index of clinical suspicion, are necessary to diagnose CO poisoning. Health workers should consider the possibility of CO exposure when people living in the same household present with similar nonspecific symptoms. Initial laboratory findings may be misleading.

The measurement of carboxyhaemoglobin levels in the blood enables the degree of exposure to be assessed. An elevated level may confirm the diagnosis of CO intoxication: low or moderately increased levels must be interpreted with caution. Baseline levels of carboxyhaemoglobin are typically 0.3–0.7% in nonsmokers, while those in smokers typically range from 3% to 8%, although higher values have been reported.

Treatment guidelines

Patients who have been exposed to CO should be removed from the source immediately. Therapy consists of the administration of 100% oxygen through a tight-fitting non-rebreather mask at a flow rate of 10 litres/min.

Registering the data

Carbon monoxide exposure and poisoning should be reported to the local health department.

Remedial action, prevention, and education

Primary prevention of CO poisoning involves prevention of exposure to known sources (39).

Smoke detectors and carbon monoxide detectors, when used properly, may provide an early warning and prevent unintentional CO-related deaths. Carbon monoxide detectors measure the amount of CO that has accumulated in the air, and sound an alarm when the CO in the air corresponds to a 10% carboxyhaemoglobin level in the blood.

Several countries, including Canada and Japan, have set guidelines for CO in indoor air. Health Canada recommends that the acceptable short-term exposure range for carbon monoxide in indoor air is less than or equal to 11 parts per million (ppm) (eight-hour average concentration), or less than or equal to 25 ppm (one-hour average concentration) (40).

The American Society of Heating, Refrigerating and Air Conditioning Engineers recommends an exposure limit of no more than 9 ppm in a living space, while Japan has an indoor standard that limits exposure to 10 ppm for any duration (40). However, these guidelines may not provide sufficient protection for infants and children.

Volatile organic compounds

Indoor concentrations of volatile organic compounds (VOCs) are greater than outdoor concentrations. Many household furnishings and products contain VOCs as residues or carriers (9, 41). These include chemicals such as aliphatic and aromatic hydrocarbons (including chlorinated hydrocarbons), alcohols, and ketones, in products such as finishes, rug and oven cleaners, paints and lacquers, and paint strippers. Formaldehyde is found primarily in building materials and home furnishings (9–10, 43). Since product labels do not always specify the presence of organic compounds, the specific chemicals to which a product user may be exposed can be difficult to discern. At room temperature, VOCs are released as gases or vapours from furnishings or consumer products. In the United States, consumer surveys conducted by the Environmental Protection Agency (EPA) and measurements of VOCs in residential and nonresidential buildings showed that exposure to VOCs is widespread and highly variable. In general, VOCs are likely to be higher in recently constructed or renovated buildings than in older buildings. Once building-related emissions decrease, consumer products are the predominant source of exposure.

Formaldehyde is one of the most common indoor air contaminants. It is used in hundreds of products, such as urea-formaldehyde and phenol-formaldehyde resin, which are used to bond laminated wood products and to bind wood chips in particle board; as a carrier solvent in dyeing textiles and paper products; and as a stiffener, wrinkle resistor, and water repellant in floor coverings (e.g. rugs and linoleum) (9, 10). Toxicology reports indicate that exposure to VOCs may result in dermal, mucocutaneous, and nonspecific effects. Epidemiological studies delineating the acute and chronic health effects of residential exposure to low levels of VOCs are limited, reflecting the difficulty of characterizing exposures and identifying effects of components of complex mixtures.

Depending on the dominant compounds and route and level of exposure, signs and symptoms may include upper respiratory tract and eye irritation, rhinitis, nasal congestion, rash, pruritus, headache, nausea, and vomiting. These effects are drawn from limited studies of occupationally exposed adults. It is unlikely that exposures of the same magnitude would be found in a typical home environment.

Volatile organic compounds have only recently attracted study, and it is still largely unknown which VOCs are associated with specific health effects. Data on children are extremely limited.

The effects of exposure to formaldehyde have received more attention. Exposure to airborne formaldehyde can result in conjunctival and upper respiratory tract irritation (i.e. burning or tingling sensations in eyes, nose, and throat);

these symptoms are temporary and resolve when exposure stops. Formaldehyde may exacerbate asthma in some infants and children.

Several questions may help to identify exposure to VOCs. These include: Does the family live in a new home with large amounts of pressed wood products? Is there new pressed wood furniture? Have household members recently worked on craft or graphic materials? Are chemical cleaners used extensively? Has the home recently been renovated? Has anyone recently used paints, solvents, or sprays in the home?

Prevention strategies include increasing ventilation and avoiding storage of opened containers of paint and similar materials within the home. If formaldehyde is thought to be the cause of the problem, the source should be identified and, if possible, removed. Measuring levels of formaldehyde in the air is usually not necessary. If it is not possible to remove the source, exposure can be reduced by coating cabinets, panelling, and other furnishings with polyurethane or other nontoxic sealants, and by increasing the amount of ventilation in the home. Formaldehyde concentrations decrease rapidly over the first year after a product is manufactured.

Moulds

Moulds are ubiquitous in the outdoor environment, and can enter the home through doorways, windows, heating and ventilation systems, and air conditioning systems. Moulds also develop in damp indoor environments, and proliferate where there is excessive moisture, such as from leaks in roofs, walls, plant pots, or pet urine. The most common indoor moulds are *Cladosporium, Penicillium, Aspergillus*, and *Alternaria* (44).

Moulds have been associated with both allergic reactions and toxic effects. Some children who are exposed to moulds have allergic effects manifesting as persistent upper respiratory tract symptoms, such as rhinitis, sneezing, and eye irritation, and lower respiratory tract symptoms such as coughing and wheezing (45–47).

Toxic effects may be produced by inhalation of mycotoxins, lipid-soluble toxins that are readily absorbed by the airways (48). Species of mycotoxin-producing moulds include *Fusarium, Trichoderma*, and *Stachybotrys* (49). *Stachybotrys* has been associated with acute pulmonary haemorrhage in young infants in Ohio (48, 50), Missouri (51), and Delaware (52), and with pulmonary haemosiderosis in a 7-year old child in Texas (53).

Several questions may help to identify exposure to moulds. They include: Has the home been flooded? Is there any water-damaged wood or cardboard in the house? Has there been a roof or plumbing leak? Have occupants seen any mould or noticed a musty smell?

Although no indoor guidelines for fungi have been set, experts have suggested that even 150 colony-forming units (CFU) per m^3 is considered to be high if there are dominant species of mould along with a few other species (54, 55).

The "tolerable" levels for airborne fungi are around 200 CFU/m^3 (56). This is exclusive of the toxigenic fungi, which are considered unacceptable in indoor air (57).

Prevention includes cleaning up water and removing all water-damaged items (including carpets) within 24 hours of a flood or leak. If this is done, toxic mould will not have the opportunity to grow. If some mould is already present, the affected area needs to be washed with soap and water, and then with a solution of 1 part bleach to 9 parts water. Protective gloves should be worn during these operations.

Treatment guidelines

Clinical symptoms due to exposure to indoor moulds are usually short-lived, and cease with elimination of exposure. Treatment of most mould-related illnesses includes relief of symptoms and elimination of the water source. Children with lower respiratory symptoms may need to be evaluated for possible allergies and asthma.

Registering the data

Data on health problems due to biological agents are rarely reported to the local health department, primarily because it is very difficult to pinpoint the specific cause.

Mercury vapour

Mercury vapour is a potentially dangerous indoor air pollutant.

Routes of exposure

Elemental mercury is used in sphygmomanometers, thermometers, and thermostat switches. Elemental mercury is also used in some folk rituals, such as Santeria, which is practised in some parts of the Caribbean. Because of its attractive appearance, schoolchildren may bring home mercury from science classes.

Mechanism of action and clinical effects in children

Elemental mercury is liquid at room temperature and readily volatilizes to a colourless and odourless vapour. When inhaled, elemental mercury vapour easily passes through the pulmonary alveolar membranes and enters the blood, where it is distributed primarily into red blood cells and the central nervous system. Inhalation of the vapours from heated mercury can be very dangerous. At high concentrations, mercury vapour produces an acute necrotizing bronchitis and pneumonitis, which can lead to death due to respiratory failure. Fatalities have resulted from heating elemental mercury in inadequately ventilated areas.

Long-term exposure to mercury vapour primarily affects the central nervous system. Early nonspecific signs include insomnia, forgetfulness, loss of appetite, and mild tremor, and may be misdiagnosed as psychiatric illness. Continued exposure leads to progressive tremor and erethism, a syndrome characterized by red palms, emotional lability, and memory impairment. Salivation and excessive sweating are accompanying autonomic signs. The child's developing brain may be especially vulnerable to mercury vapour toxicity.

Mercury also accumulates in the kidneys. Renal toxicity includes proteinuria and nephrotic syndrome, alone or in addition to other signs of mercury exposure. Isolated renal effects may be immunological in origin.

Acrodynia (painful extremities) is a hypersensitivity response to mercury that has been reported in children exposed to mercury from interior latex paint containing phenylmercury as a preservative (58, 59). Since the carbon-mercury chemical bond of phenylmercury is relatively unstable, elemental mercury can be released from painted walls.

Diagnosis

Mercury should be measured in a 24-hour urine collection, using a special mercury-free container from an environmental laboratory. In sensitive individuals, effects may already be seen at urine mercury values of around 100 micrograms per litre (3).

Treatment guidelines

The most important step is to identify the source of the child's exposure and remove it.

Registering the data

Children with documented mercury poisoning should be reported to the health authorities.

Remedial action, prevention, and education

Although there are no standards for indoor air, the Agency for Toxic Substances and Disease Registry suggests that residential air mercury levels should be not higher than 0.5 micrograms per cubic metre (37).

OUTDOOR AIR
Overview

Outdoor air pollutants typically exist as part of a complex mixture of multiple pollutants. In many countries, however, only a few air pollutants are regularly monitored to assess air quality. WHO has developed and published guidelines for air quality (3) covering about 50 compounds with noncarcinogenic health endpoints and 30 compounds with carcinogenic health endpoints, including respirable particulate matter, sulfur compounds, carbon monoxide, lead, nitrogen oxides, and ozone.

Key pollutants
Particulate matter

Particulate matter is a generic term for a variety of materials with many different characteristics. Both solid particles and liquid droplets are included, and the particle or droplet size can range from slightly above the molecular level (invisible to the naked eye) to dust particles several hundred microns in diameter. Solid particulate matter is generated by the incomplete combustion of organic matter, or can come from the mechanical breakdown of solid matter (such as rocks and soil). Fine and ultra-fine particulate matter is emitted by diesel engines and power plants, and can be found in the smoke of forest fires.

Particle size is the major factor determining where in the respiratory system the particles will be deposited. Particles larger than 10 µm in diameter are filtered out as air passes through the nose, while smaller particles reach the lower airways. Children, however, frequently breathe through their mouths, thus bypassing the nasal filtration mechanism. Particles smaller than 2.5 µm are able to penetrate deeply into the lungs. The particles that reach the alveoli (the terminal air pockets of the lungs) stay there permanently. Thus an adolescent who has lived in a polluted city for many years has "blacker" lungs than one who has lived in a polluted city for a shorter time. Particulate matter with a diameter smaller than 10 µm is called PM_{10}. The fine particles are often the most toxic.

Diesel automobile exhaust generates particles smaller than 1 µm;

Respiratory illness among children in São Paulo, Brazil

The city of São Paulo, Brazil, is one of the largest in the world, with over 40 000 industries and nearly 6 million registered vehicles. In the 1970s and 1980s, industries sprang up, many of which were indiscriminately situated in residential areas. By 1980, respiratory diseases were the second largest cause of death in the city. A series of public policies, including the establishment of clean air regulations, and programmes to promote control of air pollution and industrial zoning, have since led to reduced health risks in the city (Case study 12, page 316).

Air pollution and pregnancy outcome

There is widespread concern over the health effects of ambient air pollution. Support is growing for the idea that several adverse pregnancy outcomes may be the result of maternal or paternal exposure to airborne pollution. A consistent relationship between maternal exposure to fine particles in early gestation and intrauterine growth retardation was recently observed in a highly polluted district of Northern Bohemia in the Czech Republic. One possible explanation for this finding is that some associated copollutants, such as polycyclic aromatic hydrocarbons, may interfere with fetal development. Read about this, in Case study 13, page 320).

these remain suspended in the atmosphere for long periods of time and are more likely to be inhaled.

Sulfur compounds

Sulfur-containing compounds include sulfur dioxide (SO_2), sulfuric acid aerosol (H_2SO_4), sulfate particles, and hydrogen sulfide (H_2S). The primary source of sulfur dioxide is from burning coal; thus, major emitters of sulfur dioxide include coal-fired power plants, smelters, and pulp and paper mills. Sulfuric acid aerosol is formed in the atmosphere from the oxidation of sulfur dioxide in the presence of moisture. Facilities that either manufacture or use acids can also emit sulfuric acid aerosol. Hydrogen sulfide is emitted from a variety of industrial processes, including oil refining, wood pulp production and wastewater treatment, as well as from the operation of geothermal plants and landfills. Hydrogen sulfide, which has an odour similar to that of rotten eggs, is easily detected at levels that are far below those associated with physiological effects.

Childhood asthma in China, Hong Kong, Special Administrative Region

Childhood asthma is common in Hong Kong, SAR. High levels of ambient air pollution are now thought to be an important factor contributing to asthma morbidity. The main sources of outdoor pollution in Hong Kong include automobile exhaust and burning of fossil fuels by various factories. The incidence of asthma in children was reduced after fuel regulations were established in 1990 (Case study 14, page 323).

Carbon monoxide

Large amounts of carbon monoxide enter the outdoor air primarily through the incomplete combustion of motor vehicle fuels.

Lead

The use of leaded petrol in motor vehicles is an important source of lead exposure for children. In the absence of stringent controls on automobile emissions and volume of traffic, the use of leaded petrol in some major cities of the developing world creates the potential for serious risks to children (3). Paint and soil are generally the most common sources of lead exposure for children in countries that have eliminated lead from petrol, but industrial operations, such as battery recycling or lead smelters, can also generate potentially harmful lead emissions.

Nitrogen oxides

Motor vehicle emissions contribute to outdoor levels of nitrogen oxides. However, the levels of nitrogen oxides outdoors are generally lower than those found indoors.

Ozone

Ozone (O_3) is a pervasive outdoor air pollutant (59). Outdoor ozone and other photochemical oxidants are secondary pollutants formed in the atmosphere from a chemical reaction between volatile organic compounds and nitrogen oxides in the presence of sunlight. The primary sources of these precursor compounds include motor vehicle exhaust fumes, chemical factories and refineries. Ozone is the principal component of urban summer smog. Levels of ozone are generally highest on hot summer days, reaching a maximum in the late afternoon. It is common for outdoor air pollutants to occur together; for example, when ozone levels are high, levels of fine particles and acid aerosols may also be high.

Routes of exposure

The main pathway of exposure to air pollution is through inhalation. Substances (such as mercury) released into the atmosphere can, however, enter the hydrological cycle as a result of atmospheric dispersion and precipitation. Similarly, deposition of suspended particulate matter occurs. Thus, material that was originally released into the atmosphere can be ingested as a result of the subsequent contamination of water, soil, or vegetation.

Mechanism of action and clinical effects in children

Children are especially vulnerable to outdoor air pollution for several reasons. First, the lungs are growing rapidly during the first year of life and the number of air sacs increases until the fourth year of life. Exposure to pollutants during infancy and childhood can decrease the rate of lung development (61). Second, because children tend to spend more time outside than adults, and are often physically active, they have a greater likelihood of exposure to pollutants. Because of their higher metabolic rate, children breathe more rapidly and inhale more pollutants per kg of body weight than adults (37). In addition, because airway passages in children are narrower than those in adults, irritation caused by air pollution can result in proportionally greater airway obstruction. Unlike adults, children may not cease vigorous outdoor activities when bronchospasm occurs.

Infants and children have an increased susceptibility to CO toxicity because of their higher metabolic rate (62–64). Carbon monoxide in the bloodstream causes a leftward shift of the oxyhaemoglobin dissociation curve, resulting in reduced oxygen delivery to the tissues. Tissue hypoxia from exposure to carbon monoxide preferentially affects organ systems with a high metabolic rate and high oxygen demand.

In children, acute health effects associated with outdoor air pollution include respiratory symptoms, such as wheezing and cough, serious lower respiratory tract infections, and exacerbation of asthma (65, 66). Increases in the number of admissions to hospital emergency departments have been observed when air pollution levels are elevated, which commonly occurs in major urban areas (67, 68). Historically, episodes of very heavy air pollution (such as the London smog of 1952) have been linked with increased death rates among adults and children (69–71). Most of the short-term respiratory effects of outdoor air pollution, such as cough or shortness of breath, are thought to be reversible.

Because children with asthma have increased airway reactivity, the effects of air pollution on the respiratory system can be more serious for them (72). Some evidence suggests that exposure to ozone can increase bronchial reactivity to inhaled allergens (73, 74). New diagnoses of asthma are associated with strenuous exercise by children in communities with high concentrations of ozone (75).

The effects of repeated or long-term exposures to outdoor air pollution on the developing lungs of children are not well understood, primarily because of the methodological difficulties of long-term studies. Long-term exposure to ozone is linked to chronic respiratory symptoms and small deficits in pulmonary function tests. A study of 17–21-year-old college students in California demonstrated that lifetime exposure to ambient ozone was negatively associated with lung function measures reflecting small-airway physiology (forced expiratory flow rate between 25% and 75% of forced vital capacity ($FEF_{25-75\%}$) and forced expiratory flow rate at 75% of forced vital capacity ($FEF_{75\%}$)) (76). These pulmonary function measures are considered early indicators of pathological changes that could progress to chronic obstructive lung disease. A similar study of Connecticut college students detected an association between living for four or more years in areas of the United States with high levels of ozone, diminished forced expiratory volume in 1 second (FEV_1), and diminished $FEF_{25-75\%}$ (77). The study also demonstrated that chronic phlegm, wheezing, and a higher composite respiratory symptom index were more common in students who had lived for a long period in areas with high ozone concentrations (78).

Chronic exposure to ozone pollution has been associated with *de novo* development of chronic lung disease, mild pulmonary fibrosis, and modest increases in small airway obstruction (79, 80). Some evidence has linked ozone to chronic lung scarring, especially at the broncho-alveolar junction (66, 81).

Long-term intermittent exposure to acid aerosols is associated with a higher probability of reported bronchitis among 8–12-year-old children. Asthma, persistent wheeze, chronic cough and chronic phlegm were not associated with higher levels of acid aerosols. Long-term exposure to acid aerosols was associated with statistically significant decrements in forced vital capacity (FVC) and FEV_1 (82–84).

Several studies have noted an association between particulate air pollution and mortality among persons of all ages (85), as well as low birth weight, intrauterine growth retardation and postneonatal infant death. Table 10.2 shows results of a recent meta-analysis of the health effects of particulates (86).

Table 10.2 **Increase in health-related parameters associated with a $10\,\mu g/m^3$ increase in PM_{10}**

PARAMETER	INCREASE
Total mortality rate	1%
Cardiovascular mortality rate	1.4%
Respiratory mortality rate	3.4%
Respiratory-related hospitalizations	0.8%
Asthma-related hospitalizations	1.9%
Asthma-related emergency department visits	3.4%
Asthma exacerbations	3%

Source: ref. 86.

Diagnosis

A specific etiology for respiratory illness may be difficult to establish because most signs and symptoms are nonspecific and may occur only in association with significant exposure. The effects of low-level exposure may be mild. Furthermore, multiple outdoor air pollutants may be involved. Establishing the environmental cause of a given respiratory illness is further complicated by the similarity of effects to those associated with allergies and respiratory infections. Diagnosis of an environmentally related disease requires a high index of suspicion and a thorough environmental history. While health workers cannot always assess the causal association between outdoor air and health effects, they should consider a possible environmental cause when a child's illness does not follow usual patterns. Ways to reduce exposure should be recommended.

Treatment guidelines

The treatment of symptoms and the use of medication should be based on the usual clinical indications. A therapeutic regimen should not be changed in response to periods of poor air quality unless there is a clear indication of a change in a patient's respiratory symptoms. However, it might be advisable to recommend restriction of strenuous physical activity during periods of poor air quality.

Registering the data

There are no standard ways of reporting illnesses and deaths thought to be due to outdoor air pollution to the local health department. In some areas affected by severe temperature inversions, public health officials review and record emergency department records during temperature inversions to see if morbidity and mortality from respiratory and other causes increase. It has to be kept in mind that a causal link between a given disease episode and exposure to air pollutants may not be established.

Remedial action, prevention, and education

In many countries, national environment or health ministries have the authority to set standards for air pollutants to protect the health of people. In some cases, such as in the USA, these standards take into account people with specific sensitivities, including children and those with asthma in the standard-setting process. The WHO ambient air quality guidelines for selected pollutants are shown in Table 10.3. As another example, the US ambient air quality standards are given in Table 10.4.

Table 10.3   Guideline values for individual substances based on effects other than cancer or odour/annoyance

SUBSTANCE	TIME-WEIGHTED AVERAGE	AVERAGING TIME
Cadmium	$5 \, ng/m^3$	annual
Carbon disulfide	$100 \, \mu g/m^3$	24 hours
Carbon monoxide	$100 \, mg/m^3$	15 minutes
	$60 \, mg/m^3$	30 minutes
	$30 \, mg/m^3$	1 hour
	$10 \, mg/m^3$	8 hours
1,2-Dichloroethane	$0.7 \, mg/m^3$	24 hours
Dichloromethane	$3 \, mg/m^3$	24 hours
	$0.45 \, mg/m^3$	1 week
Fluoride	—	—
Formaldehyde	$0.1 \, mg/m^3$	30 minutes
Hydrogen sulfide	$150 \, \mu g/m^3$	24 hours
Lead	$0.5 \, \mu g/m^3$	annual
Manganese	$0.15 \, \mu g/m^3$	annual
Mercury	$1 \, \mu g/m^3$	annual
Nitrogen dioxide	$200 \, \mu g/m^3$	1 hour
	$40 \, \mu g/m^3$	annual
Ozone	$120 \, \mu g/m^3$	8 hours
Particulate matter	Dose–response	—
Platinum	—	—
PCBs	—	—
PCDDs/PCDFs	—	—
Styrene	$0.26 \, mg/m^3$	1 week
Sulfur dioxide	$500 \, \mu g/m^3$	10 minutes
	$125 \, \mu g/m^3$	24 hours
	$50 \, \mu g/m^3$	annual
Tetrachloroethylene	$0.25 \, mg/m^3$	annual
Toluene	$0.26 \, mg/m^3$	1 week
Vanadium	$1 \, \mu g/m^3$	24 hours

Source: ref. 3.

SECTION III: SPECIFIC ENVIRONMENTAL THREATS

Table 10.4   US national ambient air quality standards (NAAQS) 1997

POLLUTANT	AMBIENT AIR LIMIT	AVERAGING TIME
Ozone	0.08 ppm	8 h
PM$_{10}$	50 µg/m^3 150 µg/m^3	Annual arithmetic mean 24 h
PM$_{2.5}$	15 µg/m^3 65 µg/m^3	Annual arithmetic mean 24 h
Sulfur dioxide	0.03 ppm 0.14 ppm	Annual arithmetic mean 24 h
Nitrogen dioxide	0.053 ppm	Annual arithmetic mean
Carbon monoxide	9 ppm 35 ppm	8 h 1 h
Lead	1.5 µg/m^3	24 h

Many countries have adopted WHO's guidelines as national standards. In countries that enforce air quality standards, the ambient concentrations of the pollutants listed in Table 10.4 have decreased overall over the past decade, although fine and ultra-fine particulate matter has increased, and ozone has not decreased significantly. Large numbers of people are still exposed to potentially unhealthy levels of all these pollutants. Table 10.5 shows an example of standard index values with corresponding pollutant concentrations and health effects.

Prevention efforts have largely focused on the short-term effects of air pollution. Short-term exposure to ozone aggravates childhood asthma, leading to increased emergency visits to health facilities for acute asthma attacks. Recent research has explored whether dietary antioxidant supplementation (400 IU of vitamin E and 500 mg of vitamin C) affects ozone-induced bronchial hyper-responsiveness in persons with asthma. In several, but not all, studies of adults, dietary supplementation was associated with higher lung function values during periods of ozone pollution (87, 88). It is not yet known whether dietary antioxidant supplementation is helpful in reducing symptoms among children with asthma exposed to ozone. Future research efforts should therefore include children.

In his 1962 report on motor vehicles, air pollution, and health (89), the United States Surgeon General stated:

"As in other problems affecting the public health, it is important that, as needed research proceeds on the problem of pollution emissions from motor vehicles, all practicable steps be taken to minimize such pollution rather than waiting until the results of all the needed research are available."

This remains as true today as it was over 40 years ago.

Table 10.5 Pollution standard index values with corresponding pollutant concentrations and health effects

INDEX VALUE	AIR QUALITY LEVEL	POLLUTANT LEVELS					HEALTH EFFECT DESCRIPTOR	GENERAL HEALTH EFFECTS	CAUTIONARY STATEMENTS
		PM (24-h) $\mu g/m^3$	SO$_2$ (24-h) $\mu g/m^3$	CO (8-h) ppm	O$_3$ (1-h) ppm	NO$_2$ (1-h) ppm			
500	Significant harm	600	2620	50	0.6	2.0	—	Premature death of ill and elderly. Healthy people will experience adverse symptoms that affect their normal activity.	All persons should remain indoors, keeping windows and doors closed. All persons should minimize physical exertion.
400	Emergency	500	2100	40	0.5	1.6	Hazardous	Premature onset of certain diseases in addition to significant aggravation of symptoms and decreased exercise tolerance in healthy persons.	The elderly and persons with existing disease should stay indoors and avoid physical exertion. General population should avoid outdoor activity.
300	Warning	420	1600	30	0.4	1.2	— Very unhealthy	Significant aggravation of symptoms and decreased exercise tolerance in persons with heart or lung disease, with widespread symptoms in the healthy population.	The elderly and persons with existing heart or lung disease should stay indoors and reduce physical activity.
200	Alert	350	800	15	0.2	0.6	— Unhealthy	Mild aggravation of symptoms in susceptible persons, with irritation symptoms in the healthy population.	Persons with existing heart or respiratory ailments should reduce physical exertion and outdoor activity.
100	NAAQS[1]	150	365	9	0.12		— Moderate		

NAAQS: National Ambient Air Quality Standards.

SECTION III: SPECIFIC ENVIRONMENTAL THREATS

References

1. Bruce N, Perez-Padilla R, Albalak R. Indoor air pollution in developing countries: a major environmental and public health challenge. *Bulletin of the World Health Organization*, 2000, 78:1078–1092.

2. Smith KR, Mehta S. The burden of disease from indoor air pollution in developing countries. Comparison of estimates. *Paper presented at the USAID/ WHO Global Technical Consultation on the Health Impacts of Indoor Air Pollution and Household Energy in Developing Countries, 3–4 May 2000, Washington, DC.*

3. *Air quality guidelines for Europe*, 2nd ed. Copenhagen, WHO Regional Office for Europe, 2000 (European Series, No. 91).

4. Gordon B, Mackay R, Rehfuss E. *Inheriting the world: the atlas of children's health and the environment.* Geneva, World Health Organization, 2004.

5. Parikh J, Pandey V. Biofuels, pollution and health linkages. *Economic and Political Weekly*, 2000, 35:4125–4137.

6. Saksena S et al. Patterns of daily exposure to TSP and CO in the Garhwal Himalaya. *Atmosphere and Environment*, 1992, 26A :2125–2134.

7. Albalak R et al. Assessment of PM_{10} concentrations from domestic biomass fuel combustion in rural Bolivian highland villages. *Environmental Science and Technology*, 1999, 33:2505–2509.

8. Balakrishnan K et al. Daily average exposures to respirable particulate matter from combustion of biomass fuels in rural households of Southern India. *Environmental Health Perspectives*, 2002, 110:1069–1075.

9. Spengler JD. Sources and concentrations of indoor air pollution. In: Samet JM, Spengler JD, eds. *Indoor air pollution. A health perspective.* Baltimore, MD, Johns Hopkins University Press; 1991.

10. US Environmental Protection Agency. *Indoor air pollution: an introduction for health professionals.* Washington, DC, US Government Printing Office, 1994 (EPA 523–217/81322).

11. Smith KR. *Biomass fuels, air pollution and health. A global review.* New York, Plenum Press, 1987.

12. Lambert WE, Samet JM. Indoor air pollution. In: Harber P, Schenker MB, Balmes JR, eds. *Occupational and environmental respiratory disease.* St Louis, MO, Mosby, 1996:784–807.

13. Parikh J et al. Exposure from cooking with biofuels: pollution monitoring and analysis for rural Tamil Nadu, India. *Energy*, 2000, 26:949–962.

14. Balakrishnan K et al. Exposure assessment for respirable particulates associated with household fuel use in rural districts of Andhra Pradesh, India. *Journal of Exposure Analysis and Environmental Epidemiology*, 2004, 14(suppl 1): S14–S25.

15. Smith KR, Liu Y. Indoor air pollution in developing countries. In: Samet JM, ed. *Epidemiology of lung cancer.* New York, Marcel Dekker, 1994.

16. Smith KR et al. Indoor air pollution in developing countries and ALRI in children. *Thorax*, 2000, 55:518–532.

17. Ezzati M, Kammen DM. Quantifying the effects of exposure to indoor air pollution from biomass combustion on acute respiratory infections in developing countries. *Environmental Health Perspectives*, 2001, 109:481–489.
18. Samet JM et al. Nitrogen dioxide and respiratory illnesses in infants. *American Review of Respiratory Disease*, 1993, 148:1258–1265.
19. Robin LF et al. Wood-burning stoves and lower respiratory illnesses in Navajo children. *Pediatric Infectious Disease Journal*, 1996, 15:859–865.
20. *International consultation on environmental tobacco smoke (ETS) and child health*. Geneva, World Health Organization, 1999 (WHO/NCD/TFI/99.10).
21. American Academy of Pediatrics, Committee on Environmental Health. Environmental tobacco smoke: a hazard to children. *Pediatrics*, 1997, 99:639–642.
22. Colley JR, Holland WW, Corkhill RT. Influence of passive smoking and parental phlegm on pneumonia and bronchitis in early childhood. *Lancet*, 1974, 2:1031–1034.
23. Fergusson DM, Horwood LJ, Shannon FT. Parental smoking and respiratory illness in infancy. *Archives of Diseases in Children*, 1980, 55:358–361.
24. Harlap S, Davies AM. Infant admissions to the hospital and maternal smoking. *Lancet*, 1974, 1:529–532.
25. Rantakallio P. Relationship of maternal smoking to morbidity and mortality of the child up to the age of five. *Acta Paediatrica Scandinavica*, 1978, 67: 621–631.
26. Etzel RA et al. Passive smoking and middle ear effusion among children in day care. *Pediatrics*, 1992, 90:228–232.
27. Ey JL et al. Passive smoke exposure and otitis media in the first year of life. *Pediatrics*, 1995, 95:670–677.
28. Chilmonczyk BA et al. Association between exposure to environmental tobacco smoke and exacerbations of asthma in children. *New England Journal of Medicine*, 1993, 328:1665–1669.
29. Martinez FD, Cline M, Burrows B. Increased incidence of asthma in children of smoking mothers. *Pediatrics*, 1992, 89:21–26.
30. Weitzman M et al. Maternal smoking and childhood asthma. *Pediatrics*, 1990, 85:505–511.
31. Murray AB, Morrison BJ. The decrease in severity of asthma in children of parents who smoke since the parents have been exposing them to less cigarette smoke. *Journal of Allergy and Clinical Immunology*, 1993, 91:102–110.
32. Anderson HR, Cook DG. Health effects of passive smoking. 2. Passive smoking and sudden infant death syndrome: review of the epidemiologic evidence. *Thorax*, 1997, 53:1003–1009.
33. Taylor JA, Sanderson M. A reexamination of the risk factors for the sudden infant death syndrome. *Journal of Pediatrics*, 1995, 126:887–891.
34. Tamburlini G, von Ehrenstein O, Bertollini R, eds. *Children's health and environment: a review of evidence*. Luxembourg, Office for Official Publications of the European Communities (on behalf of the European Environmental Agency and WHO Regional Office for Europe), 2002.

35. Fiore MC et al. *Smoking cessation: information for specialists. Clinical practice guideline. Quick reference guide for smoking cessation specialists, No. 18.* Rockville, MD, Centers for Disease Control and Prevention, 1996 (Publication AHCPR 96-0694).

36. Baker MD, Henretig FM, Ludwig S. Carboxyhemoglobin levels in children with nonspecific flu-like symptoms. *Journal of Pediatrics*, 1988, 113:501–504.

37. Heckerling PS et al. Occult carbon monoxide poisoning in patients with neurologic illness. *Clinical Toxicology*, 1990, 28:29–44.

38. Etzel RA, ed. *Pediatric environmental health*, 2nd ed. Elk Grove Village, IL, American Academy of Pediatrics 2003.

39. Samet J. Environmental controls and lung disease. Report of the ATS Workshop on Environmental Controls and Lung Disease. *American Review of Respiratory Disease*, 1990, 142:915–939.

40. Health Canada. *Exposure guidelines for residential indoor air quality: a report to the federal–provincial advisory committee on environmental health.* Ottawa, Health Canada, 1989 (Publication #H46-2/90-156E).

41. American Society of Heating, Refrigerating, and Air Conditioning Engineers (ASHRAE). *Ventilation for acceptable indoor air quality.* Atlanta, GA, ASHRAE, 1989 (ASHRAE Standard 62-1989).

42. Wallace LA. Volatile organic compounds. In: Samet JM, Spengler JD, eds. *Indoor air pollution: a health perspective.* Baltimore, MD, Johns Hopkins University Press, 1991:252–272.

43. Molhave L. Indoor air pollution due to organic gases and vapours of solvents in building materials. *Environment International*, 1982, 8:117–127.

44. American Academy of Pediatrics, Committee on Environmental Health. Toxic effects of indoor molds. *Pediatrics*, 1998, 101:712–714.

45. Dales RE et al. Respiratory health effects of home dampness and molds among Canadian children. *American Journal of Epidemiology*, 1991, 134:196–203.

46. Jaakkola JJK, Jaakkola N, Ruotsalainen R. Home dampness and molds as determinants of respiratory symptoms and asthma in pre-school children. *Journal of Exposure Analysis and Environmental Epidemiology*, 1993, 3:129–142.

47. Verhoeff AP et al. Damp housing and childhood respiratory symptoms: The role of sensitization to dust mites and molds. *American Journal of Epidemiology*, 1995, 141:103–110.

48. Dearborn DG et al. Overview of investigations into pulmonary hemorrhage among infants in Cleveland, Ohio. *Environmental Health Perspectives*, 1999, 107 (Suppl 3):495–499.

49. Croft WA, Jarvis BB, Yatawara CS. Airborne outbreak of trichothecene toxicosis. *Atmospheric Environment*, 1986, 20:549–552.

50. Etzel RA et al. Acute pulmonary hemorrhage in infants associated with exposure to *Stachybotrys atra* and other fungi. *Archives of Pediatrics and Adolescent Medicine*, 1998, 152:757–762.

51. Flappan SM et al. Infant pulmonary hemorrhage in a suburban home with water damage and mold (*Stachybotrys atra*). *Environmental Health Perspectives*, 1999, 107:927–930.

52. Weiss A, Chidekel AS. Acute pulmonary hemorrhage in a Delaware infant after exposure to *Stachybotrys atra*. *Delaware Medical Journal*, 2002, 74:363–368.

53. Elidemir O et al. Isolation of *Stachybotrys* from the lung of a child with pulmonary hemosiderosis. *Pediatrics*, 1999, 104:964–966.

54. Flannigan B, McCabe EM, McGarry F. Allergic and toxigenic microorganisms in houses. *Society for Applied Bacteriology, Symposium Series*, 1991, 20:61S.

55. Gravesen S, Frisvad JC, Samson RA. *Microfungi*. Copenhagen, Munksgaard, 1994:473.

56. Wilson CE. Sudden infant death syndrome and Canadian Aboriginals: bacteria and infections. *FEMS Immunology and Medical Microbiology*, 1999, 25:221–226.

57. Miller JD et al. Fungi and fungal products in some Canadian houses. *International Biodeterioration*, 1988, 24:103–120.

58. Agocs MM et al. Mercury exposure from interior latex paint. *New England Journal of Medicine*, 1990, 323:1096–1101.

59. Hirschmann SZ, Feingold M, Boylen G. Mercury in house paint as a cause of acrodynia: effect of therapy with N-acetyl-D,L-penicillamine. *New England Journal of Medicine*, 1963, 269:889–893.

60. US Environmental Protection Agency. *1997 National air quality: status and trends*. Office of Air and Radiation, 1998 (http://www.epa.gov/oar/aqtrnd97/brochure/no2html).

61. Dietert RR et al. Workshop to identify critical windows of exposure for children's health: immune and respiratory systems work group summary. *Environmental Health Perspectives*, 2000, 108(Suppl 3):483–490.

62. Koren G et al. A multicenter prospective study of fetal outcome following accidental carbon monoxide poisoning in pregnancy. *Reproductive Toxicology*, 1991, 5:397–403.

63. Longo LD. The biological effects of carbon monoxide on the pregnant woman, fetus, and newborn infant. *American Journal of Obstetrics and Gynecology*, 1977, 129:69–103.

64. Vreman HJ, Mahoney JJ, Stevenson DK. Carbon monoxide and carboxyhemoglobin. *Advances in Pediatrics*, 1995, 42:303–325.

65. Bates DV. The effects of air pollution on children. *Environmental Health Perspectives*, 1995, 103(Suppl. 6):49–53.

66. Committee of the Environmental and Occupational Health Assembly of the American Thoracic Society. Health effects of outdoor air pollution. *American Journal of Respiratory and Critical Care Medicine*, 1996, 153:3–50.

67. World Health Organization and United Nations Environment Programme. *Urban air pollution in megacities of the world*. Cambridge, MA, Blackwell, 1992.

68. Schwela D. Air pollution and health in urban areas. *Reviews on Environmental Health*, 2000, 15:13–42.

69. Dockery DW, Pope CA. Acute respiratory effects of particulate air pollution. *Annual Review of Public Health*, 1994, 15:107–132.
70. Smithard HER. The 1952 fog in a metropolitan borough. *Monthly Bulletin of the Ministry of Health*, February 1954:26–35.
71. Etzel RA, French JG. Air pollution. In: Noji EK, ed. *The public health consequences of disasters*. New York, Oxford University Press, 1997:336–353.
72. American Academy of Pediatrics, Committee on Environmental Health. Ambient air pollution: respiratory hazards to children. *Pediatrics*, 1993, 91:1210–1213.
73. Hanania NA et al. Effect of exposure to low levels of ozone on the responses to inhaled allergen in allergic asthmatic patients. *Chest*, 1998, 114:752–756.
74. Molfino NA et al. Effects of low concentrations of ozone on inhaled allergen responses in asthmatic subjects. *Lancet*, 1991, 338:199–203.
75. McConnell R et al. Asthma in exercising children exposed to ozone: a cohort study. *Lancet*, 2002, 359:386–391.
76. Kunzli N et al. Association between lifetime ambient ozone exposure and pulmonary function in college freshmen—results of a pilot study. *Environmental Research*, 1997, 72:8–23.
77. Galizia A, Kinney PL. Long-term residence in areas of high ozone: associations with respiratory health in a nationwide sample of nonsmoking young adults. *Environmental Health Perspectives*, 1999, 107:675–679.
78. Gilliland FD et al. The effects of ambient air pollution on school absenteeism due to respiratory illnesses. *Epidemiology*, 2001, 12:43–54.
79. Abbey DE et al. Long-term ambient concentrations of particulates and oxidants and development of chronic disease in a cohort of non-smoking California residents. *Inhalation Toxicology*, 1995, 7:19–34.
80. Abbey DE et al. Long-term ambient concentrations of total suspended particulates, ozone, and sulfur dioxide and respiratory symptoms in a non-smoking population. *Archives of Environmental Health*, 1993, 48:33–46.
81. Berglund D, Abbey D. Long-term effects of air pollution. *Western Journal of Medicine*, 1996, 165:140.
82. Spengler JD et al. Health effects of acid aerosols on North American children: air pollution exposures. *Environmental Health Perspectives*, 1996, 104:492–499.
83. Dockery DW et al. Health effects of acid aerosols on North American children: respiratory symptoms. *Environmental Health Perspectives*, 1996, 104:500–505.
84. Raizenne M et al. Health effects of acid aerosols on North American children: pulmonary function. *Environmental Health Perspectives*, 1996, 104:506–514.
85. Dockery DW et al. An association between air pollution and mortality in six US cities. *New England Journal of Medicine*, 1993, 329:1753–1759.
86. Dickey J et al. Part VII. Air pollution: overview of sources and health effects. *Disease of the Month*, 2000, 46:566–589.
87. Romieu I et al. Antioxidant supplementation and respiratory functions among workers exposed to high levels of ozone. *American Journal of Respiratory and Critical Care Medicine*, 1998, 158:226–232.

88. Trenga C, Koenig JQ, Williams PV. Dietary antioxidants and ozone-induced bronchial hyperresponsiveness in adults with asthma. *Archives of Environmental Health*, 2001, 56:242.

89. United States Division of Air Pollution. *Motor vehicles, air pollution and health: a report of the Surgeon General to the U. S. Congress.* Washington, DC, US Public Health Service, Division of Air Pollution, 1962.

SECTION III: SPECIFIC ENVIRONMENTAL THREATS

CHAPTER 11
Foodborne hazards of particular concern for the young

D. B. Mahoney
International Food Safety Consultant, Canberra, Australia

G. C. Moy
Food Safety Department, World Health Organization,
Geneva, Switzerland

Introduction
While the nutritional adequacy of the diets of infants and children is a major concern for much of the world, there is also concern in many countries about the safety of the foods they consume. Indeed, the International Conference on Nutrition declared that ". . . access to nutritionally adequate and safe food is a right of each individual (1). Notwithstanding the advances in the knowledge and tools to ensure food safety, foodborne diseases are widespread and have considerable impact on communities in both developing and developed countries.

For many foodborne hazards, the susceptibility of the host is all-important. Generally the young, pregnant women, persons over 60 years, and those who are ill or immunocompromised are the most vulnerable to foodborne illness. This chapter discusses the foodborne risks for three subgroups, namely: (1) the developing fetus; (2) breastfed and bottle-fed infants; and (3) children and infants receiving complementary food. In general, foodborne illness can be reduced by preventing contamination, through improved production, processing and handling, and by educating people to avoid high-risk foods and to prevent contamination during food preparation. Success in educating consumers requires an understanding of who is most at risk, and techniques that motivate consumers to change their behaviour and follow food safety recommendations. This chapter presents specific measures that can be taken by those responsible for infants and children to help reduce their risk of foodborne disease.

Foodborne hazards
The agents responsible for foodborne disease include bacteria, viruses and parasites, as well as a range of chemicals, including biotoxins and heavy metals. The adverse health effects of foodborne illness range from mild gastroenteritis (including diarrhoea and vomiting) to life-threatening neurological, renal or hepatic syndromes, congenital anomalies and cancer. The risks posed by the

presence of microorganisms and chemicals in the food supply are of concern worldwide. However, consumers' judgement of hazards and perception of food safety risks are often at variance with those of the scientific community. Consumers' perceptions in particular are shaped by a number of factors, including personal experience, access to information about food safety, trust in sources of information, and baseline food safety risk levels. Hence, while the public may be concerned about food additives and new technologies, they may fail to recognize the major risks resulting from food contaminated by pathogenic microorganisms.

Infant exposure to organochlorine contaminants in breast milk

The benefits of breastfeeding infants from birth for at least six months are beyond question. At the same time, certain chemicals, in particular organochlorines, can enter the food chain and be stored in fatty tissue. In breastfeeding women, these chemicals can then contaminate the breast milk, and can have adverse health effects in the child. While breastfeeding is optimal and should be promoted, steps can be taken to reduce exposure to harmful chemicals. Case study 15, page 325 describes what governments, professionals and individuals can do to avoid exposure of mothers and children to harmful chemicals and to respond to health concerns.

In terms of acute illness, foodborne disease caused by pathogenic microorganisms or their toxins is more significant for children than is generally acknowledged, even among health care professionals. Even mild bouts of gastroenteritis pose serious threats to children, as they can lead to dehydration and even death if not treated properly. This is especially significant in children who are malnourished.

The duration of foodborne disease may vary from a few days in the majority of infections, to weeks or months with agents such as hepatitis A virus or *Brucella*. In the case of toxoplasmosis, infants may experience irreversible developmental and neurological deficits.

Noninfectious foodborne illness arises from exposure to raw and processed food contaminated by toxic chemicals. Such toxic chemicals include residues of pesticides and veterinary drugs, industrial pollutants, heavy metals, biotoxins, and certain substances used improperly in food processing. While illness may be acute, the effects of particular concern are generally chronic and irreversible, such as developmental deficiencies and cancer.

Magnitude of the food safety problem

Unfortunately, data on the incidence and severity of foodborne illness in the general population are limited in most countries. Where such data are collected through surveillance programmes, most cases of foodborne illness are not reported, either because medical treatment is not sought or, when treatment is sought, specimens are not taken to allow diagnostic tests to identify the food-

SECTION III: SPECIFIC ENVIRONMENTAL THREATS

borne pathogen. Also, certain pathogens transmitted via food may also be spread through water or by person-to-person contact, and this may obscure the role of food as a vehicle for transmission. In addition, some foodborne illness is caused by hitherto unknown pathogens, and thus cannot be diagnosed. Many pathogens, such as *Campylobacter jejuni*, *Escherichia coli* O157:H7 and *Cyclospora cayetanensis*, were not recognized as causes of foodborne illness twenty years ago.

Foodborne illnesses that are nationally reportable in certain developed countries include typhoid fever, cholera, hepatitis A, *E. coli* O157:H7 infection, haemolytic uraemic syndrome, salmonellosis, and shigellosis. Reporting requirements are stipulated by local and national regulations. In developing countries (excluding China), foodborne pathogenic microorganisms are estimated to cause up to 70% of the roughly 1.5 billion annual episodes of diarrhoea, and a related 3 million deaths in children under the age of five (2). In the United States it is estimated that 76 million illnesses, 325 000 hospitalizations and 5000 deaths result each year from foodborne illnesses (3). While the figure for morbidity suggests that one in three persons becomes ill each year, foodborne disease is expected to be more prevalent among the young.

Risk analysis

An important tool for the control and prevention of foodborne illness is accurate and reliable data on the risks. Such information is essential for food safety managers to develop countermeasures.

Risk analysis has three components: risk assessment, risk management, and risk communication. Risk assessment involves a scientifically based process designed to identify hazards and their adverse health effects, estimate likely risk and provide an indication of the uncertainties. The risk assessment should inform the selection of risk management options, such as establishing food standards, defining food processing and handling guidelines, and developing food safety messages to protect consumers. While there are good data on chemical risks to consumers, microbiological risk assessment is a developing science.

Specific hazards of particular concern
Foodborne protozoa
Toxoplasma gondii

Toxoplasmosis is a widespread parasitic disease that usually causes no symptoms in healthy human hosts. In pregnant women the organism *T. gondii* may infect the fetal brain, eyes and other tissues, even if the woman is asymptomatic. The infection can trigger miscarriage, stillbirth and preterm birth, or lead to mental retardation and blindness in the infant. The fetus is presumed to be at risk only if the mother has a primary, active infection during the pregnancy.

The birth prevalence of congenital toxoplasmosis throughout the world ranges from less than 1 to 10 per 10 000 live births (4–6). The age of the fetus may be a factor in maternal transmission, with the risk of fetal infection low during the first 8 weeks of pregnancy, and infection resulting mainly in spontaneous termination of the pregnancy. In one study, up to 90% of infected infants did not exhibit overt clinical signs of disease at birth (7). Of those with symptoms, many had severe neurological and development problems. In another study, visual impairment was observed in all children with congenital toxoplasmosis, while 74% had severe visual impairment (8). Of those with subclinical congenital infection at birth, up to 85% may develop chronic recurring eye disease and learning difficulties. The long-term impact carries high economic and societal costs.

Toxoplasmosis can be contracted by eating raw or undercooked meat or from exposure to the faeces of infected cats. Cats are an important host, with the parasite infecting the cells lining the cats' intestines. Farm animals may become infected when they ingest food or water contaminated by faeces from infected cats.

Giardia lamblia

G. lamblia is spread through the faecal–oral route, either directly by person-to-person contact or through contaminated food or water. The parasite infects the small intestine and may cause diarrhoea, abdominal cramps and bloating, and result in malabsorption and weight loss.

Children are infected more frequently than adults, and the parasite is commonly found in day-care centres. The Centers for Disease Control and Prevention in the USA reports that giardiasis has been identified in 10–15% of children who have not been toilet-trained attending these centres. Approximately 20–25% of day-care staff and family contacts of infected children also become infected.

Foodborne bacteria
Listeria monocytogenes

L. monocytogenes may cause a mild form of gastrointestinal illness in healthy adults. While such infections are uncommon and cause few or no symptoms in healthy people, they may be very serious for pregnant women. Women infected with *L. monocytogenes* during pregnancy may transmit the infection to the fetus, possibly leading to spontaneous abortion, fetal death, or subsequent visual, mental, or other health problems in the infant. Outbreak data show that the incubation period ranges from 2 to 6 weeks for the invasive disease. Listeriosis results in an estimated 2500 serious illnesses and 500 deaths in the United States each year (9).

Pregnant women are about 20 times more likely than other adults to get sick from *L. monocytogenes*. The organism is typically found in raw meat, delicatessen products, including processed ready-to-eat meat products, soft cheeses, unpasteurized dairy products and chilled smoked seafood.

Salmonella species

Salmonellosis results from consuming food contaminated by *Salmonella* spp. Infected persons develop diarrhoea, fever, and abdominal cramps between 12 and 72 hours after eating the contaminated food. The illness usually lasts 4–7 days, and most people recover without treatment. In vulnerable groups, such as the young, *Salmonella* infection may spread beyond the intestine to the bloodstream and cause a more severe systemic disease.

Salmonellae are found in the intestinal tracts of animals and humans, and some individuals are chronic carriers of the organism. Humans usually become infected by eating food contaminated with animal faeces, especially raw and undercooked foods of animal origin, such as beef, poultry, milk, and eggs. Food may also become contaminated through cross-contamination and poor hygiene of food handlers.

Escherichia coli O157:H7

E. coli O157:H7 is an emerging cause of foodborne illness, and has rapidly become a major cause of bloody diarrhoea and acute renal failure. The infection can be fatal, especially in children. The largest outbreak recorded so far was in Japan in 1996 (see Box).

In some people, particularly children under 5 years of age and the elderly, the infection can lead to the development of haemolytic uraemic syndrome. Between 2% and 7% of infections in the United States led to this complication. Haemolytic uraemic syndrome is the principal cause of acute kidney failure in children, and most cases are caused by *E. coli* O157:H7.

E. coli O157:H7 infection has been associated with eating under-cooked, contaminated minced beef. Because the organism lives in the intestines of healthy cattle, preventive measures on cattle farms and during meat processing are being investigated. Infection has also occurred after consumption of unpasteurized milk, unpasteurized apple cider, sprouts, lettuce, and salami. Person-to-person transmission is important in families and child care centres, especially among toddlers who are not toilet-trained.

> #### Escherichia coli O157:H7 outbreak in Japanese schoolchildren
> School lunch programmes in Japan were to blame for several outbreaks of *Escherichia coli* O157:H7 infection in 1996. Several problems were found in growth, distribution and management of food that could have been the cause of nearly 10 000 children becoming ill and five dying in more than eight outbreaks over a six-month period. Changes to the school lunch programme management led to improved food safety and reduced the incidence of foodborne illness (Case study 16, page 330).

Clostridium botulinum

Botulism is a rare, acute, descending flaccid paralysis caused by the neurotoxin produced by *C. botulinum*. Intoxication results from ingestion of food contaminated with the preformed toxin. Typical food vehicles include low-acid canned foods that have been improperly heat-processed, such as asparagus, green beans, and corn; more unusual sources have included chilli peppers, chopped garlic, tomatoes stored in oil, and smoked vacuum-packed fish.

Infant botulism is a recognized variant first described in 1976. The illness in infants is caused by ingestion of *C. botulinum* spores, which subsequently germinate, multiply, and release toxin in the infant's large intestine. A unique epidemiological feature of infant botulism is that all cases occur in children less than one year of age, with 95% of cases occurring in the first 6 months of life. Honey is a reservoir for *C. botulinum* and epidemiological studies have implicated honey consumption as a risk factor.

The clinical features include constipation, poor feeding, weakness, hypotonia, dysphasia and, in severe cases, flaccid paralysis and respiratory failure. All forms of botulism can be fatal and are considered medical emergencies.

Other pathogenic bacteria

A range of other bacteria are responsible for outbreaks of foodborne disease. Organisms such as *Campylobacter jejuni*, *Staphylococcus aureus*, *Bacillus cereus*, *Clostridium perfringens*, *Shigella* spp. and *Vibrio* spp., especially *Vibrio cholerae*, are commonly implicated in outbreaks associated with specific foods.

Foodborne viruses
Rotaviruses, hepatitis A, and noroviruses

Hepatitis A and gastroenteritis viruses, such as rotaviruses, noroviruses, astroviruses, and other caliciviruses are more often transmitted via food than other viruses. Viruses are considered the most common cause of infectious gastroenteritis (*10*), but except for rotaviruses, they are rarely identified. All foodborne viruses are shed in faeces and infect by being ingested.

The main symptoms of viral gastroenteritis are watery diarrhoea and vomiting. Patients may also have headache, fever and abdominal cramps. Symptoms occur 1 or 2 days after infection and last for 1–10 days. People with viral gastroenteritis almost always recover without long-term problems. However gastroenteritis can be serious for infants and young children, who are at risk of dehydration from loss of fluids through vomiting or diarrhoea.

Food may be contaminated by food handlers who have viral gastroenteritis, especially if their personal hygiene is poor. Raw and undercooked shellfish grown in polluted waters are also an important vehicle for viral gastroenteritis.

Rotavirus infection is the most common cause of severe viral diarrhoea in infants and young children under 5 years old, resulting in the hospitalization of approximately 55 000 children each year in the United States. The incubation period for rotavirus disease is approximately 2 days, followed by vomiting and watery diarrhoea for 3–8 days. The primary mode of transmission is faecal–oral. The virus is stable in the environment, and transmission occurs through ingestion of contaminated water or food and contact with contaminated surfaces.

HIV and other viral infections

Breast milk may be a source of viral infection in nursing infants whose mothers have acquired HIV or cytomegalovirus (11) infections. Mother-to-child transmission of HIV can occur *in utero*, at delivery, or after birth through breastfeeding. Data from various studies estimate transmission rates, without antiretroviral intervention, of 15–30% in the absence of breastfeeding, 25–35% if there is breastfeeding up to 6 months, and 30–45% if breastfeeding is continued for 18–24 months (12).

Policies and strategies are evolving as more evidence becomes available from research, but more needs to be known about the factors that influence transmission rates and the risks associated with alternative feeding strategies. For women who know they are HIV-positive and where infant mortality is high, exclusive breastfeeding may still result in fewer infant deaths than feeding breast-milk substitutes. A WHO Technical Consultation (13) recommended the following approaches to prevention of mother-to-child transmission:

- When replacement feeding is acceptable, feasible, affordable, sustainable and safe, avoidance of all breastfeeding by HIV-infected mothers is recommended. Otherwise, exclusive breastfeeding is recommended during the first months of life.
- To minimize HIV transmission risk, breastfeeding should be discontinued as soon as feasible, taking into account local circumstances, the individual woman's situation and the risks of replacement feeding (including infections other than HIV and malnutrition).
- When HIV-infected mothers choose not to breastfeed from birth or stop breastfeeding later, they should be provided with specific guidance and support for at least the first 2 years of the child's life to ensure adequate replacement feeding. Programmes should strive to improve conditions to make replacement feeding safer for HIV-infected mothers and families.

Countries should have in place a comprehensive national infant and young child feeding policy which includes information on HIV and infant feeding. Such a policy should lead to guidelines for health workers on how to protect, promote and support breastfeeding in the general population, while giving adequate support to HIV-positive women to enable them to select the best feeding option for themselves and their babies. The policy and guidelines should be based on the local situation, including an assessment of feeding options.

Chemical contaminants

Infants and children have a special vulnerability to acute, subacute and chronic effects of chemicals present in their food. There is an urgent need for recognition, evaluation and action to address potential contaminant problems. This is especially important in developing countries, where the likelihood of toxic exposures is magnified by the unsafe use of chemicals, increased pollution, and sometimes a lack of awareness of environmental hazards.

The distinctive diet and physiological immaturity of infants and children make them particularly susceptible to the toxic effects of certain chemicals. Another important factor is their greater exposure. Compared with adults, children consume more food and water and breathe more air per kg of body weight. The skin surface area of an infant per unit of body weight is double that of adults. The normal respiratory volume of a resting infant in relation to body weight is twice that of a resting adult. Food consumption by infants per unit of body weight is approximately twice that of adults. In addition, a child's diet is usually less varied than an adult's, with children consuming larger proportions of milk, fruit and fruit juices.

Pesticides

Pesticides perform an important role in maximizing agricultural production and protecting the food supply. But because of their inherent toxicity and widespread use, pesticides also pose a threat to public health, particularly to infants and children.

Epidemiological studies and laboratory studies in animals contribute to a growing body of evidence linking pesticide exposure to adverse health effects including cancer, birth defects, reproductive harm, neurological and developmental toxicity, immunotoxicity and disruption of the endocrine system. A major concern for the young is that, during the first six years of life, the child's central nervous system is still developing and is likely to be vulnerable to neurotoxic pesticides.

Most major classes of pesticides, including the organochlorines, organophosphorus compounds, carbamates, chlorophenoxy herbicides, and pyrethroids, have been shown to adversely affect the developing nervous system of laboratory animals, altering neurological function and causing subtle neurobehavioural impairments. Many of these pesticides share a common mechanism of toxicity, but their cumulative impact on children's health has not yet been fully assessed.

Persistent organic pollutants

Persistent organic pollutants (POPs) are a group of toxic chemical substances that persist in the environment, bioaccumulate along the food-chain, and are a risk to human health. Twelve substances were initially classified as

POPs under the Stockholm Convention (14): aldrin, chlordane, dichlorodiphenyl-trichloroethane (DDT), dieldrin, endrin, heptachlor, mirex, toxaphene, poly-chlorinated biphenyls (PCBs), hexachlorobenzene, dioxins and dibenzofurans. Most of these, with the exception of DDT used for malaria control, have been, or are in the process of being, phased out.

POPs resist biodegradation and are insoluble in water, but are readily stored in fatty tissue where concentrations can reach 70 000 times the background level. Long-lived species of fish, birds and mammals, including humans, have the greatest concentrations. These pollutants may accumulate in fatty tissues in the human body for many years, and may be passed to infants in breast milk.

The potential health effects of POPs include cancer, allergies, hypersensitivity and disorders of the nervous and immune systems. Of particular concern are dioxins (including dibenzofurans and dioxin-like PCBs) which may function as endocrine disrupters. Low-level exposure to such substances is particularly critical for the fetus and infants, because of their very low levels of circulating hormones. Dioxins can pass through the placenta directly to the fetus, and may cause developmental problems. Breastfeeding infants can receive up to 14% of their lifetime exposure to dioxins through breast milk. Because reproductive and developmental processes are extremely sensitive to endocrine-disruptive compounds, there is an urgent need for better risk characterization and improved evaluation procedures (15). In any case, it may be prudent to reduce the use and emissions of these substances and to establish limits for their presence in food and animal feed. An assessment of the current knowledge on endocrine disrupters has been prepared by WHO through the International Programme on Chemical Safety (16).

Mercury

Mercury occurs naturally in soils and rocks but is also used in a number of industrial applications. Organic mercury, principally in the form of methylmercury, is the most hazardous form.

Food is the main source of exposure to methylmercury and, for the fetus, the main source of exposure is the maternal diet. The highest levels of mercury in food are typically found in fish, particularly the long-lived, large, predatory fish at the top of the food chain, e.g. shark, swordfish, and tuna.

For the vast majority of consumers, the level of mercury in fish does not pose any significant health risk. However, the fetus and young children are more vulnerable to the harmful effects of mercury than adults. Mercury is toxic to the developing fetal brain, and exposure in the womb may lead to neurobehavioural effects such as deficits in motor skills, attention, language, visual-spatial skills and memory. The Codex Alimentarius Commission has established guideline levels for total mercury in predatory and non-predatory fish. In some countries, pregnant women are advised to limit their consumption of certain fish.

Lead

Lead occurs naturally in the environment and has many industrial uses. Small amounts of lead can be harmful, especially to the fetus, infant and young child. During pregnancy, especially in the last trimester, lead can cross the placenta. Cognitive and growth defects may occur in infants whose mothers are exposed to lead during pregnancy. Lead exposure is also serious for young children because they absorb it more easily than adults and are more susceptible to its harmful effects. Even low-level exposure may reduce intelligence, result in learning disabilities and behavioural abnormalities, and cause kidney damage.

Airborne lead from automobile exhaust may contaminate crops or soil; lead may also be introduced into water by certain household water systems. Lead can enter food, especially acidic food such as fruit juice, from lead-based glazes and lead-soldered cans. Infants may also ingest lead in breast milk.

There is no threshold level believed to be safe for infants and young children. However, the Joint FAO/WHO Expert Committee on Food Additives (JECFA) has established a provisional tolerable weekly intake (PTWI) for lead of 0.025 mg/kg of body weight (17).

Nitrate and nitrite

The major acute toxic effect of nitrate and nitrite poisoning is development of methaemoglobinaemia, a condition in which more than 10% of the haemoglobin is transformed into methaemoglobin, thereby reducing the oxygen-carrying capacity of the blood. When transformation exceeds 70%, the condition can be fatal.

Neonates are at special risk because of a transient deficiency in methaemoglobin reductase and the greater susceptibility of haemoglobin F (fetal haemoglobin) to oxidation. Near-adult levels of methaemoglobin reductase and haemoglobin A are reached by 4 months of age.

Most clinical cases of neonatal methaemoglobinaemia occur from drinking water or water-based formulations with high nitrate or nitrite content, i.e. nitrate levels in drinking-water of more than 100 mg per litre. Cases of methaemoglobinaemia have also been reported in infants fed with vegetable preparations in which nitrate has been converted to nitrite through bacterial action.

Mycotoxins

The growth of moulds on agricultural commodities may result in the production of mycotoxins. For example, aflatoxins are produced by *Aspergillus flavus* growing on corn, peanuts and other nuts. These toxins are human carcinogens and considered one of the most dangerous contaminants of food and animal feed. Patulin is a mycotoxin produced by certain species of *Penicillium*, *Aspergillus*, and *Byssochlamys* moulds, and has been found in high levels in apple juice made from damaged and bruised apples. On the basis of adverse effects observed in animal studies, the Codex Alimentarius Commission has proposed a limit for patulin of 50 µg/kg in apple juice and apple juice ingredients in other beverages. In deriving this limit, apple juice consumption by children was considered because they consume higher amounts relative to their body weight than other age groups. Avoiding consumption of bruised apples can also reduce exposure to patulin.

Ethyl alcohol can also be considered a mycotoxin, because it is produced by microorganisms and is toxic to humans. In particular, intake of ethyl alcohol by pregnant women can seriously injure the fetus. Ethyl alcohol is present in many fermented beverages, such as beer and wines, and is used as an ingredient in various foods.

Food additives and dietary supplements

Public health concerns about the use of food additives, such as preservatives, artificial colouring agents, flavour enhancers, sweeteners, and antimicrobials, are generally unfounded. Most developed countries have registration and approval processes which are designed to ensure that only substances that have met exacting safety assessments are used. JECFA provides reference intakes for a range of direct and indirect food additives. An acceptable daily intake (ADI) may be established for a chemical and its toxicologically significant degradation and metabolic products if data demonstrate that exposure to the chemical under its proposed conditions of use would pose no appreciable risk to the consumer over a lifetime. JECFA has, however, stated that ADIs should not be considered applicable to neonates and infants up to the age of 12 weeks (18). In addition, there is some evidence to suggest that certain food additives may produce specific effects in children, such as attention and hyperactivity disorders.

The consumption of supplementary vitamins and minerals is indicated in certain situations, but excessive use may pose health problems. Commercial fortified products include vitamin D fortified milk, iodized salt, and iron-supplemented cereals. In addition, there is widespread promotion of the use by pregnant women of folic acid supplements to prevent spina bifida, vitamin K to prevent haemorrhagic disease of the newborn, and vitamin A to reduce the risk of xerophthalmia in infants. However, there are also dangers associated with excessive intake of vitamins and minerals. For example, excess vitamin A can result in bone disease and increased intracranial pressure, while excess vitamin D can cause kidney disease. Such excesses are unlikely to be a result of dietary intake, but rather of excessive use of supplements. Consequently, it is best to seek a physician's advice before taking such supplements.

Protecting the young

The appropriate advice on how to minimize or avoid food safety risks depends on the type of hazard, the nature of the food, the age of the consumer, environmental conditions and other factors. Here, we consider three groups, namely: (a) the developing fetus, (b) breastfed and bottle-fed infants, and (c) infants receiving complementary foods, and children. The principal foodborne hazards and risk reduction strategies for each of these three groups are described.

The developing fetus

The developing fetus is at risk from infectious agents and toxic chemicals that may cross the placenta. Obviously, the exposure of the fetus is a result of exposure of the woman during pregnancy and, in some cases, before pregnancy. Because of the potential adverse health outcome for the developing fetus, women should be informed about these foodborne hazards. Table 11.1 lists the hazards, adverse health effects and possible risk reduction strategies.

Breastfed and bottle-fed infants

Breast milk is the most nutritious and safest food for the newborn infant. Exclusive breastfeeding minimizes exposure of the infant to foodborne and waterborne pathogenic microorganisms, and confers protection to the infant through the anti-infective properties of breast milk. However breastfed infants can be at risk from a range of chemicals that may be present in breast milk. These may come from the maternal diet during nursing, but may also come from the release of substances that had accumulated in the mother's adipose tissue. Certain infectious agents may also be transmitted through breast milk.

Bottle-fed infants may be exposed to a range of food- and waterborne pathogens. Bacterial contamination of bottles is an important source of diarrhoea in infants. This is particularly a problem in developing countries and in other situations where environmental sanitation is poor. Breast-milk substitutes, such as powdered infant formula, may contain viable pathogenic microorganisms. Infections in infants fed with contaminated formula products containing *Salmonella* spp. and other bacteria from the family Enterobacteriaceae have been reported. In some countries, teats contaminated with N-nitrosamines can still be found. Table 11.2 lists the hazards, adverse health effects and possible risk reduction strategies.

Infants receiving complementary food, and children

When infants reach the age of about 6 months, they should normally be given complementary foods to meet their evolving nutrient requirements. With the introduction of such foods, infants may be exposed to a range of contaminants. These include pathogenic microorganisms and their toxins, and various chemical contaminants of foodstuffs, e.g. lead, mercury and pesticides. Diarrhoea is a leading cause of death in children under the age of five. In developing countries, diarrhoeal disease may be responsible for over 40% of all deaths in children (24). Contaminated complementary foods account for a substantial proportion of diarrhoeal illness among infants and young children (25). Such

Table 11.1 Foodborne hazards for the developing fetus

DISEASE/AGENT	HAZARD	RISK REDUCTION MEASURES
Toxoplasmosis (***Toxoplasma gondii***)	Women infected during pregnancy may transmit the infection to the fetus, possibly leading to stillbirth or birth defects, e.g. hearing or visual impairments, mental retardation.	• Avoid raw and undercooked meat. • There is currently insufficient evidence to confirm that treating mothers who seroconvert during pregnancy can prevent fetal infection and improve infant outcomes (*19*).
Listeriosis (***Listeria monocytogenes***)	Women infected during pregnancy may transmit the infection to the fetus, possibly leading to spontaneous abortion or infants born with visual, mental, or other problems. The increased use of refrigeration to prolong the shelf-life of food has contributed to the emergence of *L. monocytogenes* as a food hazard.	Listeria is destroyed by cooking, but will grow at refrigeration temperatures. • Do not eat refrigerated pâtés, meat spreads, or cold meats. • Do not drink unpasteurized milk or eat foods that contain unpasteurized milk. • Do not eat soft cheese or blue-vein cheese. • Do not eat prepared or stored salads. • Do not eat refrigerated smoked seafood such as salmon, trout, tuna, or mackerel. • Do not eat raw fish such as sashimi, sushi, ceviche, roe, mussels or oysters. • Do not eat refrigerated foods that are past their expiry dates.
Heavy metals (lead, mercury)	Heavy metals may cross the placenta resulting in exposure of the developing fetus. These substances can be neurotoxic, result in reduced intelligence, and lead to behavioural problems.	Methylmercury: • Avoid consuming large amounts of fish that bioaccumulate methylmercury, such as large predatory fish. Lead: • Avoid ceramic dishes and canned food with lead-soldered seams. • Wash vegetables and fruit thoroughly. • Avoid food produced or prepared near busy roads.

Table 11.1 *continued*

DISEASE/AGENT	HAZARD	RISK REDUCTION MEASURES
Persistent organic pollutants including dioxins and polychlorinated biphenyls	POPs may cross the placenta resulting in exposure of the developing fetus. POPs may cause behavioural problems, hormone disturbances, and cancer.	Pregnant women should avoid foods that may contain high levels of POPs. *NOTE: It is important to reduce the use and emissions of POPs and to establish limits for food and animal feed.*
Ethyl alcohol	Drinking of alcohol during pregnancy can cause birth defects and developmental disabilities. Children exposed to alcohol in the womb can suffer an array of disorders, from subtle changes in intelligence to profound mental retardation. They may also suffer growth retardation and be born with birth defects. One of the most severe outcomes is **fetal alcohol syndrome** (FAS), which includes three abnormalities —disorder of the brain, growth retardation, and facial malformation.	Fetal alcohol syndrome and other alcohol-related conditions can be prevented by avoiding alcohol use and food containing alcohol during pregnancy.

SECTION III: SPECIFIC ENVIRONMENTAL THREATS

Table 11.2   Foodborne hazards for breastfed and bottle-fed infants

DISEASE/AGENT	HAZARD	RISK REDUCTION MEASURES
Pathogenic microorganisms	Exposure to pathogenic organisms such as *Salmonella* spp., *E. coli* O157 : H7, *Campylobacter jejuni*, *Staphylococcus aureus*, *Bacillus cereus*, *Clostridium perfringens*, *Shigella* spp., *Vibrio* spp., *Giardia lamblia*, and foodborne viruses, resulting in gastroenteritis and associated illnesses. Such agents have high rates of morbidity and mortality, with mortality directly due to dehydration and indirectly due to reduced resistance to disease.	● Breast milk is the safest food for infants. ● Select good quality infant formula (20). ● Use safe or boiled water when preparing formula. ● Do not store prepared formula. ● Wash and boil bottles and teats after every feeding. If possible, use a cup instead. ● Wash hands after changing the baby, using the toilet, handling raw food or touching animals. ● Follow safe food handling practices (see Table 11.3).
POPs including dioxins and PCBs	Exposure of the infant can lead to behavioural problems, hormone disturbances, and cancer. Human breast milk may contain lipophilic POPs.	● Avoid excessive weight loss during breastfeeding. **NOTE**: *It is important to reduce the use and emissions of POPs and to establish limits for food and animal feed.*
Heavy metals (lead, mercury)	Exposure of the infant to substances such as methylmercury and lead. Heavy metals can be neurotoxic, result in reduced intelligence, and lead to behavioural problems.	**Methylmercury**: ● Lactating mothers should avoid consuming large amounts of fish that bioaccumulate methylmercury, such as large predatory fish. **Lead**: ● Lactating mothers should avoid ceramic dishes and canned food with lead-soldered seams. ● Wash vegetables and fruit thoroughly. ● Avoid food produced or prepared near busy roads.
Infant botulism	Ingested *Clostridium botulinum* spores may germinate, grow and produce toxin. Spores have been found in honey.	Children less than 12 months old should not be fed honey.
HIV	Breast milk may be a vehicle for transmission of HIV.	HIV-positive mothers should seek advice (21–23).
Methaemo-globinaemia	Ingestion of nitrate and nitrite by infants results in the formation of methaemoglobin which reduces the oxygen-carrying capacity of blood.	Ensure well-water and water used to prepare breast-milk substitutes is low in nitrate.

POPs, Persistent organic pollutants; PCBs, polychlorinated biphenyls; HIV, human immunodeficiency virus.

foods may also expose infants to toxic chemical substances. Table 11.3 lists the hazards, adverse health effects and possible risk reduction strategies.

Conclusions

Protecting the health of fetuses, infants, and young children requires vigilance over the types of food consumed by pregnant mothers, special precautions for bottle-fed infants, care in selection and preparation of complementary foods, and supervision of food consumed by young children.

Pregnant women should avoid consumption of high-risk foods. Bottle-fed infants should be provided with good quality breast-milk substitutes that have been prepared and stored in a hygienic manner. Good hygienic practices are essential in the preparation of complementary foods, and infants and children should not be exposed to high-risk foods and ingredients.

Good hygienic practices should be employed in all food handling and preparation activities. Refrigeration is necessary for most foods, as food should not be kept for more than two hours at room temperature. This is especially important for meats, seafood, and dairy products. The food handler's hands, equipment and preparation surfaces must be clean. All fruits and vegetables should be thoroughly washed and the outer leaves of leafy vegetables should be removed, especially if they are to be eaten raw. Cross-contamination must be avoided, with ready-to-eat foods kept separate from raw foods. Finally, thorough cooking, especially of meats, poultry, eggs and fish, is indispensable to avoid foodborne illness. Meats should have an internal temperature of at least 70 °C. This is especially important for minced meat products. Leftover foods and ready-to-eat foods should be heated until they are steaming before being consumed. As a simple guide for consumers, WHO's *Five keys to safer food* (27) should be promoted.

It is important that food safety strategies focus upon improving knowledge and effectively communicating with consumers, including mothers, about the risks associated with specific foods and eating habits. Education to prevent foodborne illnesses should target pregnant and nursing mothers, as well as doctors, public health nurses and nutritionists in health clinics. Children themselves might also be considered targets for food safety messages (28).

SECTION III: SPECIFIC ENVIRONMENTAL THREATS

Table 11.3 Foodborne hazards for infants receiving complementary food, and children

DISEASE/AGENT	HAZARD	RISK REDUCTION MEASURES (26)
Pathogenic microorganisms	Exposure to pathogenic organisms such as *Salmonella spp.*, *E. coli* O157:H7, *Campylobacter jejuni*, *Staphylococcus aureus*, *Bacillus cereus*, *Clostridium perfringens*, *Shigella spp.*, *Vibrio spp.*, *Giardia lamblia*, and foodborne viruses, resulting in gastroenteritis and associated illnesses. Such agents have high rates of morbidity and mortality, with mortality directly due to dehydration and indirectly due to reduced resistance to disease.	● Cook all food thoroughly. ● Avoid storing cooked food. ● Avoid contact between raw foodstuffs and cooked foods. ● Wash fruits and vegetables. ● Use safe water. ● Wash hands repeatedly. ● Protect food from insects, rodents and other animals. ● Store non-perishable foodstuffs in a safe place. ● Keep all food preparation premises meticulously clean. ● Purchase food from reliable sources. ● Practise good personal hygiene during food handling and preparation activities. ● Do not eat or drink foods containing raw eggs, or raw unpasteurized milk and fruit juice. ● Avoid keeping food at room temperature for more than 2 hours. ● Ensure that persons with diarrhoea, especially children, wash their hands after using the toilet.
Haemolytic uraemic syndrome	Ingestion of *E. coli* O157:H7 in food may lead to infection and in severe cases to the development of haemolytic uraemic syndrome in infants and young children.	● Avoid eating salami, raw milk, and hard-to-clean vegetables, like sprouts and lettuce. ● Cook all meat thoroughly. ● Practise good personal hygiene during food handling and preparation activities. ● Drink only pasteurized fruit juice.

Table 11.3 *continued*

DISEASE/AGENT	HAZARD	RISK REDUCTION MEASURES (26)
POPs including dioxins and PCBs	Exposure of infants and young children can lead to behavioural problems, hormone disturbances, and cancer.	Select food likely to be low in these substances.
Organophos- phorus pesticides	Neurotoxicity, with young children at risk because of high consumption on body weight basis of certain foods.	Wash fruits and leafy vegetables, and peel other vegetables to avoid ingesting pesticides.
Heavy metals (lead, mercury)	Exposure of infants and young children to substances such as methylmercury and lead. These substances can be neurotoxic, result in reduced intelligence, and lead to behavioural problems.	Methylmercury: ● Avoid consuming large amounts of fish that bioaccumulate methylmercury, such as large predatory fish. Lead: ● Avoid ceramic dishes and canned food with lead-soldered seams. ● Wash vegetables and fruit thoroughly. ● Avoid food produced or prepared near busy roads.
Patulin	Mycotoxin found in apple juice. Codex limit of 50 µg/kg of apple juice is proposed.	● Avoid eating bruised apples. ● Avoid apple juice made from damaged or mouldy apples.
Methylhaemo- globinaemia	Ingestion of nitrate and nitrite by infants results in the formation of methaemoglobin which reduces the oxygen-carrying capacity of blood.	● Ensure well-water and water used in food contains low levels of nitrate.

POPs, Persistent organic pollutants; PCBs, polychlorinated biphenyls.

SECTION III: SPECIFIC ENVIRONMENTAL THREATS

References

1. *World Declaration on Nutrition. A plan of action for nutrition adopted on 11 December 1992 by the International Conference on Nutrition.* Rome, Geneva, Food and Agriculture Organization of the United Nations and World Health Organization, 1992.

2. Käferstein FK. Food safety: a commonly underestimated public health issue. *World Health Statistics Quarterly*, 1997, 50:3–4.

3. Mead P et al. Food-related illness and death in the United States. *Emerging Infectious Diseases*, 1999, 5:607–625.

4. Gilbert RE. Epidemiology of infection in pregnant women. In: Petersen E, Amboise-Thomas P, eds. *Congenital toxoplasmosis: scientific background, clinical management and control.* Paris, Springer-Verlag, 2000.

5. Evengard B et al. Low incidence of toxoplasma infection during pregnancy and in newborns in Sweden. *Epidemiology and Infection*, 2001, 127:121–127.

6. Neto EC et al. High prevalence of congenital toxoplasmosis in Brazil estimated in a 3 year prospective neonatal screening study. *International Journal of Epidemiology*, 2000, 29:941–947.

7. Wallon M et al. Toxoplasma infections in early pregnancy: consequences and management. *Journal of Gynecology and Obstetrics and Biology of Reproduction*, 2002, 31:478–484.

8. Lipka B et al. Visual and auditory impairment in children with congenital cytomegalovirus and *Toxoplasma gondii* infection. *Przegl Lek*, 2002, 59(Suppl. 1):70–72.

9. Multistate outbreak of listeriosis—United States, 2000. *Morbidity and Mortality Weekly Report*, 2000, 49:1129–1130.

10. Wilhelmi I, Roman E, Sanchez-Fauquier A. Viruses causing gastroenteritis. *Clinical Microbiology and Infection*, 2003, 9:247–262.

11. Hamprecht K et al. Epidemiology of transmission of cytomegalovirus from mother to preterm infant by breastfeeding. *Lancet*, 2001, 357:513–518.

12. De Cock KM et al. Prevention of mother-to-child HIV transmission in resource-poor countries—translating research into policy and practice. *Journal of the American Medical Association*, 2000, 283:1175–1182.

13. *New data on the prevention of mother-to-child transmission of HIV and their policy implications.* WHO Technical Consultation on Behalf of the UNFPA/ UNICEF/WHO/ UNAIDS Inter-Agency Task Team on Mother-to-Child Transmission of HIV. Geneva, World Health Organization, 2001 (WHO/RHR/ 01.28).

14. *Stockholm Convention on Persistent Organic Pollutants.* Nairobi, United Nations Environment Programme, 2001 (www.pops.int).

15. Cooper RL, Kavlock RJ. Endocrine disrupters and reproductive development: a weight-of-evidence overview. *Journal of Endocrinology*, 1999, 152:159–166.

16. *IPCS global assessment of the state-of-the-science on endocrine disrupters.* Geneva, World Health Organization, 2002 (http://www.who.int/pcs/emerg_site/edc/ global_edc_TOC.htm).

17. *Safety evaluation of certain food additives and contaminants.* Geneva, World Health Organization, 2000 (WHO Food Additives Series No. 44).

18. IPCS. *Principles for evaluating health risks from chemicals during infancy and early childhood: the need for a special approach.* Geneva, World Health Organization, 1986 (Environmental Health Criteria, No. 59).

19. Peyron F et al. *Treatments for toxoplasmosis in pregnancy (Cochrane review).* Oxford, Update Software, 2001 (The Cochrane Library, Issue 4).

20. FAO/WHO. *Codex Alimentarius. Codex Standard for Infant Formula.* Rome, FAO/WHO Codex Alimentarius Commission, 1997 (CX-STAN 072).

21. *HIV and infant feeding. Guidelines for decision-makers.* Geneva, World Health Organization, 1998 (WHO/FRH/NUT/CHD/98.1).

22. *HIV and infant feeding. A guide for health care managers and supervisors.* Geneva, World Health Organization, 1998 (WHO/FRH/NUT/CHD/98.2).

23. *HIV and infant feeding. A review of HIV transmission through breastfeeding.* Geneva, World Health Organization, 1998 (WHO/FRH/NUT/CHD/98.3).

24. Fikree F et al. Time to focus child survival programs on the newborn: assessment of levels and causes of infant mortality in rural Pakistan. *Bulletin of the World Health Organization*, 2002, 80:271–277.

25. Motarjemi Y et al. Contaminated weaning food: a major risk factor for diarrhoea and associated malnutrition. *Bulletin of the World Health Organization*, 1993, 71:79–92.

26. *Basic principles for the preparation of safe food for infants and young children.* Geneva, World Health Organization, 1996 (WHO/FNU/FOS/96.6).

27. *Five keys to safer food.* Geneva, World Health Organization, 2001 (http://www.who.int/fsf/Documents/5keys-ID-eng.pdf).

28. Williams T et al. *Food, environment and health: a guide for primary school teachers.* Geneva, World Health Organization, 1990.

CHAPTER 12
Poisonings and envenomings[1]

I. Makalinao
Department of Pharmacology and Toxicology, University of
the Philippines, College of Medicine, Manila, Philippines

A. Woolf
Harvard Medical School and American Association of
Poison Control Centers, Boston, USA

POISONING
Overview

Poisonings extract an enormous toll worldwide, not only in terms of human suffering and death, but also in terms of social and economic losses associated with premature death, reduced human functioning, lost potential and productivity, and the costs of treatment. Exposures can be categorized according to the circumstances: (i) acute, one-time events; (ii) subacute or time-limited exposures; and (iii) chronic poisoning. While the chronic effects of toxicants such as tobacco, nicotine, chemical inhalants, alcohol, and illegal drugs are major public health concerns and often have their roots in childhood and early adolescence, they are outside the scope of this chapter. Likewise suicide by poisoning, often with pharmaceuticals, is a serious phenomenon, and is especially common among adolescent women in developed countries. However, such exposure will not be addressed here.

Incidence and significance

Poisonings and toxic exposures are among the most prevalent public health problems affecting children in the world today. In 1990, there were 139 million cases of poisoning, with about 242 000 deaths (1). In 2001, it was estimated that over 50 000 deaths in children under 14 years were due to unintentional poisoning (2). In Finland, more than 37 000 calls are made to the national poison centre annually, and 60% of the poisonings involve children under the age of 6 (3). In Viet Nam, over 9000 hospitalizations for poisoning were recorded annually, with a mortality of 3.3% (4). Agricultural poisonings from organophosphorus compounds and paraquat are particularly problematic, along with a new rodenticide, trifluoracetamide. In the United States, 64 poison centres reported more than 2.2 million poisonings in 2001, of which 92.2%

---

[1]Reviewed by **J. Pronczuk**, Department for the Protection of the Human Environment, World Health Organization, Geneva, Switzerland.

occurred in a residence and 51.6% involved children younger than 6 years (5). There were 1074 fatalities reported by these same centres. In Sri Lanka, the death rate from poisoning was found to be 43 per 1000 total deaths (6).

Poisonings are expensive, accounting for 1–5% of hospitalizations of children in the USA (7). Miller estimated the lifetime losses related to poisonings in the USA in 1992 alone at about US$ 50 billion, with US$ 3 billion in direct medical spending (8).

Severity and vulnerable populations

Poisonings can be graded clinically on the basis of the duration (e.g. minutes, hours, days, or years) and the dose, as well as the relative sensitivity of the host to the toxicant's harmful effects. The potency of the toxic agent, in terms of its inherent ability to cause cellular injury and the nature of its toxicity, is also a determinant of the clinical importance of an exposure. The gradation of exposure along these four axes has important clinical implications in terms of the severity of the injury and the extent of likely disability.

Developmentally, children are most vulnerable to poisoning when they start to walk and climb. At the same time, they exhibit pincer grasp and other intricate finger and hand movements, and start to explore objects orally without the cognitive ability to recognize which items are edible. As has been discussed earlier, infants and young children also differ from older children, adolescents, and adults in how they are exposed to toxicants and how they absorb, distribute, detoxify, and eliminate xenobiotics. Their diets are different, and so they may be exposed to excessive amounts of certain toxicants in contaminated foods. Their respiratory rate is faster than that of adults, so that they are exposed to higher quantities of inhaled toxicants.

There are also special paediatric populations who are particularly vulnerable to poisoning. The unborn fetus is sensitive to any toxicants that pass through the placenta, and to the direct teratogenic effects of radiation. Infants who are breast-feeding may inadvertently receive doses of harmful chemicals, such as dioxin and some mycotoxins, through breast milk.

Pesticide exposure

Rural children in developing countries come into close contact with pesticides, playing in the family fields. Children help in the fields, live in houses where pesticides are stored, and may be more exposed to pesticides in inappropriate containers, leading to accidental poisoning. Thailand, a major user of pesticides, embarked on an education programme in selected school districts to improve awareness of the hazards of pesticides, their health effects and the symptoms of poisonings (Case study 17, page 334).

Routes of exposure

Children can encounter toxic exposures in many different places. However, over 90% of early childhood poisonings reported to poison centres occur in the child's home or in that of a grandparent or other carer. The home environment often contains an assortment of medicines, cooking and heating fuels, automobile supplies, cleaning agents, paints, solvents, and chemicals useful in everyday life. Often these are accessible to infants and young children, who may poison themselves by swallowing a substance or spilling a caustic chemical on their skin or in their eyes.

Many children in developing countries work full-time to help support their families, and they may be exposed to chemical solvents, pesticides, heavy metals, and other agents in the workplace (9). For example, children working in the gold mining industry in Brazil or the Philippines risk significant mercury-related neurotoxicity, as this metal is used in the gold extraction process.

Unsanitary drinking-water contaminated with infectious agents or natural or man-made toxicants affects millions of children (see Chapter 8). The contamination of wells used for drinking-water with arsenic in areas of West Bengal and Bangladesh is a poisoning epidemic on an unprecedented scale, affecting an estimated 20 million people in Bangladesh (10).

Disasters

Environmental disasters can cause poisoning epidemics, such as the explosion in Bhopal, India, in 1984, which led to diisocyanide gas poisoning, or the radiation exposure in Ukraine related to the 1986 Chernobyl nuclear reactor disaster.

Epidemics

Epidemics from contaminated foodstuffs represent an important risk. During May and June 1981, an outbreak of pulmonary and gastrointestinal illness in Spain, affecting over 19 828 people and causing 315 deaths, was traced to an illegally marketed, rapeseed-based cooking oil (11). Gupta & Singh reported periodic outbreaks of "epidemic dropsy" in New Delhi, India, from ingestion of mustard oil contaminated by *Argemone mexicana* ("prickly poppy") oil (12). Over 1726 people, including a disproportionately high number of children, were stricken in 1998 with erythema, rashes, fever, vomiting, diarrhoea, bilateral lower limb oedema and calf tenderness, hypotension, and occasional heart failure and ocular involvement.

Poisoning epidemics have also been caused by locally formulated, unregulated and impure medications. In 1995–1996, at least 109 Haitian children suffered acute renal failure, and 85 died, from the use of locally formulated and unregulated paracetamol adulterated with diethylene glycol (13).

Health effects

Drugs and chemicals may induce injury at the organ and cellular levels, through idiosyncratic adverse reactions, an extension of their dose–response pharmacology, direct or indirect toxic interactions at the cellular level with corresponding physiological perturbations, or additive or synergistic actions with other toxic agents. Toxicants cause cellular injury through a variety of mechanisms. They may interfere with energy production (e.g. cyanide, salicylates, iron) or neurotransmission (e.g. botulin, tetrodotoxin), block receptors (e.g. organophosphorus and carbamate pesticides) or subcellular channel function (e.g. calcium channel blockers). They may interfere with essential membrane-associated electrolyte pumps (e.g. digitalis), create protein adducts or other radicals that injure cell membranes (e.g. paracetamol), promote oncological transformation (e.g. benzene), or deplete cofactors essential to normal physiology (e.g. isoniazid).

Toxicants tend to affect the gastrointestinal tract first, inducing nausea and vomiting, often accompanied by intense abdominal pain. Some ingested poisons (e.g. iron, castor bean, foodborne toxicants) can produce haemorrhagic diarrhoea. Severe poisonings affect the vital signs early. Cardiovascular changes may include tachycardia and hypertension (e.g. amfetamines, cocaine), or bradycardia and hypotension (e.g. beta blockers, calcium channel blockers). Metabolic poisons, such as salicylates, iron, and cyanide, may initially increase the respiratory rate and then produce respiratory arrest. Others, such as opiates, barbiturates, gamma-hydroxybutyrate (GHB), and muscle relaxants, induce coma and depress respiration early in the course of the poisoning. Seizures are common soon after an overdose of neurotoxicants such as isoniazid, strychnine, camphor and bupropion. Some agents, notably paracetamol and *Amanita* mushrooms, may take hours before producing signs of life-threatening toxicity.

Many environmental toxicants have multisystem effects. For example, organophosphorus pesticides affect the gastrointestinal, neurological, cardiovascular, and pulmonary systems through cholinergic stimulation, producing characteristic increased sweating, vomiting and diarrhoea, seizures, bradycardia, lacrimation, salivation, bronchorrhoea and respiratory distress, and incontinence. Such constellations of symptoms and signs reflect the physiological perturbations typically produced by a particular class of toxic agents.

Management

Early medical care for the poisoned child can prevent complications, some of which may be life-threatening. The four basic tenets in the treatment of the poisoned child are described below.

- *Supportive care.* This includes resuscitation, administration of oxygen, intravenous fluids, anticonvulsants, antiemetics, vasoactive drugs, and other critical care measures.
- *Decontamination.* This involves removing the toxicant before it can be absorbed or cause an injury. Thus, poison on the skin or in the eye should be washed off. Victims of an inhalation poisoning should be removed from the contaminated environment and given oxygen. Gastrointestinal

procedures (such as evacuating the stomach by lavage with an orogastric tube or giving activated charcoal orally) may be important for the patient who has swallowed poison if they can be performed early.

- *Enhanced elimination.* This includes advanced extracorporeal techniques, such as haemodialysis or haemoperfusion, for selected poisonings. Alkalinization of urine, in order to "trap" the ionized species of certain drugs with an acidic pK (e.g. salicylates, methotrexate or phenobarbital), can also enhance elimination. Repeated doses of oral charcoal every 2–4 hours can help eliminate certain drugs by enhancing their dialysis out of the splanchnic blood back into the lumen of the gastrointestinal tract, or by interfering with their enterohepatic circulation.
- *Antidote administration.* For a few toxicants, specific antidotes can block their injurious effects or reverse physiological disturbances.

Antidotes
Antidotes work by a variety of mechanisms:

- adsorbing the toxicant before it can be absorbed into the body (e.g. activated charcoal);
- blocking the metabolism of a nontoxic compound to a more toxic metabolite (e.g. use of ethanol or 4-methylpyrazole to block methanol or ethylene glycol metabolism);
- chelating the toxicant out of the bloodstream (e.g. sodium calcium edetate, dimercaptosuccinic acid for lead poisoning; deferoxamine for iron poisoning);
- correcting the physiological perturbations induced by a poison (e.g. atropine to treat the cholinergic effects of organophosphorus pesticide poisoning);
- supplying a cofactor needed to correct physiological functioning or detoxify a drug or chemical (e.g. acetylcysteine for paracetamol poisoning; pyridoxine for isoniazid poisoning);
- reversing the toxic effects at the receptor site in affected organ systems (e.g. flumazenil for benzodiazepine poisoning; naloxone for opiate poisoning; pralidoxime for organophosphorus poisoning);
- treating the toxic effects directly (e.g. diphenhydramine for the syndrome of dystonia associated with acute neuroleptic poisoning).

Data sources
Public health authorities need to understand local and regional variations in the causes of poisonings and toxic exposures in order to formulate regulations and other measures that meet local and regional priorities (14). Information about morbidity and mortality from toxic exposures, including the numbers of hospitalizations and deaths due to poisonings, emergency department and out-

patient visits, and telephone calls to poison centres, might be found in registries. Information about toxicants and their effects is available on several web sites (e.g. www.inchem.org).

Poisoning prevention

Both active and passive prevention measures can limit injuries from toxic exposures among children. One-time childhood poisonings can be reduced through the use of child-resistant packaging for both drugs and chemicals, and by preferring nontoxic chemicals for household use. Discouraging the use of more toxic drugs, such as propoxyphene, harmful commercial products, such as thallium-containing rodenticides, and dangerous agricultural products, such as paraquat, will also reduce the incidence of childhood poisoning.

Poison control centres are a key resource for preventing poisoning in many parts of the world. In some countries, advice from poison centres is accessible only to health care professionals; in others, the poison centre is accessible to the general public, and provides advice on both medically serious and trivial toxic exposures. Poison centres offer professional medical advice and triage designed to treat and limit the injurious effects of poisoning. They can also serve as a lead agency in public education outreach campaigns directed either to the entire population or to vulnerable groups.

Active poisoning prevention measures include education of the public in order to change their lifestyles and behaviour. The home should be made a safe environment for children, ideally with a "safe area", as well as constant vigilance and close supervision by carers. The "four Rs" of poisoning prevention are important for parents of young children:

- *Recognize* what chemicals, cleaners, plants, drugs, and other products represent a poisoning hazard and are present in the household.
- *Remove* poisonous products from the reach of children by throwing them away or locking them in high cabinets.
- Be *ready* should a poisoning event occur. This may include having the telephone number of the local poison centre on hand and knowing first aid for different types of toxic exposure.
- *Respond* appropriately to a poisoning event. This includes the basic tenets of first aid: washing the skin in the case of a dermal exposure, flushing the eyes under a stream of running water in the case of an ocular exposure, or getting the patient safely to fresh air in the case of a toxic inhalation. Where local poison centres exist, calling for information and help can be a crucial aspect of first aid.

Public health programmes

Poisoning prevention also entails disaster preparedness at local, regional, and national levels. Releases of hazardous chemicals from factories or during transport or fires can lead to a disaster. Public health agencies must develop comprehensive plans that address the multiple possible environmental toxic exposures at a programme level. Recently Carlson & Tamburlini outlined a rationale and guiding principles for the development of national policies on children's environmental health, which included various types of poisoning (e.g. lead, tobacco, pesticides) as priority health outcome and exposure indicators (14).

Regulatory measures

Many countries have yet to enact regulatory measures to safeguard children from toxic exposures and poisonings. Recently the Bangkok Statement (see Chapter 1) endorsed recommendations for poisoning prevention to include a ban on leaded petrol and increased use of child-resistant packaging. The ban on leaded petrol should be extended to all countries. The requirement that drugs be packaged in child-resistant containers and that kerosene and other fuels be kept in childproof bottles (with special taps) are measures with proven effectiveness in preventing poisoning. Restrictions on child labour, regulating the age of eligibility, types of occupations, and hours per week will also help protect children from workplace-associated toxicants.

Specific toxicants

Paracetamol

Paracetamol is a popular, nonprescription medication taken for the relief of pain or treatment of fever. The toxic one-time dose is 150 mg/kg of body weight in children or 7.5 g in adolescents. High-risk groups vulnerable to the hepatotoxic effects of paracetamol include alcohol-dependent people, suicidal adolescents, and pregnant women and their unborn children.

When taken in overdose, the normal hepatic conjugation pathways for the detoxification of paracetamol become saturated. Excess paracetamol is processed via P450 oxidative degradation to a reactive intermediate compound, N-acetylbenzoquinonimine (NAMBQI). In paracetamol poisoning, the cofactor glutathione required to detoxify NAMBQI is quickly exhausted. Without enough glutathione to detoxify it, NAMBQI destroys hepatocytes.

Patients may not show symptoms of toxicity for the first 12 hours or so, then complain of nausea, vomiting, and abdominal pain. Hepatitis supervenes within 24–36 hours post-ingestion and peaks at 72–96 hours, progressing to fulminant hepatic necrosis in severe poisoning. Complications include hepatorenal failure, acidosis, encephalopathy with cerebral oedema, severe coagulopathy, and death.

Clinical severity can be gauged using the Rumack-Mathews nomogram, in which the plasma paracetamol level is plotted against time post-ingestion to predict hepatitis. For example, a plasma paracetamol concentration of 150 µg/ml or more at 4 hours post-ingestion suggests a possible risk of hepatitis, whereas a level of 200 μg/ml or more at 4 hours warns of probable hepatitis. Other relevant blood tests include liver and renal function tests and, in severe cases, measures of coagulation. The patient's neurological status should be carefully assessed periodically over the course of the hospitalization.

Treatment of paracetamol poisoning is directed towards preventing the drug's absorption using oral activated charcoal. The antidote is acetylcysteine, which supplies more than enough glutathione and sulfur to detoxify paracetamol.

Carbon monoxide

Carbon monoxide is a colourless, odourless gas emitted as a product of combustion. Sources include furnaces, hot water heaters, propane or gasoline space heaters, barbecues, fireplaces, wood stoves, and gas dryers. In many countries, especially in rural areas, the use of charcoal in domestic heating devices is common, exposing inhabitants to carbon monoxide poisoning. House fires produce high concentrations of carbon monoxide and other toxic gases. Methylene chloride, found in chemical paint strippers, absorbed by inhalation or dermal absorption, is metabolized endogenously to carbon monoxide. The pregnant woman and her unborn child are particularly susceptible to the toxic effects of carbon monoxide exposure.

Carbon monoxide interferes with cytochrome oxidase function and disrupts cellular respiration. The gas also binds to haemoglobin and myoglobin; normal oxygen unloading cannot occur, causing hypoxic injury at the cellular level. The half-life of carbon monoxide in the blood is 4–6 hours in room air, 90 minutes in 100% oxygen, and 20 minutes in hyperbaric oxygen.

Symptoms of carbon monoxide poisoning are similar to, and may be confused with, those of influenza. Patients with mild poisoning may have poor appetite, confusion, lethargy, muscular aches, nausea, vomiting and headache. In patients with severe poisoning there may be confusion, seizures and coma. Delayed symptoms (2–3 weeks after exposure) include confusion, poor memory, behavioural changes, irritability, poor concentration, focal neurological findings, weakness, and myoclonus.

Carboxyhaemoglobin levels in blood are often above 15–20% in the poisoned patient. Levels above 60% are usually lethal. However, a history of the dose and duration of exposure ("carbon monoxide soaking") is more often prognostic of outcome than the blood carboxyhaemoglobin level. Psychometric testing of patients with carbon monoxide poisoning reveals deficits in speech, orientation, and memory, many of which persist as sequelae.

Patients suffering from carbon monoxide poisoning should be moved to fresh air as soon as possible, and receive 100% oxygen. Hyperbaric oxygen therapy has also been found to be effective.

Caustic agents

Caustic household products include drain-clearing agents, toilet bowl and oven cleaners, and chrome and metal cleaners. Cement cleaners and rust removers may contain hydrofluoric acid, an extremely potent acid that can also cause systemic hypocalcaemia, even after dermal exposure.

The alkaline corrosives stick to oesophageal tissues producing transmural liquefaction necrosis, a saponification of available tissue fats and proteins. Ingestion of acid produces a more superficial chemical burn, with eschar formation and a coagulative necrotic lesion, that can extend through the oesophagus and into the stomach.

Patients may be remarkably symptom-free, even after a significant exposure to alkali. Initial symptoms of caustic poisoning include crying, hypersalivation, drooling, and swollen red lips and gums. Young children may refuse to feed; older children may complain of throat pain and significant dysphagia. Reddish or pale areas of burning may be visible around the mouth or on the lips, tongue, oropharyngeal surfaces or palate. Splash burns may be evident elsewhere on the skin or in the eyes. Respiratory symptoms, including wheezing and hypoxia, indicate aspiration of the product.

Determination of the pH of the affected tissues or the suspect product can confirm a caustic exposure. A chest radiograph in the patient with respiratory symptoms may show free air in tissues or a pneumomediastinum or pneumothorax. Arterial blood gas analysis often reveals a respiratory acidosis and hypoxaemia if the patient has aspirated caustic material into the lungs, or a metabolic acidosis after significant acid absorption.

Patients suffering from caustic poisoning should be given nothing by mouth; vomiting should be avoided and ipecacuanha should not be given. "Neutralization" (e.g. giving vinegar to counteract an alkali) exacerbates injury and is normally contraindicated. To treat patients who have swallowed a large amount of strong mineral acid, carefully instil saline into the patient's stomach using a nasogastric tube. Endoscopy of the upper gastrointestinal tract should be performed 6–24 hours after ingestion. For severely burned patients, steroids can be given to limit in-migration of inflammatory cells and reduce the risk of later stricture formation. Some patients may require a period of total parenteral nutrition, or feeding through a gastrostomy until the oesophagus heals. Parenteral antireflux drugs are adjunctive therapy. Antibiotics may be necessary to treat subsequent bacterial oesophagitis or gastritis. Surgical revision or colonic interposition may be necessary later.

Cyanide

Cyanide is found in jewellery polish, plants (cassava, apricot pits), medications such as sodium nitroprusside, smoke from some house fires, and nitriles used in industry. It is used as an intermediate in the manufacture of paper, textiles, and plastics, in electroplating, and in extracting gold from ore.

The cyanide (CN) molecule is a potent direct vasodilator, and disrupts mitochondrial cytochrome oxidase, interfering with cellular oxidative metabolism. CN is metabolized by the enzyme rhodanase in the liver to the less toxic metabolite, thiocyanate (SCN), which is freely excreted in the urine.

Sometimes a person who has swallowed cyanide has a premonitory "feeling of dread", with an odour of bitter almonds. Nausea, vomiting, confusion, lethargy, and tachycardia are early manifestations of poisoning. These quickly progress to coma and shock; seizures and metabolic acidosis may intervene at any time. Death is from respiratory failure and cardiac arrest.

Levels of CN in serum and red blood cells are elevated in the poisoned patient. Arterial blood gases show a profound metabolic acidosis, or a mixed acidosis in patients who are in respiratory failure. The whole blood lactate level is elevated.

Management of the poisoned patient includes supportive measures, such as administration of oxygen and dextrose-containing intravenous fluids. Anticonvulsants may also be necessary.

In many countries, hydroxocobalamin or other cobalt-containing antidotes are available. An alternative treatment involves three phases: (i) inhalation of amyl nitrite pearls induces a 3–5% methaemoglobinaemia, which with free blood CN forms cyanomethaemoglobinaemia; (ii) intravenous administration of sodium nitrite induces 25–30% methaemoglobinaemia, which can capture larger amounts of free CN; (iii) intravenous administration of sodium thiosulfate, which reacts with cyanomethaemoglobin to form thiocyanate ion, which is less toxic and is excreted by the kidneys.

Ethylene glycol

Ethylene glycol is present in automobile antifreeze and refrigerants, and is used as a common commercial solvent and in photographic developing. It is sweet-tasting and can be attractive to young children. Diethylene glycol, a similar substance, has sometimes been used as a solvent in the preparation of counterfeit medicines, causing the death of a large number of children.

The parent compound is metabolized by hepatic alcohol dehydrogenase to the more toxic glycoaldehyde, glycolic acid, glyoxalic acid, and oxalate derivatives. All of these are capable of causing direct injury to cell membranes. Oxalates combine with available calcium to produce symptomatic hypocalcaemia. Calcium oxalate crystals precipitate in the neurons or in renal tubules, exacerbating cellular injury.

Patients who swallow ethylene glycol may initially appear inebriated, with ataxia and confusion. Coma and seizures also occur. A severe metabolic acidosis evolves over hours and may be accompanied by congestive heart failure, hypotension, hypocalcaemic tetany and subsequently acute oliguric renal failure.

Ethylene glycol blood concentrations are rarely available; however blood osmolality shows a gap between measured and calculated values. A urinalysis shows an active urinary sediment and calcium oxalate crystals. Hypocalcaemia and abnormal renal function tests are also often present.

Management includes supportive care and intravenous fluids. An enzyme-blocking antidote such as ethanol or 4-methylpyrazole is indicated for ethylene glycol blood levels of 20 mg/dl or above. Haemodialysis is reserved for patients with confirmed exposure, who manifest worsening acidaemia or blood ethylene glycol concentrations above 50 mg/dl.

Herbal medicines and dietary supplements

Herbal preparations contain numerous different chemicals and substances. Dietary supplements frequently contain vitamins, amino acids, ephedrine, caffeine, or hormones. Contaminants and adulterants may be present if quality control is poor. Chinese patent medicines and Ayurvedic remedies may be contaminated by heavy metals, such as arsenic or lead, or contain pharmaceuticals (e.g. corticosteroids). Some remedies, especially Asian patent medicines, may contain aconite, a cardiotoxin capable of producing severe bradyarrhythmias, or drugs such as phenylbutazone, a nonsteroidal anti-inflammatory agent capable of causing aplastic anaemia. Homeopathic medicines are usually highly diluted and thus pose little medical risk.

Different herbs may have toxicity for specific organ systems. For example "chaparral", "germander" and *jin bu huan*, are all hepatotoxic. Pyrrolizidine alkaloid-containing teas (e.g. comfrey, symphytum, heliotrope) are capable of causing hepatic venous occlusion (Budd-Chiari syndrome).

Signs of poisoning vary according to the herb or dietary supplement ingested. Agents containing ephedrine or caffeine may cause nausea and diarrhoea, tremulousness, anxiety, tachycardia and hypertension.

The identification of ingredients is key to the successful management of toxic reactions to herbal products and dietary supplements. Consulting a poison control centre or Internet site can be helpful. Treatment of inadvertent poisoning might include activated charcoal and supportive measures, depending on the nature of the toxicants.

Hydrocarbons

Many household products used as fuels, cleaners, and solvents contain hydrocarbons such as kerosene, gasoline, turpentine, or mineral spirits. Hydrocarbons that have low viscosity and high volatility are most easily aspirated into the lungs. Hydrocarbons are usually absorbed in large amounts by inhalation, because of high vapour pressures, or via dermal absorption, because of their lipid solubility and solvent properties.

Hydrocarbon-containing products can cause life-threatening chemical pneumonitis if inhaled, either accidentally or deliberately. They are often toxic to the nervous system, causing inebriation, slurred speech, ataxia, and coma. Young solvent abusers who inhale hydrocarbons may suffer "solvent encephalopathy", a chronic syndrome of behavioural changes (garrulousness, aggression), seizures, poor memory, slowed cognition, motor changes, and dementia. "Sudden sniffing death" may occur as a result of lethal arrhythmia caused by a rise in blood catecholamines after the acute inhalation of highly concentrated hydrocarbon-containing solvents (e.g. toluene).

Pulmonary symptoms and signs of hydrocarbon poisoning include tachypnoea, cough, wheezing, and cyanosis. Children who vomit after ingesting a hydrocarbon-containing product have an increased risk of aspiration. Life-threatening complications, including chemical pneumonia, hypoxaemia, adult-type respiratory distress syndrome, and respiratory failure can develop in severe poisoning.

Specific hydrocarbons may also have intrinsic, extrapulmonary toxicity. Benzene exposures are linked to the development of aplastic anaemia and later leukaemia. Toluene can cause tubular necrosis and renal failure. Carbon tetrachloride poisoning causes an irreversible hepatic necrosis. Methylene chloride (paint stripper) is converted in the liver to carbon monoxide and may produce the typical symptomatology of carbon monoxide poisoning.

Blood assays for hydrocarbons are not usually available. A chest radiograph should be obtained at presentation, if the child has respiratory symptoms, or between 4 and 6 hours post-ingestion if the child is not initially symptomatic. The blood count often demonstrates leukocytosis, even without bacterial infection. Monitoring of blood gases and neurological and pulmonary function is important for severely poisoned children. Monitoring of blood counts (e.g. in benzene poisoning), renal function (e.g. in toluene poisoning), carboxyhaemoglobin (in methylene chloride poisoning), or liver function (e.g. in carbon tetrachloride poisoning) may be necessary in selected cases.

The treatment of children with hydrocarbon poisoning includes oxygen administration and, if necessary, mechanical ventilation. Steroids and bronchodilators are not effective, unless the patient has significant bronchospasm. Bacterial secondary infection is a common complication 48–72 hours after the onset of symptoms and may require the use of antibiotics.

Iron

Multivitamins and iron supplements intended for pregnant women and adults are highly toxic to children (and attractive, as they may be colourful and sweet). The toxic dose of free iron is 40 mg/kg of body weight (155 mg of ferrous fumarate = 65 mg of free iron; 30 mg of ferrous sulfate = 6 mg of free iron). Children's multivitamins with iron do not contain, in general, enough iron to pose a risk of toxicity.

Free iron acts as an oxidizing agent and a mitochondrial poison, interfering with electron transport because of its reduction–oxidation potential. The cell reverts to anaerobic metabolism, generating organic acids. Iron also causes injury and corrosion to the gastrointestinal mucosal lining. Free iron destroys hepatic cells, with unloading of glucose and the release of histamine, bradykinin, and other vasoactive substances, which contribute to vascular injury and the development of shock.

Early signs of severe iron poisoning include nausea, vomiting, diarrhoea, and haemorrhagic gastritis. Hypotension, shock, confusion, lethargy, and coma may develop early in the course of severe poisoning. Metabolic acidosis is evident, along with an initial hyperglycaemia, giving way to hypoglycaemia later. Severe hepatitis evolves within 24–48 hours of ingestion. Complications of severe iron poisoning include hepatorenal syndrome, coagulopathy, bleeding, and encephalopathy. Septicaemia with unusual organisms, such as *Yersinia enterocolitica* or *Listeria monocytogenes*, sometimes develops on the third or fourth day after poisoning. Late sequelae in survivors include cirrhosis or gastric strictures.

Measurement of blood iron concentrations can help gauge the clinical severity of poisoning, and is best done 4 hours after ingestion. Levels greater than 500 µg/dl are associated with toxicity; those greater than 1000 µg/dl are life-threatening. Unabsorbed iron pills may be radio-opaque in abdominal radiographs. Serial blood counts, glucose, liver function, and coagulation tests are all helpful in monitoring a patient's condition.

Activated charcoal should not be given as it does not adsorb heavy metals. Ipecacuanha given orally with water produces vomiting within 20 minutes. Large numbers of iron pills in the gut can also be evacuated with whole bowel irrigation using polyethylene glycol. Coagulation defects in life-threatening cases may require supportive measures, such as vitamin K or fresh frozen plasma. Deferoxamine is an antidote for iron poisoning. When given intravenously it chelates free iron in blood to produce a soluble non-toxic product, ferrioxamine, which is excreted in the urine, giving it a pinkish hue (*vin rosé* urine).

Lead

Lead is highly toxic to children. Both acute and chronic poisoning result from exposure to different sources of lead.

Children are vulnerable to lead in painted and plastered surfaces in homes and other buildings. Lead in dust or outdoor soil may be ingested by young children through their hand-to-mouth activities. Lead in petrol is released in automobile exhaust and may be inhaled. Lead can also contaminate water supplies, canned foods, traditional medicines, cosmetics and other household products.

Lead interferes with haem synthesis and other enzyme-mediated systems, and with the normal neuronal arborealization and synaptogenesis during the development of the central nervous system. It also affects bone metabolism and causes renal injury and hypertension. The absorption of lead is increased in children with iron and calcium deficiency.

Lead poisoning is usually defined as a blood lead level of 10 µg/dl or higher. However, there is growing concern about neurodevelopmental effects resulting from exposures where the blood lead levels are below 10 µg/dl. Early signs of poisoning include a microcytic anaemia, with basophilic stippling and elevated red blood cell porphyrin levels. Neurobehavioural problems caused by plumbism in children include poor appetite and irritability, with hyperactivity and an inability to focus.

Neurodevelopmental delays and learning problems are common in lead-poisoned children, especially in relation to speech acquisition, visual–motor integration, and higher-order cognitive functions. In severe lead poisoning, encephalopathy may occur as well as complications, such as peripheral neuropathies, cerebral oedema, and deafness. Blood lead levels of 70 µg/dl and above are associated with life-threatening sequelae related to cerebral oedema and lead encephalopathy.

An abdominal radiograph may be positive if the child has recently eaten plaster or paint chips containing lead; bone films may demonstrate metaphyseal "lead" lines in chronic poisoning. Children tend to suffer abdominal colicky pain.

A singularly important aspect in the prevention of childhood lead poisoning is the abandonment of lead-containing petrol by countries around the world. Another important measure is the reduction of the lead hazard in the home, day-care centre, and other environments where children spend appreciable amounts of time. Children's hand-to-mouth behaviour should be monitored and pica should be discouraged. Measures such as frequent hand-washing, damp mopping of floors, and dusting can cut down on lead-containing interior dust. Water, old lacquer or paint on cribs and furniture, imported ceramics, pots and pans, herbal remedies, and cosmetics can be unexpected sources of lead. A diet containing high levels of iron and calcium can reduce absorption of lead by children.

Children who have been poisoned by lead can be treated with chelating medications including meso-2,3-dimercaptosuccinic acid, sodium calcium edetate, and dimercaprol (15).

Methanol

Methanol, present in some paint thinners and de-icing compounds, is still found in some household products. As little as 1 tablespoon of methanol can cause life-threatening symptoms in a young child.

Methanol is metabolized by hepatic alcohol dehydrogenase to formaldehyde and formate. These compounds injure cells in the brain and the eyes. Clinical findings of poisoning include severe metabolic acidosis with a high anion gap. Patients may complain of spots before their eyes, "snow" vision, blurring, and a narrowed visual field. Central nervous system effects include inebriation, confusion, ataxia, slurred speech, coma, seizures, and amblyopia.

Laboratory findings include a high anion metabolic acidosis. In methanol poisoning there is an osmolar gap between the measured and the calculated serum osmolality. Blood methanol levels over 20 mg/dl confirm the diagnosis. Measurement of blood methanol can be used to gauge the patient's prognosis.

Alcohol dehydrogenase blockers, including ethanol or 4-methylpyrazole, are effective antidotes for methanol poisoning. Haemodialysis is necessary for patients with blood methanol levels of 50 mg/dl or higher and for those with confirmed exposure history and severe acidaemia.

Mushrooms

Only a few species of fungi are poisonous. Small children may eat mushrooms while playing and exploring, and occasionally severe poisoning may occur. The most common circumstance leading to serious toxicity is the ingestion of misidentified fungi as food. In the majority of cases, the ingestion of non-edible mushrooms produces mild gastrointestinal effects. However, some species are highly toxic. *Amanita phalloides* is one of the most toxic species: its amatoxins produce liver, kidney, pancreatic and gastrointestinal effects, and poisoning may be lethal.

Amanita muscaria—the typical red and white, colourful and attractive mushroom—produces very mild and self-limiting gastrointestinal and hallucinogenic effects. Mushrooms of the genus *Cortinarius* are nephrotoxic and may cause renal failure. In case of suspected or known mushroom ingestion, health personnel should keep the patient under clinical observation and contact an organization that can assist in the identification of the mushroom (e.g. botanical garden, university, or poisons centre). Specific treatment is required in case of poisonous mushroom ingestion and a poisons centre should be consulted.

Plants

Poisoning by plants is very common in children, but the large majority of such exposures are medically trivial. With few exceptions, once the plant has been identified, parents whose child has swallowed a few leaves or berries can be given simple reassurance.

Many plant compounds, such as terpenes, alkaloids, phytotoxicants, saponins, and cardiac glycosides, have pharmacological properties and may be toxic.

- *Solanines* (Jerusalem cherry (*Solanum pseudocapsicum*); nightshade family) cause gastrointestinal complaints, shock, and convulsions.
- *Abrin*: The rosary pea (*Abrus precatorius*) contains a phytotoxin, abrin, which causes vomiting, tremors, delirium, shock and uraemia. Even 1 or 2 ingested castor beans (*Ricinus communis*) can result in a life-threatening episode of nausea, vomiting, diarrhoea, haemolysis, renal failure, and dehydration in a child.

- *Oxalate*: Oxalate-containing plants (Jack-in-the-pulpit, philodendron, dieffenbachia) cause mouth and throat pain, swelling, and dysphagia.
- *Aconitine*: Grayanotoxicants (andromeda, azalea) and aconitine (monkshood (*Aconitum napellus*)) cause bradyarrhythmias.
- *Glycosides*: The foxglove (*Digitalis purpurea*), oleander (*Nerium oleander*) and yellow oleander (*Thevetia peruviana*) contain cardiac glycosides that cause dysrhythmias, hypotension, hyperkalaemia, and coma.
- *Scopolamine*: *Datura stramonium* (Jimsonweed) causes an anticholinergic syndrome with hallucinations.
- Holly berries (*Ilex* spp.) produce severe vomiting and diarrhoea. Pokeweed (*Phytolacca americana*) can produce gastrointestinal cramps, visual disturbances, diarrhoea, weakness, and subsequent death.
- Water hemlock (*Cicuta maculata*) is known to contain a neurotoxin capable of producing lethal seizures, while poison hemlock (*Conium maculatum*) is an autonomic nervous system depressant, causing coma and respiratory arrest.

Decontamination of the patient may be necessary if a poisoning involves a highly toxic plant. Ipecacuanha may be useful where the plants, berries or mushrooms are known to be highly toxic and vomiting can be induced within 20–30 minutes of ingestion. Activated charcoal can also be a useful adsorbant of toxicants in plants, if administered orally in a timely fashion.

Prevention of plant poisoning requires vigilance by parents of young children. Parents should survey their land, removing any toxic mushrooms or toxic plants such as poison ivy or deadly nightshade. Indoor plants should be kept well out of reach and should be nontoxic. Parents of young children should check with their poison control centre for identification of suspect plants or for advice about which ornamental plants are safe.

Salicylates

Salicylate poisoning may occur in young children who ingest the pharmaceutical, especially when it resembles a sweet. However, the incidence of exposure seems to have decreased. Children can also be poisoned by ingesting ointments and liniments that contain methylsalicylate.

At the cellular level, salicylates uncouple oxidative phosphorylation. The cell converts to anaerobic metabolism, utilizing fat and other substrates and producing free fatty acids and lactate. This results in a high anion gap metabolic acidosis. Salicylates are also irritants, and can be potentially corrosive to gastrointestinal mucosa. Antiplatelet actions of salicylates are such that the patient can develop a bleeding diathesis. Salicylates also stimulate the central respiratory centre in the hypothalamus, which accounts for a primary respiratory alkalosis often seen early in poisoning. Salicylate poisoning also causes imbalances of both fluids and electrolytes. Electrolytes cross membranes to buffer acid–base abnormalities, resulting in total body deficits of potassium, calcium, and magnesium. Intracellular ionic shifts and fluid losses can cause severe dehydration. Occasionally a syndrome of inappropriate release of antidiuretic hormone is seen in salicylate poisoning, causing fluid to move into the interstitial spaces and metabolic derangements.

Classic findings in acute salicylism include hyperventilation, diaphoresis, tinnitus and acid–base disturbances. Other symptoms and signs of poisoning are nausea, vomiting, abdominal pain, fever, haemorrhagic gastritis, respiratory alkalosis, deep, rapid (Kussmaul-type) respirations, metabolic acidosis, hepatitis, confusion, lethargy, coma and seizures.

Blood analysis may reveal hypernatraemia, hypochloraemia, hypokalaemia and hypocalcaemia. Arterial blood gases often reveal an acidosis with a base deficit. Hyperglycaemia is evident early, hypoglycaemia later. Elevated ammonia levels, abnormal liver function tests and laboratory evidence of coagulopathy are seen in life-threatening salicylism. Blood salicylate levels can suggest the severity of toxicity: 30 to 60 mg/dl indicates mild to moderate toxicity; 60 to 100 mg/dl reflects severe poisoning; and levels above 100 mg/dl are life-threatening.

Repeated doses of activated charcoal every 3–4 hours may help prevent the absorption of salicylate and enhance its elimination. The alkalinization of urine to a pH of 7.5–8.0 enhances elimination because of the low pK of the drug. The ionized form predominates, is "trapped" in renal tubules, and then excreted in urine. Haemodialysis should be considered for the salicylate-poisoned child who develops any of the following:

- noncardiogenic pulmonary oedema;
- cerebral oedema;
- worsening coma despite decontamination;
- severe metabolic derangements;
- acute renal failure;
- seizures;
- a salicylate blood concentration of 80–100 mg/dl after a one-time overdose;
- a salicylate blood level above 60 mg/dl in a patient who is taking aspirin regularly.

ENVENOMING

Venomous animals deliver a poison from a highly developed secretory gland through a bite or sting. The venom is important for their survival, as they use it for defence, overcoming prey, and digesting food. Venomous animals can be found in all types of habitat. They may be found close to where children live, learn and play, particularly—but not exclusively—in rural areas. Although venomous species exist in all parts of the world, children living in tropical countries may have a greater chance of being exposed to venomous bites and stings.

Children may be exposed to a number of venomous creatures. While at home or in areas where they play, they may be bitten by snakes, spiders, centipedes, or millipedes, or stung by scorpions, bees or wasps. At the beach, children may be exposed to envenomation from cone shells, stinging fish, stonefish, jellyfish, sea stars and sea urchins. The American Association of Poison Control Centers (AAPCC) in 2002 (16) reported that 1305 of the 15 687 scorpion stings in the USA were in children less than 6 years old. Other exposures in this age group were to centipedes and millipedes (315 out 2051), bees, wasps and hornets (2494 out of 12 632), coelenterates (116 out of 1329) and fish (33 out of 1389) (16).

Treatment and details of specific types of envenomation will not be discussed here. In case of a bite or sting, the appropriate health care facility should be consulted (e.g. a poisons control centre); in some countries, an experienced toxicologist may be contacted for advice. Life-threatening envenomation in children may warrant admission to an intensive care unit and the administration of specific antivenin.

Diagnosis of envenomation may pose a unique challenge to the health care provider, especially when there were no witnesses to the exposure and the child is not old enough to give an accurate account of it. Patients may present with nonspecific symptoms. For instance, incessant crying in children may be one of the initial signs of a scorpion sting, even before the actual lesion becomes manifest. It is important to consider the possibility of envenoming in cases of unexplained collapse, convulsions, bleeding or coagulopathy, paralysis, myolysis, renal failure, local tissue injury, pain, increased salivation, lacrimation and sweating.

The unique vulnerability of children may increase the potential for any given exposure to be life-threatening. Some case reports suggest that the smaller volume of children may predispose them to a higher morbidity than the adults (4, 5, 8, 11). However, the existing grading scores for severity of snakebite are mostly based on adult data. Various guidelines based on adults have correlated severity with amount of oedema, which may not be accurate in children.

Children and adolescents can benefit from education on how to prevent snakebites. Preventive measures such as wearing protective clothing and not reaching blindly into areas where snakes hide, may reduce the incidence of snakebite.

Snakebites

While adults are generally wary of snakes, children may not understand the potential danger and may even attempt to pick them up. The major venomous snakes are as follows:

- Elapidae—cobras, kraits, mambas and coral snakes;
- Hydrophyidae—true sea snakes;
- Laticaudidae—sea kraits;
- Viperidae—pit vipers;
- Crotalidae—rattlesnakes, water moccasins, copperheads, American and Asian bushmasters;
- Colubridae—boomslang and birdsnake of Africa and rednecked keelback of Asia.

Snake venoms are complex mixtures of proteins with enzymatic actions. They may produce local or systemic effects. Clinical effects may range from local tissue swelling to significant neurotoxicity. Pit viper bites may produce significant disseminated coagulopathy and bleeding.

Spider bites

There are over 30 000 species of spiders in the world (17), but only a few produce venoms that cause significant injury or death in humans. However, most fatalities are among children, the elderly or individuals with a pre-existing medical condition. The spiders most commonly associated with significant envenomation are the black widow (*Latrodectus*) and the brown recluse (*Loxosceles*).

The black widow spider is found in Africa, Asia, Australia, Europe and USA. Only the female, recognized by its shiny black colour and characteristic red, yellow or orange hourglass marking on the underside of the large globular abdomen, is capable of human envenomation. Diagnosis can be challenging, especially in very young children who are not able to explain that they have been bitten. The symptoms may be misdiagnosed as acute appendicitis if the child presents with severe abdominal pain associated with abdominal rigidity, especially if the characteristic lesion or "halo" remains unnoticed.

Brown recluse spiders are usually found in uncleaned, dusty areas in the home. The bite is often not painful at the outset and may remain unnoticed for up to 24 hours, after which a painful purple papule develops. Tissue necrosis may develop up to one week later. The venom contains cytotoxic enzymes. Haemolytic anaemia may follow a *Loxosceles* bite in children.

Scorpion

Scorpions have an elongated segmented body, similar to the shrimp, with a long mobile tail. The venom is contained in a vesicle found in the telson, which is the last segment of the tail. Morbidity and mortality from scorpion stings is higher in children than adults (18). Children may have more severe signs and symptoms because severity is dependent on body weight. Diagnosis in young children with unexplained crying and agitation may be difficult because of the absence of local signs. Different species of scorpions produce different clinical syndromes. The yellow scorpion (*Leiurus quinquestriatus*) found in north Africa, Jordan, Lebanon, Saudi Arabia, Syrian Arab Republic, and Turkey may produce a hyperadrenergic state with high levels of catecholamines, cholinergic signs, cardiovascular collapse and eventually death. The South African *Tityus* scorpions may produce hypertension, cholinergic signs, convulsions and death. The only American genus of clinical significance is *Centruroides* (18).

Millipedes and centipedes

Children may pick up millipedes out of curiosity. While millipedes do not bite, when handled they discharge toxic substances that may irritate the skin or, in severe cases, produce local tissue changes and even necrosis. Some can cause conjunctival irritation by spraying a highly irritating and repugnant secretion. Children who pick up centipedes may receive a painful bite, that produces localized swelling and erythema, which may later progress to lymphangitis or lymphoedema; symptoms generally subside in 48 hours (18).

Hymenoptera

Bees, wasps, hornets and ants belong to the order Hymenoptera, characterized by a stinging apparatus situated at the end of the abdomen, in the females. Bees have a barbed stinger with lances that attaches to the skin and continues to inject venom even if the insect dies. Wasps and hornets have unbarbed stingers, and can inflict multiple stings. The stings cause local pain, redness and swelling, and rarely cause severe toxicity. However, multiple stings or stings near the mouth or neck may be life-threatening. In some children, a single sting may produce a potentially fatal anaphylactic reaction within 30 minutes. These children present with rash, itching, angio-oedema, nausea, vomiting, hypotension, bronchospasm and eventually collapse. A child may go into anaphylactic shock as a result of sensitization from a previous exposure.

Deaths from bee stings in the United States are more common than from all other venomous creatures. Treatment of local effects may require the use of antihistamines, corticosteroids, and cooling lotions. The bee sting should be removed immediately, by scraping or pinching. Anaphylactic reactions require the use of epinephrine and immediate supportive care.

Aquatic animals

There are some 100 known toxic species of coelenterates and aquatic invertebrates. The venom is often found in stinging cells called nematocysts. Most of the toxins contain a complex mixture of polypeptides and proteins, including catecholamines, histamines, hyaluronidases, kinins, fibrinolysins, and cardiotoxins.

Jellyfish stings may cause death in humans. The "true" jellyfish, the Scyphozoans, are found throughout the world, and have tentacles arranged radially round the bell and even inside the bell. The Cubozoans—the "box" jellyfish, particularly the Chirodropids—have caused many deaths in humans in tropical and subtropical waters. The tentacles arise from the corners of the box or cube. When the jellyfish touch the skin, the thread tube that is tightly coiled in each nematocyst is locked in position by a set of spines. The thread tube fires at tremendous speed through the skin in just a few thousandths of a second.

The Irukandji jellyfish, found in northern Australia, mostly lives in deep waters but can be washed onto beaches during the summer months. The bell is transparent making it almost impossible to be seen in water. On initial contact the tentacles may be just 5–7 cm long, but these can increase to 60–70 cm when the Irukandji has its prey. The initial envenomation may not be noticed, since there is hardly any mark from the jellyfish bell. The skin may then develop a "goose pimple effect", which lasts for approximately 30 minutes, and redness, which may last for several days. This latent period, called the Irukandji syndrome, ranges from 5 to 50 minutes and is followed by severe and distressing systemic symptoms, namely pain, catecholamine excess and global cardiotoxicity leading to pulmonary oedema. Low back pain is characteristic, with the victim experiencing a dull aching at the sacral area and difficulty walking. Muscle cramps are often described as unbearable and coming on in "waves". Victims are usually restless, moving continuously in an effort to get comfortable. They usually have a sense of impending doom. In severe envenomation, sweating is highly profuse and generalized and piloerection is observed.

In 1996, the last recorded death from box jellyfish (*Chironex fleckeri*) envenomation in Australia was in a 3-year-old girl from the remote Northern Territory aboriginal community. According to Currie, the last ten deaths from jellyfish stings in the Northern Territory have all been in children, which shows the greater risk for a smaller body exposed to the millions of stinging cells on jellyfish tentacles. Because the efficacy and safety of the antivenom are uncertain, prevention is of paramount importance. Children should therefore not enter the sea when there may be jellyfish present (19).

Physalia are not real jellyfish, but a hydroid of the order siphonophora. They appear on beaches during the summer months, and have a sting similar to that of jellyfish. *Physalia* have a gas-filled sac that floats in water. Common examples include the bluebottle, Portuguese man-of-war and Pacific man-of-war. Pain accompanies the initial envenomation.

Scorpion bite

A 28-month-old girl with witnessed scorpion sting to the right big toe. She cried continuously for 30 minutes. The child was tachycardic with a heart rate of 176 bpm and a respiratory rate of 36/min, and had increased salivation, agitation and wheezing. At the hospital the child presented opsoclonus or roving eye movements. The scorpion was identified as a *C. sculpturatus.* The child's clinical status improved rapidly, and she was discharged from the emergency room after 2 hours. Five weeks later she was stung again by a small scorpion, on her foot. She presented with excessive salivation and secretion from mouth and nose, wheezing, supraventricular tachycardia and gross motor agitation. One hour after envenomation, the child was noted to have a body temperature of 38.2 °C, heart rate of 150 bpm, respiratory rate of 40/min with gross motor agitation and opsoclonus and copious oral secretions. One vial of the intravenous Centruroides antivenom was given. Symptoms resolved after one hour at the emergency department and the patient was discharged after 4 hours with specific instructions to watch out for signs of serum sickness. Follow-up was conducted by telephone.

NOTE: ATROPINE IS NOT ROUTINELY RECOMMENDED IN TREATING SYSTEMIC TOXICITY FROM THE DANGEROUS SCORPIONS OF ASIA, THE MIDDLE EAST AND SOUTH AFRICA. Atropine may potentiate the sympathetic effects of the venom itself leading to an "autonomic storm" with transient cholinergic effects and a sustained hyperadrenergic state.

Spider bite

The father of a previously well child found his 8-month-old boy extremely lethargic, listless and covered with vomitus. He noticed that the child had two puncture marks over the dorsal web space of the right third and fourth fingers. A large spider was found on the bed. The child presented with cholinergic signs, increased sweating, salivation, tongue fasciculation, piloerection and progression of lethargy. During transportation to the hospital the child was given two vials of Funnel Web Spider antivenom (recommended by the on-call toxinologist at the Australian Venom Research Laboratory) and an immediate reversal of symptoms was noted. The spider was identified by the Natural History Museum of Queensland as a male *Hadronyche infensa*.

Agelenopsis aperta envenomation

Previously thought as harmless, this spider has now been shown to be dangerous. A nine-year-old boy was initially unaware that the spider had bitten him, until a red mark was noted on his neck. He suffered from neck rigidity and pharyngeal swelling with fronto-occipital headache after 10 minutes. Later there was nausea and disorientation. A red papule on the bite site was noted. He developed myalgia and arthralgia, general malaise, headache, and unsteadiness with heaviness in the legs. Because of the rarity of positive identification, all spiders caught in the act of biting should be properly identified by qualified arachneiologists. The spider in this case was caught by one of the boy's classmates while still on the neck of the victim, allowing for the recognition of this species and its potential for toxicity.

Acknowledgement

Dr Woolf's work is supported in part by funds from the Comprehensive Environmental Response, Compensation, and Liability Act (CERCLA) trust fund, through a cooperative agreement with the Agency for Toxic Substances and Disease Registry, Public Health Service, US Department of Health and Human Services. The authors assume sole responsibility for the contents of this chapter; the views expressed are not necessarily those of the Agency for Toxic Substances and Disease Registry.

References

1. Murray CJL, Lopez AD. Global health statistics. *A compendium of incidence, prevalence, and mortality estimates for over 200 conditions.* Boston, MA, Harvard School of Public Health, 1996.

2. *Mental health. New understanding, new hope. The World Health Report 2001.* Geneva, World Health Organization, 2001.

3. Hoppu K. Forty years of poison information service in Finland—what has changed and what has not. *Journal of Toxicology and Clinical Toxicology*, 2001, 39:276.

4. Du NT, Due B, Due P. Epidemiology of acute poisonings in Viet Nam. *Journal of Toxicology and Clinical Toxicology*, 2001, 39:527–528.

5. Litovitz TL, Klein-Schwartz W, Rodgers G et al. 2001 annual report of the American Association of Poison Control Centers Toxic Exposure Surveillance System. *American Journal of Emergency Medicine*, 2002:391–452.

6. Senanayake N, Peiris H. Mortality due to poisonings in a developing agricultural country: trends over 20 years. *Human and Experimental Toxicology*, 1995, 14:808–811.

7. Woolf A, Wieler J, Greenes D. Costs of poison-related hospitalizations at an urban teaching hospital for children. *Archives of Pediatric and Adolescent Medicine*, 1997, 151:719–723.

8. Miller TR, Lestina DC. Costs of poisoning in the United States and savings from poison control centers: a benefit-cost analysis. *Annals of Emergency Medicine*, 1997, 29:239–245.

9. Woolf AD. Health hazards for children at work. *Journal of Toxicology and Clinical Toxicology*, 2002, 40:477–482.

10. *The Bangladesh arsenic mitigation water supply project; addressing a massive public health crisis.* Washington, DC, World Bank, 1999 (*http://wbln1018.worldbank.org/sar/sa.nsf*).

11. Kilbourne EM et al. Clinical epidemiology of toxic-oil syndrome. *New England Journal of Medicine*, 1983, 309:1408–1414.

12. Gupta SK, Singh U. Epidemic dropsy: treatment, prevention and future planning. In: Gupta SK, ed. *Poisoning, poison control, and environmental toxicology.* New Delhi, Utkarsh Prints, 2000.

13. O'Brien KL et al. for the Acute Renal Failure Investigation Team. Epidemic of pediatric deaths from acute renal failure caused by diethylene glycol poisoning. *Journal of the American Medical Association*, 1998, 279:1175–1180.

14. Carlson J, Tamburlini G. Policy development. In: Tamburlini G, van Ehrenstein O, Bertollini R, eds. *Children's health and environment: a review of evidence*, Copenhagen, WHO Regional Office for Europe and European Environment Agency, 2002.

15. Bates N et al. eds. *Paediatric toxicology: handbook of poisoning in children*. London and Basingstoke, Macmillan Reference, 1997.

16. American Association of Poison Control Centers. *2002 Annual report of the American Association of Poison Control Centers Toxic Exposure Surveillance System*. American Journal of Emergency Medicine, 21:353.

17. Diaz JH. The global epidemiology, syndromic classification, management and prevention of spider bites. *American Journal of Tropical Medicine and Hygiene*, 2004, 71:239–250.

18. *Casarett and Doull's Toxicology: The basic science of poisons*, 5th ed. New York, McGraw-Hill, 1996.

19. Currie B et al. Jellyfish envenomation in the Northern Territory of Australia. *Toxicon*, 1992, 30:501.

CHAPTER 13

Unintentional injuries in children

T. Guthrie
Children's Institute, University of Cape Town, South Africa

K. McGee
Department of Injuries and Violence Prevention, World Health Organization, Geneva, Switzerland

M. M. Thein
Home Safety Committee, National Council of Singapore, Singapore

Overview

Childhood injuries are a major public health problem worldwide. In 2000, an estimated 973 000 children under the age of 15 were killed by an injury (1). Approximately 20% of all injuries worldwide occur in children under 15, and injuries were among the 10 leading causes of death for this age group. Injuries accounted for nearly 10% of the total burden of disease in children. Of the injury deaths among children, 84% were due to unintentional injuries, with almost 32% of these caused by drowning and almost 25% by road traffic injuries (Figure 13.1).

Until recently, injuries were frequently referred to as accidents. However, there is growing consensus that using the term accident implies a degree of inevitability. This traditional view of injuries as accidents suggests that they are random events, an unavoidable part of the world in which children live. During the past few decades, public health professionals have recognized that injuries are preventable. Injuries have been taken out of the realm of chance and placed squarely in the realm of science, where they can be studied and approaches to their prevention can be planned.

An injury is "a bodily lesion at the organic level, resulting from acute exposure to energy (mechanical, thermal, electrical, chemical or radiant) in amounts that exceed the threshold of physiological tolerance. In some cases (e.g. drowning, strangulation, freezing), the injury results from an insufficiency of a vital element" (2). Injuries are typically divided into two categories: unintentional injuries, which comprise road traffic injuries (RTIs), drowning, burns, poisoning, and falls; and intentional injuries, which arise from deliberate acts of violence against oneself or others.

In this chapter we will discuss the epidemiology and risk factors of unintentional injuries among children aged 0 to 14 years, particularly those linked

Figure 13.1 Distribution of unintentional injuries by cause among children under 15 years in 2000

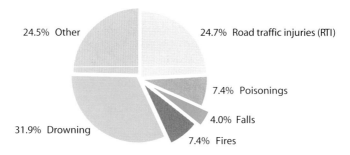

to the children's environment. We also discuss measures that can be taken to prevent injuries among children.

Magnitude of the problem

Unintentional injuries among children are a global problem; however, children and adolescents in certain regions of the world are disproportionately affected. It is estimated that 98% of all unintentional injuries in children occur in low- and middle-income countries. Children in the African, South-East Asian and Western Pacific regions account for 80% of all childhood unintentional injuries (Figure 13.2) (1).

Among high-income countries, injury continues to be a leading cause of death among children. For example, in the United States of America in 2000, unintentional injury was the leading cause of death among children aged 1–14 years (3). In Finland, between 1971 and 1996, injuries were the leading cause of death in children aged 1–14 years (4). In Australia, injuries are the leading cause of death in children aged 1–14 years, accounting for nearly half of all deaths in this age group (5). Unintentional injuries make up 90% of all child injury deaths in Australia. A recent study by UNICEF revealed that every year injuries kill more than 20 000 children aged 1–14 years in the countries of the Organisation for Economic Co-operation and Development (OECD) (6).

Figure 13.2 Distribution of unintentional injuries among children 0–15 years, by sex and region, in 2000

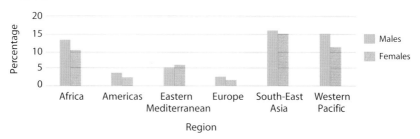

SECTION III: SPECIFIC ENVIRONMENTAL THREATS

In Bangladesh, a community-based study found that drowning accounted for between 10% and 15% of all child deaths over the 12 years of the study (7). In rural areas of the Islamic Republic of Iran, unintentional injuries are responsible for 41% of all deaths of children aged between 1 and 14 years (8). A community-based study in Jordan found that 60% of sample families lived in conditions that exposed their small children to a range of significant dangers, including exposed kerosene heaters (9). Many of the Central and Eastern European countries have significantly higher child injury mortality rates than Western European countries; for example, Latvia has a rate of 38.4 per 100 000 population versus 5.2 per 100 000 in Sweden (6). Deaths from injury account for almost the entire east–west gap in overall child mortality in Europe (10). In Croatia, injuries are responsible for 36% of all deaths in childhood and 52.5% of total mortality in the 5–14 year age group (11).

While mortality is an important indicator, it is important to realize that for each injury death, there are several thousand injury survivors who are left with permanent disabilities. Data on nonfatal childhood unintentional injuries and associated disability among children are relatively scarce. Nonetheless, a study in the Netherlands during 1991–1995 found that for every death among children under 14 caused by a home or leisure injury, there were 160 hospital admissions and 2000 visits to accident and emergency departments (12). If this proportion is extrapolated to child injury deaths in the OECD countries, there would be approximately 50 million accident and emergency department visits and 4 million hospital admissions each year (6). To measure nonfatal outcomes, WHO uses the disability-adjusted life year (DALY).[1] It is estimated that, in 2000, 32% of the DALYs lost to injury globally were among children aged 0–14 years.

A recent review of children's injuries in low-income countries revealed a good deal of consistency between WHO data and other sources with regard to common causes of childhood unintentional injuries (13). These causes are reviewed below.

Road traffic injuries

RTIs among children include injuries to pedestrians, cyclists, and motor vehicle occupants. WHO estimates that, in 2000, over 190 000 children died as a result of road traffic injuries. RTIs account for 48% of child injury deaths in the EU as a whole (14) and 41% in the OECD countries (6). RTIs cause the most serious injuries, including head and abdominal injuries, and in some places, particularly urban areas, RTIs are the most common cause of injuries that require emergency care (13). For example, in Thailand, RTIs were found to be the most common cause of injury in children over one year of age (15). The

---

[1] Disability Adjusted Life Years: the sum of years of potential life lost due to premature mortality and the years of productive life lost due to disability.

majority of children who die as a result of RTIs are not car occupants but pedestrians and cyclists. In South Africa, over 40% of children under 19 years who suffered an RTI were pedestrians (16). In Ethiopia, 84% of all persons who die in traffic crashes are pedestrians (17).

Drowning

In 2000, an estimated 229 000 children died from drowning. Half of the global mortality due to drowning occurs among children aged 0–14 years (18), with children under 5 years having the highest drowning mortality rates. There is a large disparity among children worldwide with regard to drowning; more than 90% of drowning deaths occur in low- and middle-income countries, while drowning rates in high-income countries are declining. In Uganda, a population-based community survey in a rural district found that drowning was the leading cause of injury death (19). A review of deaths among children aged 1–12 years in a rural district in India found that drowning was the single largest cause of death for this age group during the 7-year study period (20). In Mexico, from 1985 to 1990, 3408 children aged 1–4 years died as a result of drowning, making it the leading cause of death for this age group (21).

Other causes of childhood unintentional injuries

There is some evidence that falls are a common cause of childhood injury. A community survey in Brazil showed that over 46% of injuries among children aged 1–10 years were caused by falls (22). A study in the United Kingdom found that 42% of visits to emergency departments by children under 14 years were for treatment of cuts or lacerations resulting from a fall (23). In addition, a review of public hospital admissions in New Zealand over a 10-year period showed that falls were the leading cause of morbidity among children aged under 14 years (24). WHO estimates that over 32 000 children died from a fall in 2000.

Burns are also an important public health issue, particularly in terms of morbidity and long-term disability, and especially in the developing world; WHO estimates that more than 95% of fire-related burns occur in low- and middle-income countries. Burns and scalds are the third leading cause of death for children in the EU (14). A study in Kuwait found that during the 16-year study period, the majority of burn patients were children aged 0–5 years (25). An epidemiological study of childhood injury in the United Arab Emirates found that in the group under 5 years of age, the most common cause of trauma was burns and scalds (64%) (26). A four-year study in Afghanistan found that 63% of patients admitted to a Red Cross hospital for burns were children (27).

Acute unintentional poisoning also causes numerous deaths and health care visits each year. In 2000, almost 70 000 children died from unintentional poisoning. The youngest children seem to be at the greatest risk. For example, a study in Zimbabwe found that over 45% of poisoning cases occurred in children below the age of 5 years (28). In Saudi Arabia, 63% of the poisoning cases seen over the seven-year study period were in children aged 1–3 years (29). In the United States of America, children under 5 years have the highest rate of poisoning-related emergency department visits (30).

Routes of exposure and risk factors

A number of factors play a role in children's vulnerability to injury. Some of these are personal factors that are not modifiable; others are related to the children's environment and in many cases are modifiable. One personal risk factor is age; many studies show that for specific types of injuries, such as poisoning and burns, very young children are at highest risk. Sex is also a risk factor for injury among children. Boys account for most injuries in almost all studies where figures are disaggregated by sex (13). For example, boys aged 5–14 years in low- and middle-income countries are more than twice as likely to drown, more than twice as likely to be injured in falls, and about 80% more likely to be killed or injured in road traffic crashes than girls (31). Although sex and age are not susceptible to modification, awareness of the increased likelihood of specific injuries being associated with certain age and sex groups allows prevention programmes to be targeted to these high-risk groups.

Other risk factors associated with childhood unintentional injury include socioeconomic status and environmental factors, many of which are closely linked. There is evidence that children living in poverty are disproportionately affected by injuries. Economic poverty can influence injury patterns in numerous ways. For example, poor children frequently live in areas with high traffic density, are more likely to travel on foot or by bicycle than by car, and typically have inadequate play areas. Children from affluent families are more likely to sustain nonfatal injuries as passengers inside a vehicle, while poor children more frequently sustain fatal injuries as pedestrians (32). In many low- and middle-income countries, substandard housing contributes to the risk of injury. Approximately 600 million city residents in Africa, Asia and Latin America live in "life- and health-threatening homes" (33). In addition, affluent families are able to install a range of safety devices, such as smoke detectors, safety gates, and window guards, that make the home environment safer for children.

There is some evidence of rural–urban differences in injury rates, though most of this evidence is from high-income countries. In industrialized countries, such as Canada, New Zealand, and the USA, rural residents have higher rates of fatal unintentional injuries than urban residents (32). This may be particularly relevant for certain types of injuries. For example, the circumstances in which drowning occurs can differ between rural and urban settings: drowning in streams, wells, dams, cisterns or while fishing is more common in rural areas of low- and middle-income countries (34). While drowning in open bodies of water, falls from trees, burns from open fires and high-speed car crashes are important causes of death for rural residents, injuries as a pedestrian, a cyclist or as a passenger on public transport are more common for urban residents.

Remedial action, prevention and education

Overall, there are three general approaches to injury prevention: (1) education to promote behaviour change (so that individuals avoid risk and policy- and decision-makers generate informed decisions); (2) environmental modification to create safer surroundings; and (3) legal requirements and prohibitions to reduce risk (35). These are commonly known as the "three Es" of injury prevention: education, engineering, and enforcement.

Reducing deaths and disabilities from childhood unintentional injury is challenging but there are numerous examples of successful interventions. Lessons can be learned from high-income countries where the incidence and severity of childhood injuries have decreased in recent decades. Caution should be exercised, however, in transferring these interventions to low- and middle-income countries. For example, use of child safety seats in cars would be of comparatively limited value in settings where the vast majority of road traffic injury victims are pedestrians. It is important to identify the factors that contribute to the risk of injury among certain populations. For instance, childhood burns may be more commonly due to hot bath scalds, as in Japan (36), or to dropping a hot liquid while unsupervised, as in the Netherlands (37). Or the most common agent in unintentional poisoning among children may be kerosene, paraffin, or petroleum, as in many developing countries, or medicaments and household chemicals, as in many developed countries.

Modifications and improvements for avoiding specific types of injury
Road traffic injuries

There are numerous measures that can be taken to prevent RTIs among children. These include:

- reduced speed limits—in the United Kingdom, the introduction of 20 miles per hour (32 km/hour) speed limits resulted in a 70% decrease in child pedestrian collisions (14);
- traffic slowing measures such as speed bumps;
- safer vehicle car fronts—a large proportion of deaths and serious injuries among pedestrians and cyclists could be prevented this way (38);
- sidewalks and roadway barriers, such as chains and fences, designed to physically separate pedestrians from vehicles (39);
- mandatory use of safety belts and child safety seats. Where this is not feasible because of a large number of vehicles without functional safety belts, governments should ban importation of vehicles without such belts;

- use of helmets by riders on non-motorized and motorized cycles. Numerous studies have shown that helmets are effective in reducing head injuries in many settings.

Poisoning

Measures to prevent poisoning among children include:

- use of childproof caps for pesticide, medicine and fuel containers;
- establishment of poison control centres;
- community-based prevention education programmes to change storage habits in the home and improve knowledge of first aid.

Drowning

Measures to prevent drowning among children include:

- fencing and barriers around open bodies of water, and covers on wells;
- education about risks of drowning and need for closer supervision;
- training in resuscitation.

Burns

Measures to prevent burns among children include:

- raising or enclosing cooking areas;
- introduction of an electricity supply to reduce dependence on candles and kerosene;
- safe stove design;
- improved house construction;
- installation of smoke detectors and sprinkler systems;
- education about first aid for burns;
- regulation of water temperature;
- use of flame-retardant fabrics.

Falls

Measures to prevent falls by children include:

- installation of fences, roof rails, stair rails, stair gates, window bars, well covers, and window guards;
- improved recreational space for children with safe equipment and surroundings.

In addition, there are some other simple, cost-effective prevention strategies to consider:

- development of national policies on injury prevention to advocate greater resources;
- systematic surveillance for injuries;
- education for community members in first aid;
- coordinated emergency services;
- improved enforcement of existing laws.

References

1. *Global burden of disease 2000 database, Version 1.* Geneva, World Health Organization, 2001.
2. Baker SP, O'Neill B, Karpf RS. *The injury fact book.* Lexington, MA, Lexington Books, 1984.
3. National Center for Injury Prevention and Control, Centers for Disease Control and Prevention. *WISQARS leading causes of death reports, 1999–2000* (http://webapp.cdc.gov/sasweb/ncipc/leadcaus10.html).
4. Parkkari J et al. Childhood deaths and injuries in Finland in 1971–1995. *International Journal of Epidemiology*, 2000, 29:516–523.
5. Kidsafe, The Child Accident Prevention Foundation of Australia. *10 key facts about child injury in Australia* (http://www.kidsafe.com.au/tenfacts.pdf).
6. UNICEF. *A league table of child deaths by injury in rich nations.* Florence, UNICEF Innocenti Research Centre, 2001 (Innocenti Report Card No. 2).
7. Ahmed MK, Rahman M, van Ginneken J. Epidemiology of child deaths due to drowning in Matlab, Bangladesh. *International Journal of Epidemiology*, 1999, 28:306–311.
8. Soori H, Naghavi M. Childhood deaths from unintentional injuries in rural areas of Iran. *Injury Prevention*, 1998, 4:222–224.
9. Janson S et al. Accident risks for suburban pre-school Jordanian children. *Journal of Tropical Pediatrics*, 1994, 40:88–93.
10. Sethi D et al. High childhood mortality from injuries in transition countries: action is needed. *Eurohealth*, 2000, 6:47–50.
11. McKee M, Oreskovic S. Childhood injury: call for action. *Croatian Medical Journal*, 2002, 43:375–378.
12. *Deaths and injuries due to accidents and violence in the Netherlands 1998–1999.* Amsterdam, Consumer Safety Institute, 2000.
13. Bartlett SN. The problem of children's injuries in low-income countries: a review. *Health Policy and Planning*, 2002, 17:1–13.
14. *Priorities for child safety in the European Union: agenda for action.* Amsterdam, European Child Safety Alliance, 2001.
15. Ruangkanchanasetr S et al. Epidemiology and risk factors of injury in Thai children. *Southeast Asian Journal of Tropical Medicine and Public Health*, 1991, 22:127–132.
16. Child Accident Prevention Foundation of Southern Africa (Childsafe). (www.altonsa.co.za/childsafe).
17. Taft C et al. *Childhood unintentional injury worldwide: meeting the challenge.* Washington, DC, Safe Kids Worldwide, 2002.

18. Peden M, McGee K, Sharma G. *The injury chartbook: a graphical overview of the global burden of injuries.* Geneva, World Health Organization, 2002.

19. Kobusingye O, Guwatudde D, Lett R. Injury patterns in rural and urban Uganda. *Injury Prevention,* 2001, 7:46–50.

20. Bose A, George K, Joseph A. Drowning in childhood: a population based study. *Indian Pediatrics,* 2000, 37:80–83.

21. Celis A. Home drowning among preschool age Mexican children. *Injury Prevention,* 1997, 3:252–256.

22. del Ciampo LA et al. Incidence of childhood accidents determined in a study based on home surveys. *Annals of Tropical Paediatrics,* 2001, 21:239–243.

23. Laing GL, Logan S. Patterns of unintentional injury in childhood and their relation to socio-economic factors. *Public Health,* 1999, 113:291–294.

24. Kypri K et al. Child injury morbidity in New Zealand, 1987–1996. *Journal of Paediatrics and Child Health,* 2001, 37:227–234.

25. Bang RL. Burn mortality during 1982 to 1997 in Kuwait. *European Journal of Epidemiology,* 2000, 16:731–739.

26. Bener A, Al-Salman KM, Pugh RNH. Injury mortality and morbidity among children in the United Arab Emirates. *European Journal of Epidemiology,* 1998, 14:175–178.

27. Calder F. Four years of burn injuries in a Red Cross hospital in Afghanistan. *Burns,* 2002, 28:563–568.

28. Tagwireyi D, Ball DE, Nhachi CFB. Poisoning in Zimbabwe: a survey of eight major referral hospitals. *Journal of Applied Toxicology,* 2002, 22:99–105.

29. Izuora GI, Adeoye A. A seven-year review of accidental poisoning in children at a military hospital in Hafr Al Batin, Saudi Arabia. *Annals of Saudi Medicine,* 2001, 21:13–15.

30. McCraig LF, Burt CW. Poisoning-related visits to emergency departments in the United States, 1993–1996. *Journal of Toxicology—Clinical Toxicology,* 1999, 7:817–826.

31. Krug EG, Sharma GK, Lozano R. The global burden of injuries. *American Journal of Public Health,* 2000, 90:523–526.

32. Barss P et al. *Injury prevention: an international perspective. Epidemiology, surveillance and policy.* New York, Oxford University Press, 1998.

33. Global Urban Observatory and Statistics Unit, UN Human Settlements Programme. *Human settlements conditions and trends* (http://www.unhabitat.org/habrdd/introduction/html).

34. Sethi D, Zwi A. Challenges of drowning prevention in low- and middle-income countries. *Injury prevention,* 1998, 4:162.

35. Christoffel T, Gallagher SS. *Injury prevention and public health: practical knowledge, skills, and strategies.* Gaithersburg, MD, Aspen Publishers, Inc., 1999.

36. Fukunishi K et al. Epidemiology of childhood burns in the Critical Care Medical Center of Kinki University Hospital in Osaka, Japan. *Burns,* 2000, 26:465–469.

37. den Hertog PC, Blankendaal FACM, ten Hag SM. Burn injuries in the Netherlands. *Accident Analysis and Prevention*, 2000, 32:355–364.

38. *Priorities for EU motor vehicle safety design.* Brussels, European Transport Safety Council, 2001.

39. Forjuoh SN, Li G. A review of successful transport and home injury interventions to guide developing countries. *Social Science and Medicine*, 1996, 43:1551–1560.

CHAPTER 14

Ionizing radiation

L. Kheifets
M. Repacholi
Department for the Protection of the Human Environment,
Radiation and Environmental Health, World Health
Organization, Geneva, Switzerland

Introduction

Ionizing radiation is a known carcinogen to which children are particularly vulnerable. Relevant exposures include pre- and postnatal irradiation for medical reasons, radon in the home, and accidental radiation releases. In some cases, children may receive higher doses than adults because of higher intake and accumulation. Furthermore, sensitivity to radiation is highest early in life (1). Although the mechanism of greater susceptibility is not well understood, it is likely to be linked to greater cell division in growing and developing tissues. In addition, a longer expected lifetime, with a resultant increased chance of repeated exposure and accumulated damage, also leads to higher cancer risk for children. Fetuses might be particularly sensitive to ionizing radiation, since their tissue cells are not only undergoing high rates of division, but are also differentiating into mature functional cells.

Sources and exposures

All life on earth has evolved with continuous exposure to natural radiation, which was far higher in prehistoric times. Natural radiation is the major source of human radiation exposure and comes from external sources and from radionuclides accumulated within the body. External sources include cosmic radiation from remote parts of the universe and the sun, and terrestrial radiation from the ground and from building materials. Radionuclides are introduced into the body through food, water and air. In general, the highest exposure is to radon, a radioactive gas produced from the decay of uranium and radium in the earth's crust. The fact that radon is a gas means that it can diffuse into water or through soil into homes and buildings.

In addition to natural radiation, most individuals are exposed to man-made radiation. The largest source of man-made radiation is medical irradiation, which includes diagnostic X-rays and other imaging techniques. Radiation is also used therapeutically to treat cancer and, historically, enlarged tonsils, adenoids or thymus, as well as some viral and fungus infections (notably tinea capitis or infection of the scalp). Medical radiation, when used judiciously, offers enormous direct benefits to patients. Other sources of radiation include consumer products (e.g. televisions, fertilizers), nuclear weapons tests, the production of nuclear power, and the disposal of nuclear and other radioactive waste.

In terms of human exposure, the dose and risk depend on many factors. Exposure can be external or internal, for example through intake of radionuclides from air or food. The intensity of cosmic radiation depends on the altitude. The dose in the mountains is more than twice that at sea level. Still higher doses are found at altitudes used by aircraft, particularly for intercontinental flights. The level of terrestrial radiation depends on the composition of the soil and the use of certain building materials (e.g. granite). Unusually high exposures from terrestrial radiation have been reported in some areas of Brazil, India, the Islamic Republic of Iran and Kenya.

Concentrations of radon in soil exhibit a large geographical variability. In addition, the concentration of radon in buildings will depend on the amount of ventilation, with high concentrations in poorly ventilated areas, such as the basement, especially in winter, when windows are kept closed. Children may also receive relatively high doses in households that use groundwater wells with high concentrations of radon in the water.

The level of exposure to medical radiation, especially for diagnostic purposes, depends on accepted practice and varies from country to country. Procedures are checked periodically to ensure that the optimum dose is used. In addition to the frequency of use of various procedures, the doses received will depend on the equipment used. It should be noted, however, that use of medical procedures involving radiation in children is relatively rare. On the other hand, children might have a higher uptake and accumulation of radioactive isotopes (e.g. iodine 131 in the thyroid).

Types of radiation and biological effects

Ionizing radiation produces charged particles (ions) in the materials or tissues in which it is absorbed. When this happens in molecules of biological importance, it may lead to recognizable damage. There are various types of ionizing radiation: alpha, beta and gamma radiation, X-rays and neutrons. Their effects vary, but all can be damaging. Cellular damage from ionizing radiation depends on the type of radiation, the deposition rate, and the distribution through the tissue. Biological effects also depend on the radiosensitivity of the tissue exposed.

Two kinds of effects of radiation on tissues are observed. *Deterministic effects* occur when a large number of cells have been damaged, stem cells have lost their capacity to divide, or tissue structure or function is affected. These effects occur at doses above a threshold, with the probability of occurrence and the severity of effects increasing sharply above this threshold. To the extent that the organism is able to compensate for the loss of cells, the harm may be temporary. Examples of deterministic effects are nausea, diarrhoea, skin damage and cataracts.

Stochastic effects occur when cells are not killed, but are modified. Some of the changes may persist in daughter cells. Examples of stochastic effects are cancer and hereditary diseases in children or subsequent descendants of individuals who have been exposed to radiation, especially if the genital organs were exposed. Ionizing radiation is a complete carcinogen since it can act to initiate, promote and progress cellular changes that lead to cancer. The dose of radiation received by an individual affects the probability of cancer, but not its aggressiveness. Radiation-induced cancer is indistinguishable from cancer from other causes. The probabilistic nature of this risk means that children have more time to accumulate exposures and damage, and more time after exposure to develop the disease.

Health effects

With increasing dose, the severity of acute effects increases from transient pathological changes to immediate death (Table 14.1).

Much of the available evidence about the effects of ionizing radiation on human populations stems from the experiences of the survivors of the atomic bombs exploded over Hiroshima and Nagasaki in 1945 (the Life Span Study or LSS (3)), from follow-up of patients exposed to radiation for diagnostic or therapeutic reasons, and from the radiation accident that occurred in 1986 at the Chernobyl nuclear power plant in the Ukraine.

LSS includes a cohort of 85 000 survivors who received total body exposure and for whom individual estimates of radiation exposure have been calculated. This population, of all ages and both sexes, has been carefully followed up for

Table 14.1   Effects of whole body exposure to ionizing radiation

WHOLE BODY DOSE (Gy)	SYMPTOMS	SURVIVAL TIME
20	Damage to the central nervous system	Death within a few hours to a few days
8–20	Damage to the gut	Death after about two weeks
3.5	Bone marrow damage	50% of patients will survive; the rest will die in 1–2 months
0.5–3	Bone marrow damage causing transient reduction in the number of blood cells	All survive; stochastic effects, some resulting in death, may occur later in life
Under 0.5	Stochastic effects may occur later in life	All survive; stochastic effects, some resulting in death, may occur later in life

Source: ref. 2.

many years since 1950. Available data include results of numerous clinical tests, as well as a comprehensive monitoring of both cancer development and mortality. Large numbers, relatively good dose information encompassing a wide range of exposure and a broad demographic composition make this study the most important source of information on radiation risk. Of particular relevance here are two groups: children who were under 10 years of age at the time of the explosions (approximately 5% of the cohort) and 1630 people who were exposed to the bombing *in utero*.

Numerous studies of radiotherapy and diagnostic irradiation have been conducted. The most relevant findings from these studies for particular cancers are presented below. Overall the studies were limited in terms of their size, the sex and age distribution of the study populations, and the organs irradiated. Nevertheless, they provide important information complementary to the LSS study because they cover many different countries, represent a broad range of doses (high for radiation therapy and low for diagnostic procedures), and encompass various types of ionizing radiation. They are particularly valuable in providing additional information of risks for particular cancers and for particular ages.

As a result of the explosion at the Chernobyl nuclear power plant, large areas of Belarus, the Russian Federation and Ukraine were contaminated. As a result millions of people were exposed to low levels of radiation over an extended time period. Several studies of residents of the contaminated area, their offspring and clean-up workers are currently under way. Most of the information is limited by lack of reliable individual doses and difficulties in conducting studies because of population resettlement, changes in food supply, and restrictions on the activities of individuals and families. The break-up of the Soviet Union exacerbated these difficulties, through differences in registration criteria, follow-up mechanisms, dose-reconstruction methods and compensation laws. WHO established the International Programme on the Health Effects of the Chernobyl Accident (IPHECA) to support national programmes, monitor health consequences and indicate future work needed to ensure that maximum information is gained from this disaster (4).

Cancer

Epidemiological studies have shown that exposure to high levels of ionizing radiation leads to an increased risk of cancer. Exposure in childhood, in particular, increases risk of leukaemia, and breast and thyroid cancer. Age dependence for these cancers, which are among the diseases most readily induced by radiation, is complex, and generally tracks changes in background rates, i.e. increase in the risk due to radiation is proportional to the overall increase in cancer risk due to ageing.

The radiation exposure from a single diagnostic procedure is usually small. However, many people undergo radiological examinations, some of them rather frequently, making these procedures the highest man-made source of radiation exposure. Because of the increased lifetime risk per unit dose for children, the potentially higher doses, and the increasing frequency of paediatric computerized tomography (CT) examinations, diagnostic procedures that use radiation can lead to a small, but non-negligible, increase in risk of cancer (5). While these procedures are undisputedly beneficial, the magnitude of exposure of children can often be reduced without significant loss of information.

Leukaemia

Studies of survivors of atomic bomb explosions showed an increased risk in both incidence of leukaemia and associated mortality. Furthermore, the risk of leukaemia from radiation is higher than for other risk factors and occurs earlier than for solid cancers. Leukaemia risk is best described by non-linear fit; risk is higher for exposures that occur in childhood, but tends to begin to decrease 10–15 years after exposure (6). Most of the studies of radiotherapy and diagnostic irradiation confirm an increase in leukaemia risk at high doses.

The observed association between childhood leukaemia and *in utero* exposure to diagnostic X-rays has been interpreted as providing further support for the etiological role of ionizing radiation, despite methodological limitations of some of the studies.

Breast cancer

Breast cancer risk was associated with radiation exposure in the LSS cohort and among several medically exposed groups. The risk increases with dose linearly and is particularly high for those exposed at young ages. The risk of breast cancer was increased in women who were under 10 years of age at the time of the atomic bomb explosion—a time when girls have little or no breast tissue. Women who developed early-onset breast cancer might have been genetically susceptible to radiation (7). On the basis of these findings, it is recommended that breasts should be shielded when possible during diagnostic or therapeutic radiation (8).

Thyroid cancer

Thyroid gland tissue is highly susceptible to radiation during childhood. In the LSS cohort a significant association was found between radiation dose and risk of thyroid cancer for those exposed before 19 years of age. Irradiation in childhood for benign conditions, as well as therapeutic exposure, can increase the risk of thyroid cancer. Risk is highest for children and decreases with increased age at exposure. The excess risk can be observed for many years after exposure and is highest 15–30 years after exposure (6). The most dramatic finding after the Chernobyl incident was a large increase in thyroid cancers in children. Some 2000 children have now been diagnosed with thyroid cancer, and in some locations where contamination was highest, as in the Gomel region, the incidence of this cancer increased over 100-fold.

Brain cancer

Ionizing radiation is related to brain tumours, although the relationship is weaker than for the cancers described above. Most brain tumours associated with ionizing radiation are benign, but an increase in malignant brain tumours has been observed in patients who received radiotherapy. The evidence is strongest for those exposed before age 20 years (9).

Mental retardation

Fetal exposure to radiation has been associated with severe mental retardation in the LSS study. A dose-dependent relationship with reduced head circumference was reported (10). The risk depended on gestational age, and was most severe at 8–15 weeks.

As a result, it is recommended that, because of the potentially high exposure of the head of an infant during CT scans (around 100 mGy), frequent radiological examinations over short periods should be avoided, particularly when other imaging techniques are available.

Indoor radon

The evidence of carcinogenicity of radon comes largely from studies of lung cancer in uranium miners. The risk of lung cancer from radon is much higher for smokers. Ecological and analytical studies carried out in several countries have not provided any evidence of an association between indoor radon and childhood cancer risk (11). Although indoor radon exposure has been postulated to cause leukaemia, recent evidence does not support such an association (12).

References

1. *Ionizing radiation, Part 1: X- and gamma-radiation, and neutrons*. Lyon, International Agency for Research on Cancer, 2000 (IARC Monographs on the Evaluation of the Carcinogenic Risk to Humans, Volume 75).
2. *Diagnosis and treatment of radiation injuries*. Vienna, International Atomic Energy Agency, 1998 (Safety Reports Series No. 2).
3. Radiation Effects Research Foundation. *Life Span Study reports*. (www.rerf.or.jp/eigo/titles/lsstitle.htm).
4. WHO. *Children affected by the Chernobyl accident*. Geneva, World Health Organization (www.who.int/ionizing_radiation/research/children/en/index.html).
5. Brenner DJ et al. Estimated risks of radiation-induced fatal cancer from pediatric CT. *American Journal of Roentgenology*, 2001, 176:289–296.
6. United Nations Scientific Committee on the Effects of Atomic Radiation. *Report to the General Assembly, United Nations, New York, Volume II: Effects*. New York, United Nations, 2000.
7. Land CE. Early-onset breast cancer in A-bomb survivors. *Lancet*, 1993, 342: 237.

8. American Academy of Pediatrics. Risk of ionizing radiation exposure to children: a subject review. *Pediatrics*, 1998, 101:717–719.

9. Tilyou SM. NRC issues interim rule on medical use of radionuclides. *Journal of Nuclear Medicine*, 1990, 31:20A–21A.

10. Lee S, Otake M, Schull WJ. Changes in the pattern of growth in stature related to prenatal exposure to ionizing radiation. *International Radiation Biology*, 1999, 75:1449–1458.

11. Little J. *Epidemiology of childhood cancer*. Lyon, International Agency for Research on Cancer, 1999 (IARC Scientific Publications No. 149).

12. Kiriou JC et al. A comparison of doses and techniques between specialist and non-specialist centers in the diagnostic X-ray imaging of children. *British Journal of Radiology*, 1996, 69:437–450.

CHAPTER 15

Noise[1]

C. F. Bearer
Departments of Pediatrics and Neurosciences, Case Western Reserve University; Division of Neonatology, Mary Anne Sears Swetland Environmental Health Center, Rainbow Babies and Children's Hospital, Cleveland, OH, USA

What is noise?

Noise is undesirable sound. Sound is vibration in a medium, usually air. It has frequency (pitch), intensity (loudness), periodicity, and duration.

The frequency of sound is measured in cycles per second or hertz (Hz): 1 Hz = 1 cycle per second. People can hear frequencies ranging from 20 to 20 000 Hz, but are most sensitive to sounds in the range of 500 to 3000 Hz, the band that includes human speech.

The loudness of sound is measured in terms of pascals (Pa) or decibels (dB). One Pa is 1×10^5 standard atmospheres of pressure. The sound limits of human hearing are 0.00002 Pa (the weakest sound that a keen human adult ear can detect under quiet conditions) to 200 Pa (the pressure that causes pain in the adult ear). The decibel expresses the energy of a sound in comparison with a reference sound, usually 0.00002 Pa. The dB SPL (sound pressure level) of one sound (p1) is therefore: $20 \log_{10}(p1/p2)$ where p2 is 0.00002 Pa. Noise in a quiet room may be 40 dB, while a pneumatic drill may produce 130 dB. Human speech is approximately 50 dB SPL. The perceived loudness of sound varies with the frequency. For example, to match the perceived loudness of a 1000 Hz 40 dB SPL tone requires over 80 dB SPL at 50 Hz and over 60 dB SPL at 10 000 Hz. The 40 dB SPL equivalency curve is used to determine the sound intensity, referred to as the decibel weighted by the A scale, or dBA.

Periodicity refers to either continuous sound or impulse sound.

Routes of exposure

Sound waves enter the ear through the external auditory canal and vibrate the ear drum. This vibration travels through the three ossicles of the middle ear (the malleus, incus and stapes), to the oval window, causing the fluid of the inner ear, the cochlea, to vibrate. Within the cochlea, the basilar membrane covers the organ of Corti which is composed of the hair cells. Each hair cell

---

[1]Based on the Handbook of Pediatric Environmental Health of the American Academy of Pediatrics.

responds to a specific frequency and converts this signal to a nerve impulse. The impulses travel up the auditory nerve to be interpreted as sound by the brain. Loss of hearing originating in the external auditory canal, ear drum, ossicles or middle ear is called conductive hearing loss and is usually treatable. Loss of hearing originating in the cochlea or auditory nerve is called sensorineural hearing loss and is usually permanent.

Sound vibration may also be transmitted to the body directly through the skin as vibration, but this will not be discussed here.

Systems affected

Noise-induced hearing loss

Although noise pollution receives little public attention, there is evidence that current environmental levels of noise are damaging our hearing. A study on deafness among college students conducted in 1990 could find no students unexposed to loud music to serve as controls (1). Among the controls who had low exposure, noticeable hearing loss was found. Statistics from the University of Washington Occupational Medicine Clinic in Seattle show that nearly 10% of the 1424 persons evaluated between 1982 and 1987 showed noise-induced hearing loss (NIHL). Approximately 50% of these people had been exposed to hazardous noise at work. Susceptibility to NIHL is highly variable; while some individuals are able to tolerate high noise levels for prolonged periods of time, others in the same conditions will rapidly lose hearing. NIHL results from trauma to the hair cells of the cochlea. Prolonged exposure to sounds louder than 85 dBA is potentially injurious. Continuous exposure to hazardous levels of noise tends to have its maximum effect in the high-frequency regions of the cochlea. NIHL is usually most severe around 4000 Hz with downward extension toward speech frequencies with prolonged exposure. This pattern of loss of frequency perception is true regardless of the pitch of the noise exposure. Impulse noise is more harmful than continuous noise since it bypasses the body's natural protective reaction, the dampening of the ossicles mediated by the facial nerve.

Exposure to loud noise may result in a temporary decrease in sensitivity of hearing and tinnitus. This condition, called temporary threshold shift (TTS), lasts for several hours depending on the degree of exposure.

Physiological effects

Noise causes a stress response. The hypothalamic–pituitary–adrenal axis is sensitive to noise intensities as low as 65 dBA, resulting in a 53% increase in plasma 17-OH-corticosteroid levels. Increased excretion of adrenaline and noradrenaline has been demonstrated in humans exposed to noise at 90 dBA for 30 minutes.

Noise contributes to sleep deprivation. Noise at 40–45 dBA results in a 10–20% increase in awakening or EEG arousal changes. Noise at 50 dBA results in a 25% probability of arousal features on EEG.

Noise has undesirable cardiovascular effects. Exposure to noise greater than 70 dBA increases vasoconstriction, heart rate and blood pressure. A case of persistent ventricular fibrillation upon arousal from sleep by noise has been reported (2).

Psychological effects

Exposure to moderate levels of noise can cause psychological stress. Annoyance, inability to concentrate and symptoms such as headaches, tiredness and irritability are common psychological reactions to noise. The degree of annoyance is related to the nature of the sound. Intense noise can cause personality changes and a reduced capacity to cope. Sudden and unexpected noise can cause a startle reaction which may provoke physiological stress responses.

Work performance may be affected. At low levels, noise can improve performance of simple tasks. However, noise may impair complex intellectual functions and performance of complex tasks.

Paediatric exposures

Little work has been done to estimate children's exposure to noise. Available data suggest that children are routinely exposed to more noise than the 24-hour equivalent noise exposures (Leq24) of 70 dbA recommended as an upper limit by the United States Environmental Protection Agency (EPA) in 1974 (3, 4). A longitudinal study of hearing in suburban and rural Ohio children aged 6–18 years found that Leq24s varied from 77 to 84 db, and were higher for boys than girls (5).

Developmental sensitivity

There is little evidence to suggest that the organs of hearing are more sensitive to NIHL in children than adults. Children are at increased risk of exposure to noise for behavioural reasons: infants cannot remove themselves from noise, and cannot communicate if they cannot hear adult speech. Older children may play with firecrackers or cap pistols, while teenagers may listen to loud rock music.

Clinical effects

There is evidence to suggest that: (1) exposure to excessive noise *in utero* may result in high-frequency hearing loss in the newborn, and may be associated with prematurity and intrauterine growth retardation; (2) exposure to noise in the NICU may result in cochlear damage, and (3) incorporation of individualized environmental care (including reduction of noise) in the management of premature infants decreases the time they spend on the ventilator, and appears to allow more normal maturity of the central nervous system as measured by quantitative EEG (6, 7). Very few studies have been done on the clinical effects of noise on children.

NIHL

A longitudinal study of hearing was conducted in suburban and rural Ohio children aged 6–18 years. While there was no clear relationship between noise exposure and hearing loss, the hearing loss that was evident was greater at higher frequencies than lower ones, and sex differences in hearing acuity became greater with age; both observations are consistent with a developing noise-induced hearing loss (5). Auditory screening of 3322 children attending schools within 2 miles of Logan Airport in Boston, Massachusetts (USA), was conducted, and follow-up examinations performed to permit classification of the type of hearing loss (8). Children living directly under the flight paths or immediately adjacent to runways did not have a higher incidence of bilateral sensorineural or mixed hearing loss than the sample average. Hearing acuity among children without diagnosis of hearing loss was unrelated to distance from the flight path or duration of residence.

Physiological effects

A stress response consisting of acute terror and panic has been described in children exposed to sonic booms in Labrador, Canada (9), and in Germany. Biochemical evidence of the stress response was found in elevated urinary cortisol levels. Hypertension accompanied a 30-minute exposure to 100 dBA in 60 children aged 11–16 years.

School performance

In a comparison of schoolchildren aged 8–10 years living in lower or upper floors of a 32-floor apartment building, reading achievement and auditory discrimination were poorer among those living in lower-floor apartments where noise levels from adjacent highways were higher (10). The range of noise levels was not large: the interior apartment noise levels varied from 55 to 66 dBA. Reading performance is negatively affected by noise either in the classroom or in the home. Bronzaft & McCarthy (11) showed that children aged 6, 8, and 10 in classrooms on the side of the school building adjacent to elevated trains had poorer reading performance than children from the quieter side of the same building. Classroom noise varied from 59 dBA when trains were not passing, to 89 dBA when they were. Aircraft noise was inversely related to the percentage of children whose reading ability was below average in a study of children in New York City (12). In a study of children in 15 schools in California, reading level was inversely related to freeway noise (13).

Effects on parenting

There is a growing body of evidence that noise and crowding adversely affect the interactions of carers with infants and toddlers (14–16). Parents in noisy environments were less likely to be highly involved in their child's activities, and less likely to be verbally responsive to their child.

Diagnosis

The typical finding in noise-induced hearing loss is a dip in hearing thresh-old around 4000 Hz on an audiogram. Health care providers who lack the capacity to perform pure tone audiograms should refer their patients for evaluation. Audiological evaluation, including pure tone audiometry, should be performed for noise-induced hearing loss on any child with a history of:

- *in utero* exposure to excessive noise because of maternal occupation or recreational activities;
- playing with cap pistols or other loud "impulse" toys;
- an occupation with excessive noise exposure;
- poor school performance;
- short attention span;
- complaints of ringing in the ears, a feeling of fullness in the ears, muf-fling of hearing, or difficulty in understanding speech.

Adolescents should be screened yearly because of their propensity to listen to loud music.

The American Academy of Pediatrics (AAP) currently recommends objective hearing screening for high-risk newborns (*17, 18*) and at 4, 5, 12 and 18 years of age (*19*).

Treatment of clinical symptoms

There is no treatment for permanent noise-induced hearing loss.

Prevention of exposure

Questions about noise exposure should be part of routine health visits. Parents should be encouraged to reduce the noise exposure of their children by:

1. avoiding loud noises, especially loud impulse noise, whenever possible;
2. avoiding loud toys, especially cap pistols and firecrackers;
3. turning off televisions, computers, and radios when not in use;
4. reducing the volume of televisions, computers, and radios; a good rule of thumb is that volume levels should be such that one does not need to raise one's voice during normal conversation;
5. creating a "stimulus haven", the quietest room in the house for play and interactions with infants and toddlers.

When reducing noise is impossible, hearing protectors should be worn. There are two types, ear plugs and ear muffs. Ear plugs should fit properly; they should require a slight tug to remove them. Ear muffs are the most effective type of ear protector available. They have cups lined with sound-absorbing material that are held against the skull with a spring band or oil-filled ring that provides a tight seal.

Unfortunately, environmental noise is often not under the control of the hearer, which makes noise reduction and hearing protection difficult. Government regulations are needed to protect parents and children. The standard for the workplace is no more than 8 hours of exposure to 90 dBA, 4 hours to 95 dBA, 2 hours to 100 dBA, with no exposure allowed to continuous noise above 115 dBA or impulse noise above 140 dBA. In other settings, environmental noise is expressed as a day-night average sound level (DNL). For the protection of public health, the US Environmental Protection Agency proposed a DNL of 55 dB during waking hours and 45 dB during sleeping hours in neighbourhoods, and 45 dB during the day and 35 dB at night in hospitals.

Table 15.1 lists some common environmental noises and their potential effects.

Table 15.1   Decibel ranges and effects of common sounds

EXAMPLE	SOUND PRESSURE (dBA)	EFFECT OF EXPOSURE
Breathing	0–10	Threshold of hearing
Whisper, rustling leaves	20	Very quiet
Quiet rural area at night	30	
Library, soft background music	40	
Quiet suburb (daytime), conversation in living room	50	Quiet
Conversation in restaurant, average office, background music, chirping bird	60	Intrusive
Freeway traffic at 15 m, vacuum cleaner, noisy office or party, television	70	Annoying
Garbage disposal, washing machine, average factory, freight train at 15 m, dishwasher, arcade games	80	Possible hearing damage
Busy urban street, diesel truck, food blender	90	Hearing damage (8 hr exposure), speech interference
Jet take-off (305 m away), subway, outboard motor, power lawn mower, motorcycle at 8 m, farm tractor, printing plant, jackhammer, garbage truck	100	
Steel mill, riveting, automobile horn at 1 m, boombox stereo held close to ear	110	
Thunderclap, textile loom, live rock music, jet take-off (161 m away), siren, chain saw, boom stereo in cars	120	Human pain threshold

Table 15.1   *continued*

EXAMPLE	SOUND PRESSURE (dBA)	EFFECT OF EXPOSURE
Armoured personnel carrier, jet take-off (100 m away), earphones at loud level	130	
Aircraft carrier deck	140	
Jet take-off (25 m away), toy cap pistol, firecracker	150	Eardrum rupture

References

1. West PD, Evans EF. Early detection of hearing damage in young listeners resulting from exposure to amplified music. *British Journal of Audiology*, 1990, 24:89–103.
2. Kam PC, Kam AC, Thompson JF. Noise pollution in the anaesthetic and intensive care environment. *Anaesthesia*, 1994, 49:982–986.
3. DeJoy DM. Environmental noise and children: review of recent findings. *Journal of Auditory Research*, 1983, 23:181–194.
4. Von Gierke H. Noise: how much is too much? *Noise Control Engineering Journal*, 1975, 5:29–34.
5. Roche AF, Chumlea WC, Siervogel RM. Longitudinal study of human hearing: its relationship to noise and other factors. III. Results from the first five years. Aerospace Medical Research Laboratory, 1982 (Report no. AFAMRL-TR-82-68).
6. Als H et al. Individualized behavioral and environmental care for the very low birth weight preterm infant at high risk for bronchopulmonary dysplasia: neonatal intensive care unit and developmental outcome. *Pediatrics*, 1986, 78:1123–1132.
7. Buehler DM et al. Effectiveness of individualized developmental care for low-risk preterm infants: behavioral and electrophysiologic evidence. *Pediatrics*, 1995, 96:923–932.
8. Andrus WS, Kerrigan ME, Bird KT. Hearing in para-airport children. *American Space and Environmental Medicine*, 1975, 46:740–742.
9. Rosenberg J. Jets over Labrador and Quebec: noise effects on human health. *Canadian Medical Association Journal*, 1991, 144:869–875.
10. Cohen S, Glass DC, Singer JE. Apartment noise, auditory discrimination, and reading ability in children. *Journal of Experimental Social Psychology*, 1973, 9:407–422.
11. Bronzaft AI, McCarthy DP. The effect of elevated train noise on reading ability. *Environment and Behaviour*, 1975, 7:517–528.
12. Green KB, Pasternack BS, Shore RE. Effects of aircraft noise on reading ability of school-age children. *Archives of Environmental Health*, 1982, 37:24–31.
13. Lukas JS, Dupree RB, Swing JW. Effects of noise on academic achievement and classroom behavior. Office of Noise Control California Department of Health Services, 1981 (Report no. FHWA/CA./DOHS-81/01).

14. Wachs TD, Chan A. Specificity of environmental action as seen in physical and social environment correlates of three aspects of twelve month infants' communication performance. *Child Development*, 1986, 57:1464–1475.

15. Wachs TD, Camli O. Do ecological or individual characteristics mediate the influence of the physical environment upon maternal behavior. *Journal of Environmental Psychology*, 1991, 11:249–264.

16. Wachs TD. Nature of relations between the physical and social microenvironment of the two-year-old child. *Early Development and Parenting*, 1993, 2:81–87.

17. American Academy of Pediatrics, Joint Committee on Infant Hearing. Joint Committee on Infant Hearing 1990 Position Statement. *AAP News*, 1991, 7.

18. American Academy of Pediatrics, Committee on Environmental Health. Noise: a hazard to the fetus and newborn. *Pediatrics*, 1997, 100:724–727.

19. American Academy of Pediatrics, Committee on Psychosocial Aspects of Child and Family Health. *Guidelines for health supervision*, 2nd ed. American Academy of Pediatrics, 1988.

CHAPTER 16

Global environmental change and child health[1,2]

A. J. McMichael
National Centre for Epidemiology and Population Health,
The Australian National University, Canberra, Australia

S. Bunyavanich
Department of Medicine, Massachusetts General Hospital,
Harvard Medical School, Boston, MA, USA

P. R. Epstein
Center for Health and the Global Environment, Harvard
Medical School, Boston, MA, USA

Introduction

The distinctive aspect of global environmental change is its scale. For the first time, humankind is exerting sufficient pressure on the earth's biophysical systems to cause changes in some environmental processes and conditions at the global level. Several such environmental changes have now been confirmed, in particular stratospheric ozone depletion and climate change. There is also a human-induced global change in the elemental cycles of nitrogen, sulfur and potassium. Various other environmental changes are now occurring worldwide, in rather more mosaic fashion. These include depletion of fresh water, degradation of agroecosystems, depletion of fisheries, and the dissemination of persistent organic pollutants (POPs).

These large-scale environmental changes do not necessarily pose qualitatively new risks to health. Rather, they amplify and extend the health risks posed by many existing environmental hazards. These include extreme weather events, thermal stress, food and water shortages, toxic POPs, and increased ultraviolet radiation at middle to high latitudes. More important risks to health will probably come from the disruption of ecological processes or systems. For example, changes in land use, climatic conditions and surface water distribution will influence the geographical range and density of disease vectors, such as mosquitoes, ticks and water-snails. Likewise, many of these environmental changes will

---

[1] Reviewed by **D. Schwela**, Physical and Chemical Exposure Unit, Institute for Health and Consumer Protection, Joint Research Centre, Ispra, Italy.
[2] Some of the material in this chapter is adapted from Bunyavanich S, Landrigan CP, McMichael AJ, Epstein PR. The impact of climate change on child health. *Ambulatory Pediatrics*, 2003, 3:47–55.

affect crop production, fruit and vegetable production, and animal husbandry, with particular consequences for child nutrition and development.

A well-known example of these environmental changes is global climate change. This phenomenon results from the recent rapid increase in human-induced greenhouse gas emissions, altering the properties of the lower atmosphere, and thereby causing a change in world climate. This has widespread consequences for human health, and poses some particular risks to children's health.

There are three pathways by which global climate change may affect child health (1). These are via:

1. The immediate environmental consequences of the processes that cause climate change, such as burning of fossil fuels and forests. The toxic air pollutants produced can cause or exacerbate cough, asthma and some childhood respiratory infections, particularly within the urban environment.
2. The direct impact of altered climatic conditions. Heat waves may increase the incidence of heat stroke in children; a greater intensity and frequency of natural catastrophes related to weather will increase drowning, dehydration, gastrointestinal illness, and psychological trauma (e.g. from disruption of family and community social networks).
3. The indirect impacts caused by ecological disturbances. Malnutrition and childhood stunting will occur in food-insecure populations as a consequence of climatic effects on food production. Increased production of pollen and fungal spores may exacerbate allergies and asthma. Higher temperatures and increased flooding will tend to expand the geographic range of malaria, dengue, various types of encephalitis, and tick-borne diseases, leading to greater morbidity and, especially among children, mortality. Even more complex ecological disturbances underlie the increased risk of diseases such as hantavirus pulmonary syndrome, where, for example, drought followed by heavy rains disturb the balance between rodents and their predators, and increase human exposure to viruses excreted by rodents.

To date, there has been little empirical research specifically into the health impacts on children of global environmental changes (1). This may reflect the large spatial scale and rapid pace of environmental change, which mean that, as yet, there are few local, clear-cut, acute health impacts. Further, the mathematical modelling of the future health impact of climate change (and other global environmental changes) has, to date, not specifically addressed child health. Most such modelling has either encompassed the full age range or has been confined to adult health outcomes (e.g. heart attacks and strokes during heat waves). Further, there are well recognized limitations in the mathematical and statistical models that have been developed for this type of research, which is still in its early stages. The difficulties in modelling future processes include handling the various scientific uncertainties and the unavoidable demographic, economic, and technological contextual uncertainties about future human societies and behaviour.

In this chapter we focus on the impact of global climate change on child health, as an illustration of how global environmental changes in general can, or may in the future, affect children's health.

Global climate change and children's health

Human communities are accustomed to climatic conditions that vary on daily, seasonal and interannual time scales. The recent and growing concern over global climate change is caused by the accumulating evidence that the average climatic conditions, measured over extended time periods (conventionally 30 years or longer), are changing as a result of human activities that produce various greenhouse gases, especially carbon dioxide and methane.

Temperature records since the 1860s (see Figure 16.1) show that global warming has occurred, including a 0.6 °C increase in surface temperature during the twentieth century (2). The Intergovernmental Panel on Climate Change (IPCC) has concluded that most of the climate change observed since 1950 is due to human alteration of the lower atmosphere (troposphere), and that future climate change will have far-reaching effects on the environment and health. The IPCC predicts a rise in average world surface temperature of 1.4–5.8 °C by 2100 (2). The range of uncertainty in this prediction reflects both the scientific uncertainties and the societal and developmental uncertainties mentioned above.

Figure 16.1 Observed global average land and sea surface temperatures from 1860 to 2000

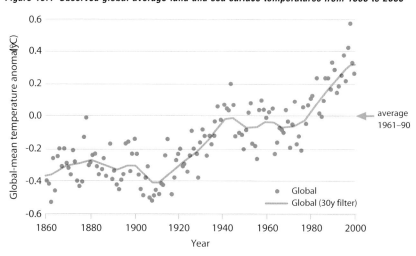

Source: Climatic Research Unit, Norwich, England.

SECTION III: SPECIFIC ENVIRONMENTAL THREATS

Such a rise in average world temperature would be faster than any since the inception of agriculture around 10 000 years ago. Predictions for precipitation and wind speed are less consistent, but also suggest significant changes. We should note also that climatologists are increasingly concerned that disruption of the climate system may exceed critical thresholds, causing abrupt rather than gradual climate change and an associated rapid shift in health effects (3, 4).

Over the past two decades, an increasing rate of changes in natural physical and biological processes, attributable to warmer temperatures, has been reported. For example, sea ice and glaciers have been diminishing in volume, bird nesting has begun earlier, and animal and insect migration patterns have changed. To date, however, there is relatively little empirical evidence of the impact of recent climatic trends on human health, and very little such evidence refers specifically to children.

Children may be an especially susceptible group, because of both their developing physiology and their anticipated lifelong exposure to altered climatic and environmental conditions. Worldwide, two-thirds of all preventable disease and premature death due to environmental concerns occurs in children (5). Global climate change will almost certainly increase the influence of environmental conditions and processes on health, especially in children.

The economic activities that cause increased emission of greenhouse gases, particularly fossil fuel combustion and the burning of forests and other vegetation, may also produce immediate local environmental hazards to health. The most obvious example is that of urban air pollution, comprising a mix of power-plant emissions, industrial smoke and gases, and traffic exhaust gases. The impact on child health of this mix of ambient air pollutants—including fine particulates, lead compounds, carbon monoxide, nitrogen oxides, sulfur oxides, and ozone—is described elsewhere in this volume. The following review focuses on the other two large-scale causal pathways, direct and indirect, that connect climate change to risks to health.

Direct health effects from altered climatic conditions
Thermal extremes: heat stroke

It is predicted that small changes in mean climate conditions will trigger relatively large changes in the frequency and severity of heat waves (2). Heat waves are therefore expected to increase in number and intensity in the future.

By extrapolation from many prior studies, any future increase in the frequency and severity of heat waves will increase the risks of death and serious illness. The very old, the very young and the sick are particularly vulnerable to thermal stress (4). Children are less able than adults to modify their local (usually domestic) climate, especially if a heat wave is sudden and severe. In children, heat stroke is the most serious outcome of central or peripheral impairment of body temperature regulation, and may result in death.

Weather disasters: drowning, dehydration, diarrhoeal disease, and psychological trauma

The hydrological cycle accelerates with global warming (6–10). As heat energy accumulates in the deep ocean, more water evaporates (2), causing increased intensity and frequency of precipitation. Evaporation from soil may also be increased, causing drought. Models indicate that there will be more heavy deluges, with flooding (11–13), and more frequent and longer droughts (14).

Extreme weather events such as heavy precipitation, severe storms, floods, droughts, and cyclones may have increased in frequency, duration, and intensity in some regions over the past century. An increase in the frequency of large floods over the twentieth century has recently been demonstrated (11), and several-fold increases in the frequency of what are currently considered extreme wet seasons are predicted for various regions, using a range of climate models (15). Recent climate catastrophes, such as Hurricane Mitch in Honduras, have had major adverse health impact. Over the past decade, floods in Bangladesh, China, various parts of Europe, Mozambique and Venezuela have taken a considerable toll on human life and well-being.

Severe weather events have many effects on child health. Studies of earthquakes indicate that women and young children are more vulnerable to the acute impacts of natural disasters (16) and famines (17). Floods cause child injuries and death by drowning, and also compromise clean water supplies, fostering epidemics of diarrhoea. In Peru, hospital admissions for paediatric diarrhoea were 50% above the seasonal norm after precipitation and flooding related to the El Niño-Southern Oscillation (ENSO). Following Hurricane Mitch, 30 000 cases of cholera occurred in Central America (18). A review of 548 reported gastrointestinal infection outbreaks between 1948 and 1994 in the United States revealed that 68% of cases were preceded by precipitation events above the 80th percentile (19).

Weather disasters devastate homes, spawning refugee communities that are likely to have poor public health. Basic life support systems, including water, forests and other natural resources, may also be undermined by climate change. Food production and availability are impaired by droughts and floods. Children are especially vulnerable to the emotional trauma caused by sudden changes in living routines and social networks, and the social disruption, economic damage and population displacement caused by weather disasters can impair their psychological and social development.

Diarrhoeal disease

Diarrhoeal disease is one of the most important causes of ill-health in the world. It is highly sensitive to climatic conditions and shows strong seasonal variations in many locations (20). The usually positive correlation of diarrhoeal disease with temperature reflects the fact that most cases in tropical developing countries are caused by bacteria, entamoebae and protozoa (21), all of which are favoured by high temperatures.

Deaths from gastrointestinal infectious disease are especially high in children. An estimated 3–4 million children die each year from diarrhoeal diseases, predominantly in poorer countries (22). Children consume more water per kg of body mass than adults, giving them an increased relative exposure to waterborne pathogens. Further, with their less well developed immune systems, children are less able to counteract microbes (23) or to compensate for a given level of dehydration.

Several recent studies have used time-series analysis to correlate measurements of temperature and relative humidity with the incidence of diarrhoeal disease in children. A 6-year study in Lima, Peru, showed, on average, an 8% increase in daily hospital admissions for each degree increase in temperature (24). This analysis controlled for seasonal variations and long-term trends, thus imparting high confidence to the observed relationship of diarrhoeal disease with temperature. A similar time-series analysis in Fiji assessed the relationship of monthly reported incidence of diarrhoea to variations in temperature and rainfall, allowing for the effects of seasonal variation and long-term trends (25). The reported incidence increased by approximately 3% for each degree increase in temperature, by 2% per unit increase in rainfall above $5 \times 10^{-5} \, kg/m^2$ per minute (average rainfall conditions), and by 8% per unit decrease in rainfall below this level.

These studies indicate that future changes in mean climatic conditions and in the occurrence of extreme weather events are likely to significantly affect the incidence of diarrhoeal disease in children. As well as meteorological influences on microbial exposures, child diarrhoeal disease may also increase because drinking-water becomes contaminated by toxins from warming-induced algal blooms.

Indirect health effects resulting from ecological alterations
Food availability: malnutrition, growth retardation, and developmental delay

Childhood malnutrition was estimated to account for 15.9% of the total burden of premature death and disabling disease in 1990 (26). A multiplicity of biological, social, political, and economic factors affect the incidence of malnutrition, but one of the fundamental determinants is the availability of staple foods, predominantly cereal grains.

Climate change has many effects on food availability (27). Because there is more carbon dioxide in the atmosphere, plants take up more CO_2 and less nitrogen (28). Plant protein content is thus reduced, with less nitrogen available as building-blocks. Although elevated atmospheric carbon dioxide may increase plant biomass, the nutritional content of the biomass may be impaired. Further, the increased carbon-to-nitrogen ratio, by reducing the synthesis of alkaloids and other nitrogen-based plant defences, may increase the eating of plants by insects, rodents and other pests (29). Increased evaporation may reduce soil moisture, while flooding may cause some arable land to become saline. Climate change can also reduce parasite resistance in livestock (30).

Figure 16.2 shows the estimated impact on cereal grain production in sub-Saharan Africa of standard scenarios of climate change, over three time periods in the coming century, as modelled by scientists at the Hadley Research Centre, United Kingdom Meteorology Office (31). Cereal grains account for around two-thirds of total food energy for human populations, and therefore represent an important index of future food supplies. This study, which incorporated esti-mates of future trends in population growth, economic development, govern-mental policies on pricing, world food trading and agricultural technological developments, found that global climate change would result in a 5–10% drop in total yield. Importantly, this deficit would occur very unevenly around the world, with most of the shortfall occurring in low-latitude countries where food insecurity is often already present, especially in South Asia, the Eastern Mediterranean, North Africa, parts of sub-Saharan Africa, parts of Central America and the northern part of South America.

The above-mentioned modelling studies, collectively, forecast that an addi-tional 40 to 300 million people will become hungry by 2060 as a result of climate change (27–32). The IPCC has concluded with "medium confidence" that "mod-elling studies have indicated that climate change would increase the number of hungry and malnourished people in the world later in the twenty-first century by 80 to 90 million" (4). Most of this hungry population would be children, who require three to four times more food than adults in proportion to their body size (33). Food shortage in critical areas will therefore contribute to child mal-nutrition and, hence, to retarded growth and development. Undernourishment

Figure 16.2 *Estimated impact of standard scenario of global climate change on production of cereal grains in sub-Saharan Africa, in the 2020s, 2050s and 2080s*

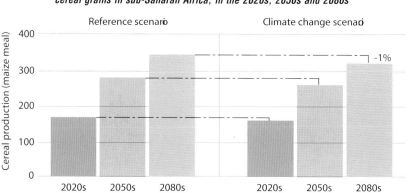

SECTION III: SPECIFIC ENVIRONMENTAL THREATS

is a well-studied fundamental cause of impaired physical and intellectual development in children, low productivity in adults, and susceptibility to infectious disease (34, 35).

Increased aeroallergens: allergies

Human allergic response to airborne plant pollens is a widespread environmental contributor to hay fever, allergenic rhinitis and allergenic asthma (36–39). Sensitization to allergens in early childhood can cause an allergic (including asthmatic) disposition (40).

Ambient pollen levels may rise in response to higher atmospheric carbon dioxide concentrations and higher temperatures (41, 42). Pollen counts have been rising, and this may be partly a result of increased carbon dioxide, warmer winters, the earlier arrival of spring, or excess of nitrogen (43). Thus, climate change may already be contributing to the increased incidence of hay fever and asthma that has occurred in many parts of the world in recent decades.

Malaria, dengue fever, and other vector-borne diseases

The reproduction and survival of blood-feeding vector organisms, such as mosquitoes and ticks, are greatly affected by climate and other ecological factors. Higher temperatures, changes in precipitation, and altered climate variability may therefore change the distribution of vector-borne diseases, both spatially and seasonally (44–48). Immunologically naive populations may thus face unfamiliar pathogens. In some locations, climate change may actually lead to decreased vector-borne disease transmission because of reduced rainfall or excessively high temperatures.

In general, without strong public health defences, the anticipated increases in range and seasonality of pathogens and their vector organisms will cause a greater incidence of various infectious diseases. Children are particularly susceptible to malaria, dengue fever and various forms of encephalitis.

Malaria

Malaria is the world's most serious vector-borne disease. Around 40% of the world's population currently lives in malaria-endemic areas. Various mathematical modelling studies have estimated that increased temperatures will expand the geographical range of conditions conducive to malaria transmission, both to higher altitudes and higher latitudes (49–51). Further, elevated temperatures, in combination with conducive patterns of rainfall and surface water, will extend the transmission season in some locations. Some data suggest that global warming may have already exacerbated malaria incidence, especially in areas where transmission is limited by low temperatures or high altitude (52).

Children experience disproportionately high levels of both morbidity and mortality from malaria. Young children have little specific immunity to malarial species and may therefore suffer yearly attacks of debilitating and potentially fatal disease. Children are also more susceptible to cerebral malaria and to the hypoglycaemia that is secondary to malaria, both of which can lead to neurological damage and, often, death (53).

While excessive heat kills mosquitoes, warmer average temperatures within their survival range increase their reproduction, biting activity, and the rate at which pathogens mature within them, including the malaria parasite, *Plasmodium*. Furthermore, warm nights and warm winters in particular favour insect maturation and survival. This is the specific warming pattern that climate change induces, and mosquitoes will therefore probably mature faster and live longer with climate change.

Dengue fever

Dengue fever is the world's most common mosquito-borne viral disease. The disease is currently endemic in much of tropical Asia, the South Pacific islands, tropical Africa, the Caribbean, and Central and South America. Dengue is characterized by fever, myalgia or arthralgia, rash, leukopenia, and lymphadenopathy. Children are more likely to experience overt, serious, disease. Dengue haemorrhagic fever is a severe, often fatal, febrile disease caused by serial infection with several strains of the dengue virus (54). Dengue outbreaks in urban areas infested with *Aedes aegypti* can be explosive, involving up to three-quarters of the population.

Aedes aegypti, a daytime biting mosquito, is the principal vector and is highly urbanized. It breeds in water stored for drinking or bathing and in collected rainwater. Increased flooding and precipitation as a result of climate change will therefore increase the presence of stagnant water breeding sites, thereby fostering dengue virus propagation. Modelling studies indicate that global warming will increase the geographical range of dengue (55).

Encephalitis and other vector-borne diseases

Greater climate variability will increase the incidence and geographical distribution of other vector-borne diseases, including mosquito-borne encephalitis, tick-borne encephalitis, and Lyme disease. Children are especially vulnerable to mosquito and tick bites, because they tend to play outside and are closer to the ground where ticks and mosquitoes can be found. The reported incidence of Lyme disease in the USA is highest among children aged 5–10 years, almost twice that among older children and adults (56).

Warm winters encourage the overwintering of ticks. Global climate change will therefore foster the geographical spread of tick-borne diseases. A recent study in Sweden showed that a decade of milder winters and earlier springs in the 1980s was related to a significant increase in the range and incidence of tick-borne encephalitis (57).

Ultraviolet exposure: sunburn, skin cancer, and immunosuppression

Global climate change does not include depletion of stratospheric ozone *per se*. However, certain gases (such as the chlorofluorocarbons) contribute to both phenomena, which interact with one another.

Stratospheric ozone provides protection to life on earth by filtering out much of the incoming solar ultraviolet (UV) radiation. In mammals and other animals, this radiation can cause oxidative damage (and hence cancer) and suppression of the immune system. Industrial activity and biomass burning have resulted in the emission of particular gases, especially halogenated fluorocarbons, that undergo photolytic release of high-energy "free radicals", which destroy stratospheric ozone. Consequently, ozone depletion has been observed since the early 1970s, and has caused a 5–10% seasonal (late winter and early spring) increase in UV radiation exposure at middle to high latitudes.

Since ozone depletion is causing greater ground-level UV radiation exposure, it can be presumed to be contributing to sunburn in children at middle to high latitudes. Children's skin and eyes burn more easily than those of adults. Childhood sunburn significantly increases the risk of malignant melanoma later in life (58–60).

UV radiation also suppresses immune system activity, both local and systemic, in animals and humans (61). Although further research is needed on this relationship, there is a theoretical possibility that such immune suppression may pose a health risk to children by increasing their susceptibility to infectious agents.

Other global environmental changes

The impact on human health has been most completely assessed for global climate change and stratospheric ozone depletion. Meanwhile, many other large-scale environmental changes will also have consequences for child health around the world.

In 2001, a network of international agencies and environmental conventions initiated the Millennium Ecosystem Assessment Project, to assess the causes and extent of ecosystem changes in the world, the projected future scenarios of such changes, and how these are affecting and will affect the well-being and health of human populations. This is a scientifically challenging task, since the scope of ecosystem disruption and biodiversity losses is broad and multifaceted. The causal connections with human health outcomes will generally be harder to discern and quantify than has been the case for climate change and ozone depletion.

It is clear, however, that such things as the loss of wetlands and the degradation of arable land will reduce the natural cleansing of freshwater supplies and the productivity of agro-ecosystems, respectively. The latter will also be affected by such things as the loss of plant pollinators, the shortage of freshwater supplies, and the encroachment of invasive introduced species. The spread of megacities in many developing countries also jeopardizes the retention of good arable land, since cities, historically, have usually been built on good land near rivers and coastlines.

We still have much to learn about the myriad ways in which global environmental changes will affect the health of human populations. In the meantime, we should remember that we are now depleting and disrupting the earth's life-support systems. In the medium to long term, this will inevitably reduce the carrying capacity of the biosphere for healthy human life.

Prevention options

Primary prevention is always preferred in public health. This applies particularly in this setting, where environmental change processes may acquire momentum and may induce irreversible changes in important components of the biosphere's life-support systems.

In relation to climate change, the prime requirement is for governments and populations everywhere to modify technological choices and economic practices, so as to greatly reduce the global emission of greenhouse gases. The IPCC and other expert commentators estimate that we need to eliminate around two-thirds of current emissions in order to stabilize the lower atmosphere and its climate at acceptable (apparently not dangerous) levels. This will not prove easy—as is already evident from the inability of most countries to achieve their Kyoto Protocol targets, agreed in 1997. This protocol was developed within the UN Framework Convention on Climate Change, originally formulated at the UN Conference on Environment and Development, Rio de Janeiro, Brazil, in 1992 (62).

Given that the process of climate change is already under way—as are other global environmental changes—and that the world is committed to the continuation of such change over at least several decades, societies must now also seek adaptations that will lessen its adverse health impacts. Many of the climate-amplified risks to children's health would be lessened by strengthening public health infrastructure and environmental management—including sanitation, fresh water provision, immunization programmes, mosquito control, improved housing quality, and better and more secure nutrition.

There is also a need for increased education of primary and secondary schoolchildren about the need for communities to think and act in ecologically sustainable ways, and about the ways of lessening personal and family exposure to environmental hazards consequent upon global environmental changes. Finally, there are some risk-reducing responses that are specific to the hazards of environmental change—such as strengthening coastal defences against rising seas, managing local and regional fisheries sustainably in order to maintain nutritional (especially protein) supplies, and altering clothing and recreational behaviour to reduce exposure of children to ultraviolet radiation.

Conclusion

The impacts of global environmental change on child health span a wide spectrum, covering respiratory health, temperature regulation, trauma, nutrition, development, allergy, infectious disease, mental health, skin cancer, and immunological changes. Nevertheless, there remains a serious lack of empirical data on how climate change specifically affects child health. Much of this knowledge gap reflects the fact that global climate change is a recent and inherently slow process. Furthermore, scientific and popular consensuses have only recently converged in recognizing that climate change and the other global environmental changes require both research and policy attention.

We need more research on how changes in temperature, precipitation and extreme weather events, and their resultant ecological changes, affect children's health. Because many aspects of the physiology and metabolism of children differ markedly from those of adults, several of the health impacts in children, of climate change and other global environmental changes are likely to be distinctive.

To protect children fully from these health consequences will require a substantial change in our pattern of economic activities and in our technology choices. By understanding better the range and extent of risks posed by climate change, stratospheric ozone depletion and other global environmental changes, we will strengthen the contribution of the health sciences to the ongoing public debate over the future, sustainable, management of the biosphere.

References

1. Bunyavanich S et al. The impact of climate change on child health. *Ambulatory Pediatrics*, 2003, 3:47–55.
2. Intergovernmental Panel on Climate Change. *Third Assessment Report* of *Working Group 1: The Science of Climate Change*. Cambridge, Cambridge University Press, 2001.
3. Broecker WS. Thermohaline circulation, the Achilles heel of our climate system: Will man-made CO_2 upset the current balance? *Science*, 1997, 278:1582–1588.
4. Intergovernmental Panel on Climate Change. *Climate change 2000. Impacts, adaptation, and vulnerability*. Third Assessment Report, Volume 11. Cambridge, Cambridge University Press, 2001.
5. McMichael AJ, Kjellstrom T, Smith K. Environment and health. In: Merson M, Black R, Mills A, eds. *International public health*. Gaithersburg, MD, Aspen Press, 2000:379–430.
6. Cubasch UG et al. Projections of future climate change. In: Houghton JT et al., eds. *Climate Change 2001: The scientific basis. Contribution of Working Group I to the Third Assessment Report of the Intergovernmental Panel on Climate Change*. Cambridge, Cambridge University Press, 2001.
7. Church J. How fast are sea levels rising? *Science*, 2001, 294:802–803.

8. Kattenberg A et al. Climate models projections of future climate. In: Houghton J et al. eds., *Climate change 1995*. Cambridge, Cambridge University Press, 1996:285–357.

9. Karl T, Knight R, Plummer N. Trends in high-frequency climate variability in the twentieth century. *Nature*, 1995, 377:217–220.

10. Whetton P et al. Implications of climate change due to the enhanced greenhouse effect on floods and droughts in Australia. *Climate Change*, 1993, 25.

11. Milly P et al. Increasing risk of great floods in a changing climate. *Nature*, 2002, 415:514–517.

12. White KS et al. Technical summary. Climate change 2001: Impacts, adaptation, and vulnerability. In: McCarthy J et al. eds., *Climate change 2001: impacts, adaptation, and vulnerability*. Cambridge, Cambridge University Press, 2001.

13. Easterling D. Climate extremes: observations, modeling, and impacts. *Science*, 2000, 289:2068–2074.

14. Epstein P. Climate change and emerging infectious diseases. *Microbes and Infection*, 2001, 3:747–754.

15. Palmer TN, Ralsanen J. Quantifying the risk of extreme seasonal precipitation events in a changing climate. *Nature*, 2002, 415:512–514.

16. Beinin C. An examination of health data following two major earthquakes in Russia. *Disasters*, 1981, 5:142–146.

17. Rivers JPW. Women and children last; an essay on sex discrimination in disasters. *Disasters*, 1982, 6:256–267.

18. Epstein P. Climate and health. *Science*, 1999, 285:347–348.

19. Curriero F et al. The association between extreme precipitation and waterborne disease outbreaks in the United States, 1948–1994. *American Journal of Public Health*, 2001, 91:1194–1199.

20. Drasar BS, Tomkins AM, Feachem RG. *Seasonal aspects of diarrhoeal disease. Seasonal dimensions to rural poverty*. Brighton, University of Sussex, 1978.

21. Black RE, Lanata CF. Epidemiology of diarrhoeal disease in developing countries. In: Blaser MJ et al. eds. *Infections of the gastrointestinal tract*. New York, Raven Press, 1995:13–36.

22. *Health and environment in sustainable development : 5 years after the Earth Summit*. Geneva, World Health Organization, 2002 (http://www.who.int/archives/inf-pr-1997/en/pr97-47.html).

23. *Children and drinking water standards*. Washington, DC, United States Environmental Protection Agency Office of Water, 1999 (815K-99-001).

24. Checkley W et al. Effect of El Nino and ambient temperature on hospital admissions for diarrhoeal diseases in Peruvian children. *Lancet*, 2000, 355:442–450.

25. Singh RB et al. The influence of climate variation and change on diarrhoeal disease in the Pacific Islands. *Environmental health perspectives*, 2001, 109:155–159.

26. Murray CJL, Lopez AD. *The global burden of disease*. Cambridge, MA, Harvard School of Public Health (on behalf of the World Health Organization and the World Bank), 1996.

27. McMichael AL. Impact of climatic and other environmental changes on food production and population health in the coming decades. *Proceedings of the Nutrition Society*, 2001, 60:195–201.

28. Campbell B et al. Impacts of atmospheric composition and climate change on temperate and tropical pastoral agriculture. In: Bouma W, Pearman G, Manning M, eds. *Greenhouse. Coping with climate change.* Melbourne, CSIRO, 1996:171–189.

29. Coley P. Possible effects of climate change on plant/herbivore interactions in moist tropical forests. *Climatic Change*, 1998, 39:455–472.

30. Coop R, Holmes P. Nutrition and parasite interaction. *International Journal of Parasitology*, 1996, 26:951–962.

31. Parry M et al. Climate change and world food security: a new assessment. *Global Environment Change—Human and Policy Dimensions*, 1999, 9:S51–67.

32. Parry M, Rosenzweig C. Food supply and risk of hunger. *Lancet*, 1993, 342:1345–1347.

33. *How EPA protects children's health.* Washington, DC, Environmental Protection Agency, 2002 (http://www.epa.gov/epahome/chm_factsheet.html).

34. Chandra R. Nutrition, immunity, and infection: present knowledge and future directions. *Lancet*, 1983, 1:688–691.

35. McMichael A, Haines A. Global climate change: the potential effects on health. *British Medical Journal*, 1997, 315:805–809.

36. *Something in the air: airborne allergens.* Bethesda, MD, National Institutes of Health, 1993.

37. D'Amato G, Liccardi G, D'Amato M. Environmental risk factors (outdoor air pollution and climatic changes) and increased trend of respiratory allergy. *Journal of Investigational Allergology and Clinical Immunology*, 2000, 10:123–128.

38. Arrighi H. US asthma mortality: 1941–1989. *Annals of Allergy, Asthma, and Immunology*, 1995, 74:321–326.

39. Wuthrich B. In Switzerland, pollinosis has really increased in the last decade. *Allergy and Clinical Immunology News*, 1991, 3:41–44.

40. Wahn U et al. Indoor allergen exposure is a risk factor for sensitization during the first three years of life. *Journal of Allergy and Clinical Immunology*, 1997, 99:763–769.

41. Ziska L, Caulfield F. The potential influence of rising atmospheric carbon dioxide on public health: pollen production of common ragweed as a test case. *World Resources Review*, 2000, 12:449–457.

42. Reekie J, Hinkleton P, Reekie E. Effects of elevated CO_2 on time of flowering in four short-day and four long-day species. *Canadian Journal of Botany*, 1994, 72:533–538.

43. Wayne P et al. Production of allergenic pollen by ragweed (*Ambrosia artemisiifolia* L.) is increased in CO_2-enriched atmospheres. *Annals of Allergy, Asthma and Immunology*, 2002, 8:279–282.

44. Patz J, Reisen W. Immunology, climate change and vector-borne diseases. *Trends in Immunology*, 2001, 22:171–172.

45. Epstein P. Emerging diseases and ecosystem instability: new threats to public health. *American Journal of Public Health*, 1995, 85:168–172.

46. Sutherst R. The vulnerability of animal and human health to parasites under global change. *International Journal of Parasitology*, 2001, 31:933–948.

47. Rogers D, Randolph S. The global spread of malaria in a future, warmer world. *Science*, 2000, 289:1763–1765.

48. Patz J et al. Effects of environmental change on emerging parasitic diseases. *International Journal of Parasitology*, 2000, 30:1395–1405.

49. Sutherst R. Arthropods as disease vectors in a changing environment. *Environmental Change and Human Health*, 1993:124–145.

50. Reiter P. Climate change and mosquito-borne disease. *Environmental Health Perspectives*, 2001, 109:141–161.

51. Martens P. How will climate change affect human health? *American Scientist*, 1999, 87:534–541.

52. Epstein P et al. Biological and physical signs of climate change: focus on mosquito-borne infectious diseases. *Bulletin of the American Meteorological Society*, 1998, 79:409–417.

53. Krause P. Malaria (*Plasmodium*). In: Behrman RE et al. eds. *Nelson textbook of pediatrics*. WB Saunders and Co., Philadelphia, 2000.

54. Halstead B. Dengue fever/dengue hemorrhagic fever. In: Behrman RE et al. eds. *Nelson textbook of pediatrics*. WB Saunders and Co., Philadelphia, 2000.

55. Hales S et al. Potential effect of population and climate changes on global distribution of dengue fever: an empirical model. *Lancet*, 2002, 360:830–834.

56. Shapiro E. Lyme disease (*Borrelia burgdorferi*). In: Behrman RE et al. eds. *Nelson textbook of pediatrics*. WB Saunders and Co., Philadelphia, 2000.

57. Lindgren E, Gustafson R. Tick-borne encephalitis in Sweden and climate change. *Lancet*, 2001, 358:16–18.

58. *Ozone depletion glossary*. Washington, DC, Environmental Protection Agency, 2002 (http://www.epa.gov/dots/ozone/defns.htmigods).

59. Fitzpatrick T. The skin cancer cascade: from ozone depletion to melanoma— some definitions and some new interpretation. *Journal of Dermatology*, 1996, 23:816–820.

60. *Skin cancer fact sheet*. Atlanta, GA, American Cancer Society, 1996.

61. *Melanoma risk factors fact sheet*. Schaumberg, IL, American Academy of Dermatology, 1997.

62. *United Nations Framework Convention on Climate Change*. New York, United Nations (www.unfccc.int).

CHAPTER 17

Emerging environmental threats: endocrine-disrupting chemicals

T. Damstra

Department for the Protection of the Human Environment, International Programme on Chemical Safety, World Health Organization, Geneva, Switzerland

Introduction

The knowledge that environmental exposures to chemicals can significantly affect children's health is not new. However, recently there has been growing concern that children may be adversely affected by exposure to a group of chemicals that have the potential to alter the normal functioning of the endocrine system in wildlife and humans. Concerns regarding exposure to these endocrine-disrupting chemicals (EDCs) are primarily related to: (1) adverse effects observed in certain wildlife, fish, and ecosystems; (2) the increased incidence of certain endocrine-related human diseases; and (3) endocrine disruption observed in laboratory experimental animals exposed to certain environmental chemicals.

Potential adverse health outcomes are mainly neurodevelopmental and neurobehavioural abnormalities, reproductive disorders, immune impairment, and certain hormone-related cancers (1). Children may be particularly susceptible to exposure to EDCs during critical periods of development. Both the nature and severity of health outcomes may depend on the developmental stage at which exposure occurs.

Although most of the concerns regarding EDCs have focused on persistent organic pollutants (POPs), a variety of chemical classes including natural and synthetic hormones, plant constituents, pesticides, compounds used in the plastics industry and in consumer products, and other industrial by-products and pollutants are potential EDCs. They are often pervasive and widely dispersed in the environment. Some are persistent, can be transported long distances, and have been found in virtually all regions of the world. Others are rapidly degraded in the environment or human body, or may be present for only short periods of time. This enormous diversity means that it is not possible to define a "typical" EDC, and each chemical or mixture must be carefully evaluated.

Mechanisms of action

Research has shown that disruption of the endocrine system can occur through various mechanisms. Some chemicals may mimic a natural hormone, whereas others may block the effects of hormones. Some may interfere with hormone synthesis, transport, or metabolism (2). Exposure to EDCs during critical developmental stages, when programming of the endocrine system is occurring, may result in changes in growth, development, reproduction, and behaviour, whereas exposure at other time periods might not result in any significant effects. Cross-talk between various components of the endocrine-system may also have different consequences at various life stages and effects may occur in systems other than the system predicted to be affected (3).

Potential health effects

A variety of field investigations and laboratory studies have shown that exposure to certain EDCs has contributed to adverse effects in some wildlife populations, including mammals, birds, reptiles, and molluscs (4). Effects range from subtle changes to permanent alterations. For example, reproductive and immune dysfunction has been reported in various species of mammals, particularly aquatic species at the top of the food chain. Exposure to polychlorinated biphenyls (PCBs) and dichlorodiphenyltrichloroethylene (DDE) has been shown to adversely impact the reproductive function of Baltic seals (5). Studies on fish have shown that exposure to certain constituents present in pulp and paper mill effluents and sewage treatment effluents may function as EDCs and contribute to alterations in reproductive development (6). Another example is masculinization in female gastropods due to exposure to tributyltin (used in antifouling paints), which has resulted in a global population decline in a number of gastropod species (7). These are but a few examples of the breadth of responses observed in a wide variety of wildlife species. For humans, evidence of causal associations between low-level exposure to EDCs and adverse health outcomes is less clear-cut.

Reproductive effects

Much of the concern about human health effects resulting from EDC exposure has focused on adverse effects on reproductive development and function, including decreased semen quality (i.e., reduced numbers, motility, and altered morphology of sperm); male reproductive tract abnormalities (e.g. hypospadias and cryptorchidism); altered sex ratio; endometriosis; precocious puberty; and early menarche. A number of studies have reported a decline in sperm counts in several countries (8–10). The available data suggest important variations in sperm count between different countries, various regions within the same country or between various districts of the same city; however, these data must be interpreted with caution. All the studies published to date have been retrospective and report data from men recruited for other purposes. There are a number of confounding factors (e.g. age, seasonal variations, methods of collecting sperm) that can influence sperm count making it difficult to compare data between locations or from one time to another. These preliminary observations require further study.

Concerns have also been raised about the effects of EDCs on female reproductive tissues and pregnancy outcomes. Exposure to certain EDCs (e.g. 2,3,7,8-tetrachlorodibenzyl-p-dioxin (TCDD) and PCBs) has been reported to be associated with endometriosis, but the studies remain equivocal (11). Concerns that EDCs may cause spontaneous abortion and affect fecundity and fertility have also been raised but studies are inconsistent and suggest only a weak association at relatively high exposure levels (12). There have also been isolated reports of precocious puberty resulting from foods possibly contaminated with estrogenic compounds (13), but the mechanisms of action are unclear, and other factors (e.g. nutrition) must also be considered.

Cancer

Increases in the incidence of certain hormone-related cancers in many parts of the world are often cited as evidence that exposure to EDCs has had adverse health effects. Of particular concern are increases in breast cancer and testicular cancer. Numerous epidemiological studies, as well as laboratory studies, have been conducted to determine whether exposure to organochlorine chemicals contributes to an increased risk of breast cancer (14–16). Overall, the current scientific evidence (including meta-analyses of human studies) does not support a direct association between exposure to environmental EDCs and increased risk of breast cancer (17); however, all the studies published to date have measured EDC exposure levels in adult women. The claim that the time of life when exposure takes place (e.g. prenatal, neonatal, childhood, adolescence) may be the most critical factor is supported by human data on radiation and smoking, and by basic research in animal models (18, 19). Adult women, currently at risk for breast cancer, may have been exposed to exogenous EDCs in utero or during infancy, childhood, or adolescence in the mid-twentieth century when contaminant levels of organochlorines were higher. Research is urgently needed to address the role of timing of exposure to environmental chemicals, as well as the contributions of diet, lifestyle, and genetic profile to the overall risk of breast cancer.

While there are marked differences in incidence of testicular cancer among countries, there have been reports that testicular cancer incidence has increased since the 1960s in certain countries (20, 21); however, there have been no epidemiological studies to examine a direct linkage between exposure to estrogenic or anti-androgenic compounds and testicular cancer (22). Unfortunately, animal models for germ cell (testicular) tumours in men do not currently exist. Although the data are limited, some evidence suggests that the incidence of cryptorchidism and hypospadias may show geographical differences similar to those of testicular cancer, and research on the etiology of this syndrome is needed.

Neurological and immunological effects

The neuroendocrine and immune systems play an integrative role in orchestrating critical physiological functions, which may be disrupted through a variety of mechanisms, including endocrine-disrupting mechanisms. Certain EDCs have been shown to cause neurotoxic and immunotoxic effects (*23, 24*). Of particular concern are the potential effects of exposure to these contaminants on the developing nervous and immune systems, since exposure during these critical periods may result in irreversible changes, which may not be apparent until later in life.

Numerous studies have investigated the effects of prenatal and early postnatal exposure to PCBs in newborn and young children (*25*). Studies in humans who consumed high amounts of contaminated fish from the Great Lakes (*26, 27*) or accidentally contaminated rice oil (*28, 29*) have shown that PCBs contribute to neurobehavioural changes in newborn children and that some of these changes persist through childhood. Changes included motor immaturity, abnormal reflexes, and low psychomotor scores. Subtle neurobehavioural alterations have also been observed in children born to mothers exposed to lower PCB levels (*30*). PCBs are known to interfere with thyroid hormones, which are critical for normal brain development (*31*).

The immune system may also be perturbed as a result of exposure to environmental contaminants, although for most chemicals the mechanism of action is unclear (*32*). Immunological changes have been observed in human populations exposed to mixtures of PCBs, dibenzodioxins, and dibenzofurans (*33*). Findings included increased susceptibility to respiratory tract infections in adults and their children (*34*), and increased prevalence of ear infections in infants (*35*). Infants exposed *in utero* or via breastfeeding appear to be particularly vulnerable. Animal data support the immunotoxicity of PCBs and dibenzodioxins (*36*). There is evidence of perturbed immune function at high exposure levels, but data at lower levels are sparse, and further research is needed.

Sources and timing of exposure

As has already been mentioned, the timing of exposure is critical to understanding the potential long-term health effects of EDC exposure in children (prenatal and postnatal). Lack of adequate exposure data is often the weakest link in attempts to determine whether exposure to EDCs poses an emerging environmental threat. Data on the magnitude and trends of EDC exposure in children, particularly in developing countries, are almost completely lacking. Potential sources of exposure in children include: transplacental migration, contaminated breast milk or food, contaminated air and groundwater, and contaminants in toys and other consumer products. Global coordinated efforts are needed to collect data on exposure.

Research needs

Data have clearly shown that POPs and EDCs are toxic at relatively high concentrations. The question remains whether adverse effects occur from low-level chronic exposures. Information on timing of exposures is critical for understanding potential effects in children, and studies are urgently needed to address the long-term effects of exposure during critical development stages. Significant data gaps remain that often limit our ability to estimate the risks of environmental exposures to POPs and EDCs. Internationally and nationally, decision-making on the possible deleterious effects of chemical exposure is increasingly governed by the precautionary principle when scientific knowledge is uncertain. The influence of endocrine disruptors on adverse health outcomes has yet to be definitely established. However, it is clear that the risk from endocrine disruptors is important at certain stages (preconception, prenatal and postnatal), and further research is required to identify the windows of exposure that are critical for children's health in terms of the irreversibility of the effects.

References

1. *Global assessment of the state-of-the-science of endocrine disrupting chemicals.* Geneva, World Health Organization, 2002.
2. McLachlan JA, Korach KS. Symposium on estrogens in the environment III. *Environmental Health Perspectives*, 1995, 103:173.
3. Olea N et al. Inadvertent exposure to xenoestrogens in children. *Toxicology and Industrial Health*, 1999, 15:151–158.
4. Ankley GT, Giesy JP. Endocrine disruptors in wildlife: a weight of evidence perspective. In: Kendall R et al. eds. *Principles and processes for assessing endocrine disruption in wildlife*. Pensacola, FL, SETAC Press, 1998:349–368.
5. Reijnders PJH. Reproductive and developmental effects of endocrine disrupting chemicals on marine mammals. In: O'Shea TJ et al. eds. *Marine mammals and persistent ocean contaminants: proceedings of the Marine Mammal Commission Workshop, Keystone, Colorado, 12–15 October 1998*. Bethesda, MD, Marine Mammal Commission, 1999:139–143.
6. Van Der Kraak G et al. A comparison of bleached kraft mill effluent, 17-b-estradiol, and b-sitosterol effects on reproductive function in fish. In: Kendall RJ et al. eds. *Principles and processes for evaluating endocrine disruption in wildlife*. Pensacola, FL, SETAC Press, 1998:249–265 (SETAC Technical Publication).
7. Matthiessen P, Gibbs PE. Critical appraisal of evidence for tributyltin-mediated endocrine disruption in molluscs. *Environmental Toxicology and Chemistry*, 1998, 17:37–43.
8. Sharpe RM, Skakkebaek NE. Are estrogens involved in falling sperm counts and disorders of the male reproductive tract? *Lancet*, 1993, 341:1392–1395.
9. Larsen SB et al. Semen quality and sex hormones among organic and traditional Danish farmers. ASCLEPIOS Study Group. *Occupational Environmental Medicine*, 1999, 56:139–144.

10. Carlsen E et al. Evidence for decreasing quality of semen during past 50 years. *British Medical Journal*, 1992, 305:609–613.

11. Lebel G et al. Organochlorine exposure and the risk of endometriosis. *Fertility and Sterility*, 1998, 69:221–228.

12. Joffe M. Time trends in biological fertility in Britain. *Lancet*, 2000, 355:1961–1965.

13. Colon I et al. Identification of phthalate esters in the serum of young Puerto Rican girls with premature breast development. *Environmental Health Perspectives*, 2000, 108:895–900.

14. Hoyer AP et al. Repeated measurements of organochlorine exposure and breast cancer risk (Denmark). *Cancer Causes and Control*, 2000, 11:177–184.

15. van't Veer P et al. DDT (dicophane) and postmenopausal breast cancer in Europe; case control study. *British Medical Journal*, 1997, 315:81–85.

16. Dorgan JF et al. Serum organochlorine pesticides and PCBs and breast cancer risk: results from a prospective analysis (USA). *Cancer Causes Control*, 1999, 10:1–11.

17. Laden F et al. 1,1-Dichloro-2,2,-bis(p-chlorophenyl)ethylene and polychlorinated biphenyls and breast cancer: combined analysis of five US studies. *Journal of the National Cancer Institute*, 2001, 93:768–775.

18. Tokunaga M, Land CE, Yamamoto T. Incidence of female breast cancer among atomic bomb survivors, Hiroshima and Nagasaki. *Radiation Research*, 1987, 112:243–272.

19. Palmer JR, Rosenberg L. Cigarette smoking and the risk of breast cancer. *Epidemiology Review*, 1993, 15:145–156.

20. Adami H et al. Testicular cancer in nine Northern European countries. *International Journal of Cancer*, 1994, 59:33–38.

21. Bergstrom R et al. Increase in testicular cancer incidence in six European countries: a birth cohort phenomenon. *Journal of the National Cancer Institute*, 1996, 88:727–733.

22. *An updating of IARC Monographs, Vols 1–42.* Lyon, International Agency for Research on Cancer, 1987 (IARC Monographs on the evaluation of the carcinogenic risk of chemicals in humans, Supplement 192).

23. International Programme on Chemical Safety. *Principles and methods for assessing direct immunotoxicity associated with exposure to chemicals.* Geneva, World Health Organization, 1996 (Environmental Health Criteria No. 180).

24. International Programme on Chemical Safety. *Neurotoxicity risk assessment for human health: principles and approaches.* Geneva, World Health Organization, 2001 (Environmental Health Criteria No. 223).

25. Schantz SL. Developmental neurotoxicity of PCBs: what do we know and where do we go from here? *Neurotoxicology and Teratology*, 1996, 18:217–227.

26. Stewart P, Darvill T, Lonky E. Assessment of prenatal exposure to PCBs from maternal consumption of Great Lakes fish: an analysis of PCB pattern and concentration. *Environmental Research*, 1999, 80:S87–S96.

27. Lonky E, Reihman J, Darvill T. Neonatal behavioral assessment scale performance in humans influenced by maternal consumption of environmentally contaminated Lake Ontario fish. *Journal of Great Lakes Research*, 1996, 22:198–212.

28. Hsu CC, Yu MLM, Chen YCJ. The Yu-Cheng rice oil poisoning incident. In: Schechter A, ed. *Dioxins and health*. New York, Plenum Press, 1994:661–684.

29. Rogan WJ, Gladen BC. PCBs, DDE, and child development at 18 and 24 months. *Annual Reviews in Epidemiology*, 1991, 1:407–413.

30. Winneke G et al. Developmental neurotoxicity of polychlorinated biphenyls (PCBs): cognitive and psychomotor functions in 7-month old children. *Toxicology Ltters*, 1998, 102/103:423–428.

31. Porterfield SP, Hendry LB. Impact of PCBs on thyroid hormone directed brain development. *Toxicological Industrial Health*, 1998, 14:103–120.

32. Van Loveren H et al. Report of the Bilthoven symposium: Advancement of epidemiological studies in assessing the human health effects of immunotoxic agents in the environment and workplace. *Biomarkers*, 1999, 4:135–157.

33. Weisglas-Kuperus N et al. Immunologic effects of background prenatal and postnatal exposure to dioxins and polychlorinated biphenyls in Dutch infants. *Pediatric research*, 1995, 38:404–410.

34. Yu ML, Hsin JW, Hsu CC. The immunological evaluation of the Yucheng children. *Chemosphere*, 1998, 37:1855–1865.

35. Muckle G et al. Prenatal exposure of the northern Quebec Inuit infants to environmental contaminants. *Environmental Health Perspectives*, 2001, 109:1291–1299.

36. Vos JG, De Heer C, Van Loveren H. Immunotoxic effects of TCDD and toxic equivalency factors. *Teratogenesis, Carcinogenesis and Mutagenesis*, 1997/98, 17:275–284.

The paediatric environmental history IV

CHAPTER 18

Paediatric environmental history-taking in developing countries[1]

J. Pronczuk
Protection of the Human Environment, World Health Organization, Geneva, Switzerland

Introduction

Over the past decade, evidence about the association between the environment and children's health has increased, as has knowledge about children's particular susceptibility to environmental exposures. The fetus, the child and the adolescent may be exposed to physical, chemical and biological risks during crucial periods of growth and development. These exposures may not only cause disease in childhood but also have an impact on health during adulthood. Health professionals are in a key position to identify children at risk, advise parents on ways to reduce the risk, and recommend actions to policy-makers. They should be able to recognize and assess the environmental health threats present in the places where children and adolescents live, learn, play, and work. They should also know that the threats are greater in low-income populations and marginalized communities, in degraded environments and when children and adolescents are living under extreme stress (e.g. during civil unrest, or in refugee camps).

Front-line health care providers dealing with children's health issues have specific roles and responsibilities: they should be able to take a detailed history of environmental exposure that will allow any resulting diseases to be detected and treated. Health care providers should be able to identify potential exposure to chemical, physical and biological agents, and should know how these could cause or trigger respiratory, gastrointestinal or neurological diseases. They should also be aware of potential reproductive, endocrine and neurobehavioural toxicity, understand the mechanisms of environmental disease and know the biomedical techniques available for the study and monitoring of environmental exposures. This knowledge will enable more effective primary care of the child and his or her family, improve the quality of medical surveillance, and contribute to the prevention of environmentally related diseases.

---

[1] Reviewed by **R. A. Etzel**, Department of Environmental and Occupational Health, School of Public Health and Health Services, George Washington University, Washington, DC, USA. Additional input provided by: C. Alonzo (Uruguay), N. Chauduri (Canada), L. Corra (Argentina), I. Makalinao (Philippines), and K. Shea (USA).

In spite of the growing concern about health and the environment, and the demands of communities for advice on environmental matters from health care professionals, environmental health is seldom taught in medical and nursing schools. Health professionals in many countries, especially developing countries, lack training in and knowledge of the clinical recognition, management and prevention of diseases linked to the environment. Few clinicians are able to elicit information about the home, the school or the playground as part of the demographic and social history.

The need to incorporate training on health and the environment into medical and nursing curricula is obvious. However, it is likely to be a lengthy process, and immediately applicable solutions are required. Taking an environmental history is one way in which health professionals can learn and apply basic environmental health concepts immediately.

The paediatric environmental history (PEH) is a tool for identifying and assessing children's exposure to environmental health threats and for responding with effective therapeutic and preventive measures. It is also a key mechanism for collecting case data in a harmonized manner and building the evidence required for interventions to eliminate or reduce environmental health threats and improve the quality of life of children within their families and communities. Furthermore, it provides an opportunity for close interaction between the health professional and parents, and also among clinicians, environmental scientists, researchers, educators, policy-makers, and members of the community.

What is the PEH?

The PEH is a series of basic concise questions that enables health professionals to identify children's risks of exposure to environmental threats and their special vulnerabilities.

Some questions cover general issues and are applicable throughout the world. Others are more specific and should be tailored to the local situation and needs and to the age group that is being addressed. The questions should be adapted to the epidemiological trends observed in the population group and the sociocultural, economic and geographic characteristics of the area where the child lives. In developing countries, the PEH requires careful consideration of the specific risk factors that are found in run-down and poor environments and also the special vulnerability factors that children may have, for example, malnutrition.

Key areas

1. *What are the potential environmental hazards?*
   - Identify the different hazards that may be present in the environments where children spend most of their time: physical, chemical and biological hazards (including their sources).

2. *How are children exposed?*
   - In the places where children spend most of their time: home and surroundings, school, playground and recreational areas, streets, fields, work and other places, in urban and rural settings. Include nearby hazardous and waste sites.
   - Through media that originate or carry the agents: water, air, food, soil and objects.
   - As a consequence of activities such as: eating, drinking, playing, exploring, learning, working, and others.
   - Through specific behaviours according to age group or circumstances (e.g. crawling, tasting and "hand-to-mouth" behaviour in a toddler; hobbies and drug-taking in adolescents).
3. *What are the main effects observed?*
   - Requires consideration of special vulnerabilities ("windows of susceptibility").
   - During different periods of development: *in utero*, postnatal period, toddler, infant, school-age and adolescence.
   - Encompasses clinical and subclinical effects on organs, systems or functions, and on the development of the child or adolescent.

Developing and using the PEH questions

The questions should be prepared locally, taking into consideration the three key areas mentioned above. They should address the main environmental threats present in the places where children spend most of their time, the toxicants and pathologies most commonly encountered, and unhealthy behaviours and conditions observed.

The harmonization of these questionnaires in the health sector offers a number of advantages. First, the comparability of the data collected offers the potential for cooperative research studies and publication of observations. Secondly, there are increased facilities for generating reports (e.g. annual reports on the status of children's environmental health, use of indicators of children's environmental health). Thirdly, increased communications, sharing of experiences and awareness about local environmental problems may facilitate action, e.g. to find common solutions.

The harmonization of the PEH requires a common terminology and case definitions. Electronic data entry offers the possibility of creating a database that could provide valuable information for interventions and for the follow-up of environmental health problems in the area.

The preparation of the harmonized questionnaire requires consultation among health professionals and agreement on the basic set of questions. It also requires close collaboration with other sectors, such as environment, education and labour, and with the community and decision-makers (in order to ensure completeness and facilitate communications). A list of the potential issues to address in the PEH questions for developing areas is provided in Appendix 18.1. This list may be used as a basis for evaluating the main environmental health risks to children in the area and for preparing a locally adapted PEH.

Who takes the PEH, when and how?

Health care professionals dealing with infants, children and adolescents can take the PEH. They may be the paediatricians, family doctors, primary health care workers or nurses dealing with children and adolescents, or the residents and medical and nursing students and midwives who care for pregnant women.

The decision on who takes charge will depend on the characteristics of the health system and the availability of health personnel. In some instances, part of the environmental history-taking may be done by a social worker or environmental officer who can visit the home, school, playground or other places where children spend their time. Environmentally trained staff in health care facilities would offer tremendous advantages, as they would be in a position to identify and assess the potential threats in the child's environment, inform the health care providers and authorities, and educate parents, teachers and communities.

A PEH may be taken when children, whether symptomatic or asymptomatic, are seen at a medical facility or during a home visit. It is crucial to take a PEH when children with acute or chronic disease come to emergency rooms, outpatient clinics, primary health care centres or private medical offices. It is also a highly significant preventive tool when used during routine health surveillance visits.

In some special cases, the PEH may be a key tool for addressing public health problems, such as clusters of paediatric disease, uncommon cases or symptoms, epidemics of unknown origin, or changes in epidemiological trends in a given area.

How much time should be devoted to the PEH?

A basic set of questions should be part of the normal medical history-taking, but in special cases, when an environmental cause or trigger of disease is suspected, more time and patience will be required.

Taking a PEH requires the clear formulation of specific questions to parents, children (depending on age) and carers. If possible, a home audit should be made by parents and carers and a simple questionnaire completed on the characteristics of the places where children spend most of their time, their activities and their behaviour.

Barriers to the PEH

The main obstacles to the use of the PEH include: (a) lack of awareness of health professionals and decision-makers about the importance of environmental factors, (b) lack of training and information on environmental health issues, (c) limited time available for the paediatric consultation, (d) overstretched health facilities and lack of personnel, and (e) lack of motivation. These barriers may be overcome by incorporating environmental health into the curricula of medical and nursing schools, increasing awareness of health authorities, disseminating information and strengthening health facilities. Also, health workers in training could carry out home visits. Many developing countries require newly graduated medical students to work for some years in a rural setting before practising in urban areas, and could use these graduates to promote the use of environmental home audits in rural areas.

South Texas Environmental Education and Research Center (STEER)

A good example of home audits is found in the South Texas Environmental Education and Research Center (STEER) training programme used by medical and nursing students at the University of Texas Health Science Center in San Antonio. The STEER programme sends students out on "environmental health house calls", targeting houses that have children with asthma. Families in the area with children who have asthma volunteer to open their homes to the students. Under professional supervision, the students visit the family home three times, observing its characteristics, identifying potential "triggers" and learning about the relationship between illness and the environment of their patient. This innovative programme is described in Case Study 20, page 345.

Taking a paediatric environmental history in developing areas

Main issues for consideration in developing a local harmonized questionnaire

Places

1. **Where does the child live?**

    Home

    Is it a separate dwelling, a multiunit dwelling, a temporary structure or something else?

    What is the family structure, how many members are there?

    Socioeconomic status of the household?

    What is the building made of? (Wood, brick, mud, cardboard, . . . ?)

    What is the age of the building?

    Is there mould on the walls?

    How well ventilated and lit is it?

    Are there any odours?

    Has there been any recent painting or refurbishing?

    Do family members smoke at home? What do they smoke? How much?

    Are pesticides used indoors? How?

    Are there cockroaches? Mites? Rats?

    Are there pets (dogs, cats, birds) or other animals?

    How often is the place cleaned?

    Which chemicals are used for cleaning?

    Where and how is the cooking done?

    How is the home heated?

    Type of stove, exhaust and fuels used (see section 12 below)

    Type of water supply (see section 11 below)

    Access to sanitation (see section 5 below)

    Does the child have a place of his/her own?

    Is it shared? With whom?

    Is the home a workplace too?

    Location

    Is the home in an urban, periurban or rural area?

    Is it in a shanty town?

    Is it next to a sea, lake or water extension?

    Is it near a waste site? industrial site? mining area? transformers? high-tension electric line?

    Is it in an area of high-density traffic?

If in a rural area, are pesticides used locally? How and when?
Where are agrochemicals stored?
Are there any particular poisonous animals?

Street
If the child lives on the street—where does he/she sleep?
Who else lives in the group?
What are the characteristics of the living place?

2. **Where the child plays**
Outdoors
Where is the outdoor playground?
Is there protection from excessive sun radiation? Are there trees?
Is it a high-risk area? (e.g. near a creek, pond, ravine . . .)
Is it near an industrial area? Mining area? High-traffic area? Agricultural area
    where pesticides are being applied?

Indoors
The indoor playground—same questions as for Home—see section 1 above)
Hobbies (see section 15)

3. **Where the child learns**
Same questions as for Home (section 1) applied to:
    — child care centres;
    — school;
    — community house;
    — workshop.

4. **Where the child works**
Characteristics of the place/activity:
    — cottage industry;
    — factory;
    — rural area, plantation, farm;
    — street (street vendors);
    — waste sites (scavengers);
    — manufacturing processes;
    — mining;
    — textiles;
    — chemicals used.

5. **Sanitation and hygiene (in all places covered by sections 1–4)**
Sanitation facilities
Latrines

Wastewater irrigation
How is hygiene maintained?
Type of water treatment plant

Risks (chemical, physical, biological)

6. **Exposure to chemicals**
   Pesticides?
   Lead, mercury, arsenic, fluoride?
   Solvents?
   Gases and fumes?
   Persistent organic pollutants?
   Others (see section 24 below).

7. **Exposure to radiation**
   Is the child overexposed to ultraviolet radiation? Are there any effects on the
     skin? On the eyes? Phototoxicity? Photoallergy?
   Is the child exposed to ionizing radiation: X-rays, gamma rays, radon?
   Did the child receive X-rays while in the womb?
   What are the possible sources of exposure (including diagnostic proce-
     dures)?
   Is the child exposed to electromagnetic fields?

8. **Noise exposure**
   Is the child exposed to undesirable sounds? During the day or night? At
     school? Home? Work? Recreational area?
   Have the sounds affected the child's health and well being?
   Possible sources of noise:
   — traffic;
   — work, industry;
   — music;
   — airport.

9. **Exposure to adverse and extreme environmental conditions**
   Is the child stressed by extreme conditions?
   — extreme/adverse climatic conditions (e.g. mountains, hot or cold
     weather, storms, weather disaster);
   — drought ;
   — floods;
   — environmental degradation;
   — technological disasters;
   — war;
   — social conflict and postconflict circumstances;

— refugee camp;
— imprisonment.

10. Exposure to vector-borne diseases
Is the child exposed to parasitic or infectious diseases?
— malaria;
— filariasis;
— onchocerciasis;
— schistosomiasis;
— trypanosomiasis;
— leishmaniasis;
— dracunculiasis;
— hookworm;
— *Toxocara canis;*
— trachoma;
— ringworm;
— arboviral diseases (dengue, yellow fever, encephalitis, other).

Media

11. Water
Is there access to a safe water supply?
What are the water pipes made of?
Is there a home treatment system?
How are the water sources protected?
Is drinking-water stored in the house? How?
Are there potential sources of contamination? (chemicals, germs, parasites, radionuclides)
Specific problems: nitrites and nitrates, arsenic, fluorides, lead.
Are there risks posed by recreational waters?
Is the recreational water near an industrial site? A petrochemical plant?
Is there pesticide pollution?
Water quality of ponds, dams and pools
Exposure to algal blooms.

12. Air quality
Sources of indoor air pollution:
— combustion products (carbon monoxide, nitrogen dioxide, sulfur dioxide);
— household materials (volatile organic compounds, hydrocarbons, alcohols, ketones);
— moulds (indoor);
— allergens (cockroaches, dust mites);

— pets and other animals;
— environmental tobacco smoke;
— asbestos, polyurethane, flame-retardants;
— ventilation and air-conditioning.

Sources of outdoor air pollution:
— coal use, power generation, motor vehicles;
— haze (e.g. from forest fires);
— burning in the open;
— incinerators;
— waste sites;
— use of pesticides.

Types of pollutants: sulfur compounds, ozone, particulate matter, carbon monoxide, nitrogen dioxide, volatile organic compounds, lead, etc.

13. Food and diet

Is the child exposed to chemical food contaminants?
— pesticides and persistent organic pollutants;
— food additives and preservatives (colouring, flavouring and other agents added intentionally);
— breast milk contaminants;
— toxins (mycotoxins, pyrrolizidine alkaloids, aquatic microorganisms, toxins in fish and seafood);
— pathogens (viruses, bacteria, toxins, parasites);
— hormones;
— pesticides.

Are dietary supplements used, such as vitamins and minerals?
Is food genetically engineered?

14. Clothing and objects

Quality and materials of:
— plastic toys;
— wooden painted toys;
— furry toys;
— pacifiers;
— clothing (textiles, colour, flame retardants);
— diapers;
— school and art materials (paint, crayons).

Activities

15. Hobbies

Painting—paint and solvents used?
Model-building—glue and solvents used?
Pottery—pigments, paints used?

Gardening—pesticides used?
Woodwork—chemicals used?

16. Activities
Eating habits (type of diet, food quality).
Drinking habits (alcohol use and abuse, soft drinks)
Playing habits
Learning habits
Working habits
Scavenging (time spent near garbage)
Exploring
Testing (trying drugs, eating unknown berries, pica)

17. Sports
Type of sport
Sports area (see section 2)
Injuries (see section 23)
Toxic exposures (see section 24)
Use of energizing drugs, application of poultices?

Behaviour
18. Personal hygiene and habits
How often does the child bathe? How? Where? With what (type of soap/cleansing product)?
How often are the hands and face washed?
Are the clothes washed regularly?
What type of diapers are used?
Does the child have lice? How is the infestation treated?
Does the child play on the floor? Carpet?
How and how often is the child's bedroom and play area cleaned?
Which chemicals are used to clean the home?
Does the child have pica? Does the child have hand-to-mouth activities?

19. Cultural history
Use of alternative medicines or cosmetics
Cultural practices
Religious practices
Traditions involving the use of chemical substances.

20. Transport
What transport does the child use?
— individual or collective;
— bicycle;

— motorcycle;

— horse;

— other.

Characteristics of bus (street or school)? Bus stop? Characteristics of car, truck?

Vulnerability (during different periods of development)

21. Special vulnerability

Age: "windows of vulnerability"—*in utero*, postnatal period, toddler, infant, school-age, adolescence.

Previous diseases (respiratory, gastrointestinal, neurological, renal, hepatic, other).

Clinical effects

22. Specific health problems that may have an environmental cause or trigger

Asthma

Bronchitis, bronchiolitis

Pneumonia

Allergies

Immune disorders

Diarrhoea

Polyneuropathy

Attention deficit disorders

Learning disorders

Altered behaviour

Skin effects: neurodermatitis, eczema

Urinary infection

Early puberty

Cancer (brain, leukaemia, other)

Multiple chemical sensitivity syndrome

Sudden infant death syndrome

Poisoning (lead, mercury, pesticides, carbon monoxide) (see section 23)

Drug abuse, overdose

Silicosis

Arsenicosis

Fluorosis

Home accidents: lesions, sequelae

Malformations

Sterility in adolescents and young adults

Repeated abortions in adolescents and young adults

23. Accidents and injuries

Has the child suffered from the following?
- — Traffic-related injuries and diseases
- — Home accidents
- — Risk of drowning and water-related accidents
- — Exposure to fire and fumes; burns
- — Exposure to electricity
- — Sports-related injuries
- — Exposure to violence (in the home)
- — Animal bite (cat, dog, other).

24. Poisonings

Has the child been poisoned? When?
Was the poisoning accidental, intentional or occupational?
Was the exposure acute or low-level and chronic?
Where did it occur? (home, school, street, workplace, ...)
What was the cause?
- — pesticide (organophosphorus, organochlorine, rodenticide, herbicide, fungicide);
- — metal (lead, arsenic, mercury, cadmium, iron);
- — household product (solvent, kerosene, detergent);
- — pharmaceutical (analgesic, cough syrup, psychoactive drug, adulterated medicine);
- — drug abuse;
- — alcohol;
- — traditional medicine (herbal and other preparations).

25. Envenoming

Has the child been stung or bitten? When? Where?
- — snake
- — scorpion
- — spider
- — bee or wasp.

CHAPTER 19

The clinical environmental history: experience in the USA[1]

S. J. Balk
Children's Hospital, Montefiore, New York, USA

A child's surroundings—the physical environment—may have an impact on his or her health. Numerous chemical toxicants have been shown to affect children's health and development. Paediatricians and other clinicians who give medical care to infants, children and adolescents should enquire about the child's surroundings in order to uncover potential chemical and physical hazards, and to provide guidance about avoiding or reducing them. Questions about the child's environment should be an integral part of the routine health history, along with questions about nutrition, sleep, development, and injury prevention.

Paediatricians can include environmental health questions during routine health care visits (check-ups). In addition, when a child presents with symptoms of illness, clinicians should consider environmental etiologies as part of the differential diagnosis (1).

Integrating environmental health questions into the routine health visit

A few basic questions about the child's surroundings (the dwelling, child care setting or school setting) are integral to a complete health history. These are outlined below.

1: Where does the child live or spend time?

Children may spend time in their own home or the home of a child care provider or babysitter, and at school. Playtime may be spent in a playground. Infants and young children often spend 80–90% of their time indoors, either in their own home or in a child care (day-care) setting.

Important aspects of the indoor setting are described below.

Type of dwelling

Children generally live with their family in an individual home, apartment, or mobile home. In private homes, children may be exposed to lead or asbestos.

---

[1]Based on the *Handbook of Pediatric Environmental Health of the American Academy of Pediatrics*.

They may encounter radon in basements or the ground floor. Children living in mobile homes may be exposed to formaldehyde, a respiratory and dermal irritant commonly found in particle board and pressed wood materials used in these dwellings.

Age and condition of the dwelling

Homes and apartment buildings, especially those built many years ago, may contain lead paint. As paint ages, it may peel, flake or "chalk", particularly from poorly maintained surfaces and those that are subject to friction, such as windows. Young children may be exposed to deteriorated lead paint through normal hand-to-mouth activity. Homes that have been damaged by floods or leaks may have problems with growth of mould. Homes built to conserve energy ("tight" homes) may have poor ventilation, exposing occupants to high levels of indoor air pollutants.

Ongoing or planned renovation

Often parents renovate a room in preparation for the birth of a baby, or shortly after the baby's birth, possibly exposing the pregnant woman, or the infant, to lead or asbestos.

Sources and uses of heat

Parents may heat the home, fully or in part, using wood burned in a wood stove or fireplace. Respiratory irritants such as nitrogen dioxide (NO_2), particulates and polycyclic aromatic hydrocarbons are found in wood smoke. Children exposed to smoke may experience the onset or worsening of respiratory symptoms especially when there is poor ventilation or the stove or fireplace is poorly maintained.

Natural gas cooking stoves are used in over half of homes in the USA. Parents whose homes are inadequately heated may use the stove for supplemental heat in the winter, exposing children to nitrogen dioxide released during the combustion of natural gas.

Carbon monoxide (CO) may be released from improperly functioning stoves, fireplaces and furnaces, with potentially fatal results.

Pesticides

Pesticides may be used to control indoor infestations of insects such as ants and cockroaches. Outdoors, pesticides may be used to control insects, herbicides to control weeds and unwanted plants, and fungicides to control moulds. Children are exposed through inhalation, ingestion and dermal absorption of these chemicals as they crawl or play on treated surfaces. Health workers should determine whether parents use pesticides and similar products, make them aware of potential dangers, and encourage them to use safer methods of pest and weed control.

Outdoor environment—proximity to hazards in the community

Health workers should be aware of outdoor hazards in their community. Lakes and streams used for fishing may be contaminated with chemicals; children may play near contaminated dump sites and waste sites or be exposed to pesticides in fields. Renovations may result in the release of toxic contaminants.

Cultural uses of toxic materials

Health workers should take into account patients' cultural backgrounds. For example, some children from Central America may be exposed to elemental mercury, which is sprinkled in the home during a religious ritual performed by practitioners of Santeria.

School exposures

Pollutants may be present in school buildings, especially those that are old and deteriorating. Pollutants may be released during school renovations. In addition, children may be exposed to toxic materials during certain school activities, such as arts and crafts.

Populations particularly at risk

In the USA, certain communities may be disproportionately at risk for environmental exposures. These are likely to be members of ethnic minority groups and low-income populations. Because children are also disproportionately affected by environmental exposures (see Chapter 2), children from poor and minority groups may be the most affected by environmental toxicants. For example, in 1991–94, 10% of children under 6 years from low-income families had elevated blood lead levels (greater than 10 μg/dl), compared with 1% of children from high-income families; more than 11% of African-American children had elevated lead levels compared with 4% of Hispanic children and 2.3% of white non-Hispanic children (2).

Some ethnic minorities may be more exposed to certain contaminants in food because of dietary habits. For example, Native Americans and subsistence fishers are likely to be more exposed to contaminants in fish, such as mercury and polychlorinated biphenyls. Children of agricultural workers may be more exposed to pesticides, either directly in fields or brought home on parents' clothing and shoes.

2: Is the child exposed to environmental tobacco smoke through parental smoking? Is the child or teenager a smoker?

In the USA, over 40% of children aged between 2 months and 11 years live with a parent who smokes (3). Environmental tobacco smoke (ETS, or "second-hand smoke") comprises the smoke exhaled by the smoker ("mainstream smoke") and the smoke from the smouldering end of a cigarette, pipe or cigar ("sidestream smoke"). ETS is composed of more than 3800 chemical compounds. It contains fine particulates (less than 2.5μm in diameter, a size that reaches the lower airways) in concentrations that may be 2–3 times that of the outside air. ETS primarily affects the respiratory tract of children. Children exposed to ETS have higher rates of lower respiratory infections, more persistent middle-ear effusions, and more frequent and more severe asthma exacerbations. Infants exposed to ETS have a higher incidence of sudden infant death syndrome ("cot death"). Children whose parents smoke are more likely to become smokers themselves.

Paediatricians, or other physicians who care for children, can play an important role in counselling parents who smoke. They may be the only medical staff that parents visit regularly. Thus they have opportunities to help eliminate or decrease children's exposure to ETS by helping parents to quit smoking. The first step is to ask about smoking habits; these questions should become an integral part of the routine paediatric health history.

In 2000, the US Public Health Service published its clinical practice guideline, *Treating tobacco use and dependence*, which describes how even brief counselling (3 minutes or less) can be effective in increasing quit rates (4). A "5 As" approach ("ask, assess, advise, assist, arrange follow-up") is suggested:

- Paediatricians should *ask* parents about smoking habits.
- If parents smoke, paediatricians should *assess* willingness to quit smoking and should *advise* parents who smoke to quit.
- If the parents are willing, paediatricians should *assist* them by providing counselling and information about medications, such as nicotine replacement therapies (NRT).
- They should *arrange follow-up* for this issue on future visits; the issue should be addressed at every visit.

Pharmacotherapies, including NRT (such as nicotine patches and gum) and oral amfebutamone, have been shown to increase quit rates. Paediatricians should become familiar with these approaches in order to discuss them with parents.

All smokers should be encouraged to quit. It is important to ask about reasons for tobacco use (such as for energy, tactile sensation, because smoking is pleasurable, to relax, to relieve cravings, or because it is a habit) in order to suggest specific coping strategies. The paediatrician can then ask questions directed towards determining whether the smoker is ready to quit. These questions involve the "stages of change". In the *pre-contemplative phase*, the smoker talks about quitting in an abstract way, without having any plans to do so. In the *contemplative phase*, the smoker begins to seriously consider quitting within the next six months, but has no plans to quit, and has not had one tobacco-free day within the past year. In the *preparative phase*, the smoker plans to quit in the next 6 months, and has had a 24-hour quit attempt in the past year. Strategies appropriate to each phase have been summarized (4).

Some 90% of smokers begin to smoke as teenagers. The average smoker begins to smoke at age 12; 3000 children and adolescents in the USA begin smoking each day. Obtaining accurate smoking histories from children and teenagers is often more challenging than obtaining similar histories from adults. They may be reluctant to discuss smoking with paediatricians. Their concerns about maintaining confidentiality must be addressed. With children and young teenagers, a direct approach to questioning may be awkward; clinicians may first have to ask about other lifestyle matters, such as hobbies, sports activities and friends, before asking about smoking. It may help to ask first about the peer group—"Do any of your friends smoke?"—before asking directly if the patient smokes. For patients who are not yet smokers but have a favourable attitude towards smoking, clinicians can point out the influence of tobacco advertise-ments on young people, using magazines with cigarette advertisements as teaching aids. High school students usually have the capacity to understand the short-term and long-term health consequences of smoking. Short-term conse-quences include cough and sputum production; shortness of breath; reduced athletic performance; recurrent upper respiratory infections; stained teeth and fingers; bad breath; risk of fires; and exposing others, including younger sib-lings, to ETS. The cost of cigarettes may also serve as a deterrent to the teenage smoker (5).

Strategies adopted at the consultation can aid in history-taking and smoking cessation efforts. Such interventions include the following:

(1) *Systematic assessment of patient's or parent's smoking*: smoking status can be added as an item on the office intake form filled out by the parent or teenage patient. Office systems, such as tobacco-use status stickers or adding tobacco use as a vital sign, are helpful in reminding clinicians to gather this information.

(2) *Involving staff members in smoking cessation history-taking and education*: because cessation rates increase with the number of contacts a patient has with staff, the goal is to have all professionals, including receptionists, ask about smoking as part of the visit. Nurses and health educators can be a vital part of this effort.

(3) *Providing patient education materials*: materials are available free or at low cost from local affiliates of the American Cancer Society, American Heart Association, American Lung Association, and the National Cancer Institute's Cancer Information Service. Many agencies also provide self-help materials.

(4) *Utilizing local resources*: paediatricians can compile a list of local agencies or programmes to be given to motivated patients.

(5) *Office policy*: the office should have signs indicating that the office has a no-smoking policy. Staff should not smoke in or near the office. There should be no literature with pro-smoking messages in the waiting room.

3: Is tap water or well-water used?

Whether the supply of water is safe is generally well known locally. Most industrialized countries provide universal access to safe drinking-water. Many developing countries, however, do not have the necessary infrastructure and have not overcome the barriers to providing adequate supplies of safe water to their citizens. Often, water is safe in the cities but not in rural or periurban sites. In addition, even where water is considered safe, contamination, for example with lead and nitrates, is still a potential hazard. Paediatricians should enquire about the source of water. Tap water used to reconstitute infant formula, or given directly to the infant, may be contaminated with bacteria or chemicals, such as lead from pipes. To avoid possible contamination, parents can consider boiling water or testing it for specific contaminants. Alternatively, in the morning or whenever the water has been standing for hours in the pipes, parents may run the water for two minutes, or until cold, before giving it to an infant.

Well-water or water in rural sites, in particular, may be contaminated with high levels of nitrates, which may result in methaemoglobinaemia in young infants. Parents who use well-water should be advised to have the water tested for nitrates before using it to reconstitute infant formula.

Boiling water for one minute is sufficient to kill microorganisms. Over-boiling of water should be discouraged as this will concentrate contaminants such as lead and nitrates.

4: Is the child protected from excessive sun exposure?

The incidence of all skin cancers, including squamous cell carcinoma, basal cell carcinoma, and cutaneous malignant melanoma, has risen dramatically in the USA in recent years. The incidence is highest in persons with light skin and light eyes, those who burn easily rather than tan, and those living closer to the equator where the sun's rays are strongest. The ultraviolet (UV) spectrum of sunlight is implicated in the development of skin cancer. Squamous cell and basal cell carcinomas appear to be related to chronic cumulative sun exposure. Malignant melanoma is related to the occurrence of blistering sunburn in child-hood. As 80% of lifetime sun exposure occurs during the first 18 years of life, paediatricians should enquire about sun exposure in order to advise about preventive measures.

Prevention advice

(1) Avoid exposure. Young infants should be kept out of direct sunlight when-ever possible because of the possibility of heat stroke. Infants and children should be dressed in clothing that is cool and comfortable, such as light-

weight cotton shirts and trousers, which offer some protection. Lycra shirts, which let in little light, are gaining popularity in Australia, which has the world's highest incidence of melanoma. A hat with a brim, facing forwards, offers some protection for the face and eyes. For older children and adolescents, activities should be timed to avoid peak sun exposure hours (10h00 to 16h00).

(2) Consulting the Ultraviolet Index. The Ultraviolet (UV) Index was developed in 1994 by the US National Weather Service in consultation with the US Environmental Protection Agency and the Centers for Disease Control and Prevention. The UV Index predicts the intensity of UV light for the following day. The UV Index may be found in the weather section of newspapers, and is sometimes discussed during weather reports on the radio and television.

(3) Use sunscreen. Sunscreens prevent or diminish sunburn. There is controversy about the ability of sunscreens to prevent melanoma; some studies suggest that sunscreen use, by allowing increased time in the sun, increases the risk of melanoma. Nevertheless, using sunscreen with frequent reapplications is still recommended as part of a programme of sun avoidance for children and adults.

(4) Protect eyes. A hat with a brim can reduce exposure to UV by 50%. Sunglasses should be worn when the sun is strong enough to cause sunburn. Parents should choose sunglasses that block out 99% of UV rays.

5: Are there any hazards relating to occupation of adolescent or parent?
Parental occupations

Chemicals and dusts in the workplace may be brought into the home on parents' skin, clothes, shoes and belongings if the parent does not shower and change clothes at work. These substances may also contaminate cars. Pesticides may be brought home by agricultural workers. Lead poisoning has been described in children whose parents worked in the lead industry (6); elevated mercury levels were found in children whose parents were employed in a mercury thermometer plant (7); asbestos-related lung diseases, including fatal malignant mesothelioma, have been reported in family members of asbestos workers (8). Paediatricians should ask about mothers' and fathers' occupations (9). They should encourage parents employed in dangerous occupations to shower before leaving the work site and to leave potentially contaminated items there. In addition, children should not be allowed to play in areas where parents work with toxic substances, such as artists' paints that may contain lead or other harmful substances.

Employment among adolescents

Teenagers may be employed, allowing them to accumulate skills, earn money, and assume responsibility. More than 80% of high school students in the USA are employed as part of their normal schedule. These teenagers may be exposed to hazardous work conditions, including chemical exposures (10).

Many countries have established laws that regulate employment of children. These laws often set standards for minimum ages for employment, maximum daily and weekly work hours permissible, prohibition of certain types of work, prohibition of night work, and registration of minors for employment. Often, children must visit a physician to obtain a certificate of physical fitness before becoming employed. This provides the paediatrician with the opportunity to inquire about the nature of employment, whether paid or voluntary. In the informal sector, children work without such support and infrastructure. Questions about employment should also be part of the complete adolescent health history.

Children and teenagers should be asked about where they work, how many hours, and whether they are exposed to any chemicals, dusts or metals. Those with chronic illnesses may be susceptible to hazards in certain job situations (such as a previously well-controlled patient with asthma working as a server in a restaurant, whose condition is exacerbated after exposure to cigarette smoke in the restaurant).

Paediatricians should talk to parents about the potential risks and benefits of their child's employment. Parents may be unaware of the nature of the child's job, especially possible hazards.

How to understand children's medical history, the surroundings, and the link between observed effects and potential environmental causes

Because illnesses or symptoms may result from environmental exposures, health care workers should consider environmental etiologies in their differential diagnoses (Goldman, Shannon & Wolff, Personal Communication, 1999).

Asthma, upper respiratory symptoms and middle-ear effusion can result from exposure to environmental tobacco smoke. Asthma and allergies can result from exposure to certain indoor air pollutants. Recurrent abdominal pain, constipation, irritability, seizures and unexplained coma can result from lead poisoning. Headaches may be the result of acute or chronic exposure to carbon monoxide from improperly vented heating sources, formaldehyde, or chemicals. Idiopathic pulmonary haemorrhage in young infants has been linked to exposure to certain toxigenic moulds.

When faced with an illness or symptom that may have an environmental etiology, the health worker should give careful consideration to all aspects of the child's physical surroundings, incorporating the areas detailed in question 1 above. The environmental etiology of illness is not always obvious. For example, an 8-month-old girl with persistent hypertonicity was initially thought to have cerebral palsy. Her paediatrician, not satisfied with the diagnosis, discovered that her symptoms were related to chronic poisoning with diazinon, an organophosphorus insecticide that had been sprayed inside the home. Symptoms resolved when the family moved out of the home (11). In another instance, acrodynia (painful extremities, a syndrome in children associated with mercury exposure) was found to be associated with exposure to latex paint to which mercury had been added as a fungicide (12).

Symptoms may be nonspecific or common to other medical problems. A history of environmental exposure may be missed unless the clinician seeks a specific history (13). It is particularly important to obtain this history if the condition is not typical or is unresponsive to usual treatment. Questions should cover:

- **Location**: whether symptoms are worse or better in a particular location such as home, school or child care setting.
- **Time**: whether symptoms are worse or better at certain times, such as at weekends (when the child is at home), or during the week (when the child may be out of the home in a child care setting, school or work).
- **Particular activities**: symptoms may be worse when the child engages in a hobby or other activities that result in certain exposures.
- **Common symptoms**: whether other children or adults are experiencing similar symptoms, suggesting a common exposure.

References

1. Etzel RA, Balk SJ, eds. *The handbook of pediatric environmental health.* Elk Grove Village, IL, American Academy of Pediatrics, 1999.
2. Centers for Disease Control and Prevention. Update: blood lead levels—United States; 1991–1994. *Morbidity and Mortality Weekly Report*, 1997, 46:141–146.
3. Centers for Disease Control and Prevention. Strategies for reducing exposure to environmental tobacco smoke, increasing tobacco use cessation, and reducing initiation in communities and health care systems. *Morbidity and Mortality Weekly Report*, 2000, 49(RR12):1.
4. Treating tobacco use and dependence. A clinical practice guideline. *Journal of the American Medical Association*, 2000, 283:3244–3254.
5. Heymann RB. Tobacco: prevention and cessation strategies. *Adolescent Health Update*, 1997, 9:1–8.
6. Watson WN, Witherell LE, Giguerre GC. Increased lead absorption in children of workers in a lead storage battery plant. *Journal of Occupational Medicine*, 1978, 20:759–761.
7. Hudson PJ et al. Elemental mercury exposure among children of thermometer plant workers. *Pediatrics*, 1987, 79:935–938.
8. Kilburn KH et al. Asbestos disease in family contacts of shipyard workers. *American Journal of Public Health*, 1985, 75:615–617.
9. Chisolm JJ. Fouling one's own nest. *Pediatrics*, 1978, 62:614–617.

10. Pollack S et al. Pesticide exposure and working conditions among migrant farm-worker children in western New York State. *1990 American Public Health Association Annual Meeting Abstracts*: 317.

11. Wagner SL, Orwick DL. Chronic organophosphate exposure associated with transient hypertonia in an infant. *Pediatrics*, 1994, 94:94–97.

12. Centers for Disease Control and Prevention. Mercury exposure from interior latex paint. *Morbidity and Mortality Weekly Report*, 1990, 39:125.

13. Agency for Toxic Substances and Disease Registry. *Case studies in environmental medicine: taking an exposure history.* Atlanta, GA, US Department of Health and Human Services, 1992.

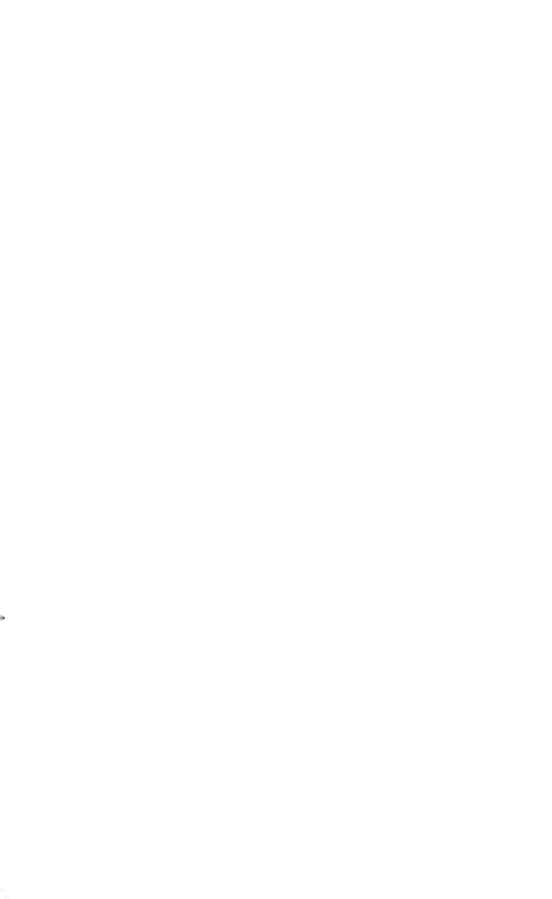

CHAPTER 20

Taking action to protect children from environmental hazards[1]

S. Boese-O'Reilly
Children's Environmental Health Professional, Munich,
Germany

M. K. E. Shimkin
MShimkin Consulting, Alexandria, USA

In protecting children's environmental health, every level has a role to play, from members of the family and community to local, regional, national and international bodies. Everyone has a part in offering children the best chances in life, and in making a difference in how they live, grow, play, learn, develop and eventually work and become productive members of society. While note-worthy accomplishments at all levels reach a variety of people, much remains to be done to sustain progress and intensify change. Certain countries have leapt into action while others hardly know of the concern. Global movements will narrow gaps between countries in the level of effort and involve progres-sively more regions of the world, enhancing opportunities for children in all countries to have healthy and productive lives.

Families, carers and teachers

Parents, child care providers and teachers can make a tremendous differ-ence in the health of children through actions at home, in the child care setting and at school. These adults can provide role models for healthy behaviour and teach and guide children to create healthy environments. Efforts to motivate teachers in Chinese schools to refrain from smoking, for example, have improved the quality of indoor air in the schools and may influence children not to smoke. "Tools for Schools" is a programme in the USA that teaches children, teachers and administrative staff to conduct indoor air audits in schools and take action to remedy sources of pollution. In Australia, many schools are joining the SunSmart Schools Program, which involves the whole school com-munity in protecting children from overexposure to the sun. Parents, child care providers and teachers can find success acting alone or with others to improve

[1]Reviewed by **M. Berger**, Office of Children's Health Protection, Environmental Protection Agency (EPA), Washington, DC, USA; **I. Corra**, Asociación Argentina de Medicos por el Medio Ambiente (AAMMA), Buenos Aires, Argentina; **J. Pronczuk**, Department for the Pro-tection of the Human Environment, World Health Organization, Geneva, Switzerland.

children's environmental health. Individual and local level effort will make a difference for children and may have greater impact than anticipated.

Ideas for action at the local level

The United States Environmental Protection Agency has developed "Tips to protect children from environmental risks" (1), which have been disseminated through doctor's offices, schools and on the Internet. These are practical, action-oriented steps that parents and carers can take to protect children. Any individual or group could develop similar tips and share them as part of a community education effort, focusing on local issues of greatest concern for children's well-being. WHO has put together messages for creating healthy environments for children as shown in Fig. 20.1 (2).

Tips to protect children from environmental risks[a]
Help children breathe easier
- Don't smoke and don't let others smoke in your home or car.
- Keep your home as clean as possible. Dust, mould, certain household pests, second-hand smoke, and pet dander can trigger asthma attacks and allergies.
- Limit outdoor activity on "ozone alert" days when air pollution is especially harmful.
- Walk, use bicycles, join or form carpools, and take public transportation.
- Limit motor vehicle idling.
- Avoid open burning.

Protect children from lead poisoning
- Get kids tested for lead by their doctor or health care provider.
- Test your home for lead paint hazards if it was built before 1978.
- Wash children's hands before they eat; wash bottles, pacifiers, and toys often.
- Wash floors and window sills to protect kids from dust and peeling paint contaminated with lead—especially in older homes.
- Run the cold water for at least 30 seconds to flush lead from pipes.

Keep pesticides and other toxic chemicals away from children
- Store food and trash in closed containers to keep pests from coming into your home.
- Use baits and traps when you can; place baits and traps where kids can't get them.
- Read product labels and follow directions.
- Store pesticides and toxic chemicals where kids can't reach them—never put them in other containers that kids can mistake for food or drink.
- Keep children, toys, and pets away when pesticides are applied; don't let them play in fields, orchards, and gardens after pesticides have been used for at least the time recommended on the pesticide label.
- Wash fruits and vegetables under running water before eating—peel them before eating, when possible.

Box continued
Protect children from carbon monoxide (CO) poisoning
- Have fuel-burning appliances, furnace fluids, and chimneys checked once a year.
- Never use gas ovens or burners for heat; never use barbecues or grills indoors or in the garage.
- Never sleep in rooms with un-vented gas or kerosene space heaters.
- Don't run cars or lawnmowers in the garage.
- Install a CO alarm that meets UL, IAS, or Canadian standards in sleeping areas.

Protect children from contaminated fish and polluted water
- Be alert for local fish advisories and beach closings. Contact your local health department.
- Take used motor oil to a recycling centre; properly dispose of toxic household chemicals.
- Learn what's in your drinking-water—call your local public water supplier for annual drinking water quality reports; for private drinking-water wells, have them tested annually by a certified laboratory. Call 1-800-426-4791 or contact www.epa.gov/safewater for help.

Safeguard children from high levels of radon
- Test your home for radon with a home test kit.
- Fix your home if your radon level is 4 pCi/L or higher. For help, call your state radon office or 1-800-SOS-RADON.

Protect children from too much sun
- Wear hats, sunglasses, and protective clothing.
- Use sunscreen with SPF 15+ on kids over six months; keep infants out of direct sunlight.
- Limit time in the midday sun—the sun is most intense between 10 and 4.

Keep children and mercury apart
- Eat a balanced diet but avoid fish with high levels of mercury.
- Replace mercury thermometers with digital thermometers.
- Don't let kids handle or play with mercury.
- Never heat or burn mercury.
- Contact your state or local health or environment department if mercury is spilled—never vacuum a spill.

[a]Developed by the US Environmental Protection Agency.

Figure 20.1 Messages for creating healthy environments for children (WHO)

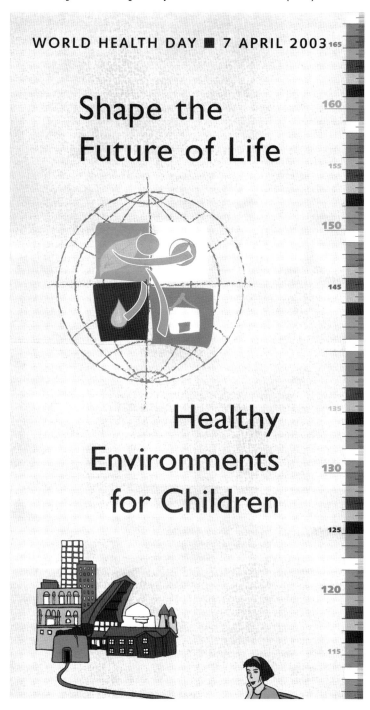

Figure 20.1 Continued

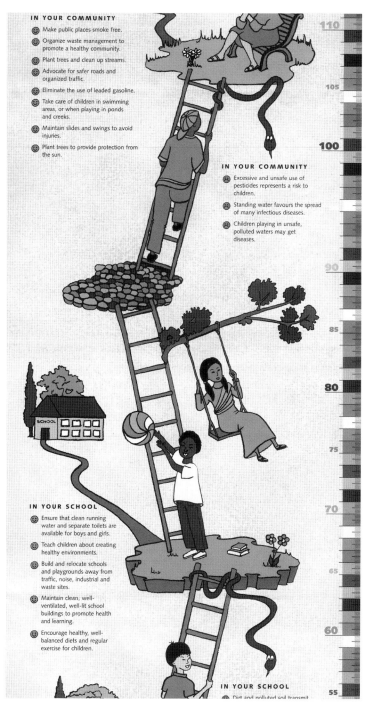

IN YOUR COMMUNITY

- Make public places smoke free.
- Organize waste management to promote a healthy community.
- Plant trees and clean up streams.
- Advocate for safer roads and organized traffic.
- Eliminate the use of leaded gasoline.
- Take care of children in swimming areas, or when playing in ponds and creeks.
- Maintain slides and swings to avoid injuries.
- Plant trees to provide protection from the sun.

IN YOUR COMMUNITY

- Excessive and unsafe use of pesticides represents a risk to children.
- Standing water favours the spread of many infectious diseases.
- Children playing in unsafe, polluted waters may get diseases.

IN YOUR SCHOOL

- Ensure that clean running water and separate toilets are available for boys and girls.
- Teach children about creating healthy environments.
- Build and relocate schools and playgrounds away from traffic, noise, industrial and waste sites.
- Maintain clean, well-ventilated, well-lit school buildings to promote health and learning.
- Encourage healthy, well-balanced diets and regular exercise for children.

IN YOUR SCHOOL

- Dirt and polluted soil transmit

110
105
100
90
85
80
75
70
65
60
55

Figure 20.1 Continued

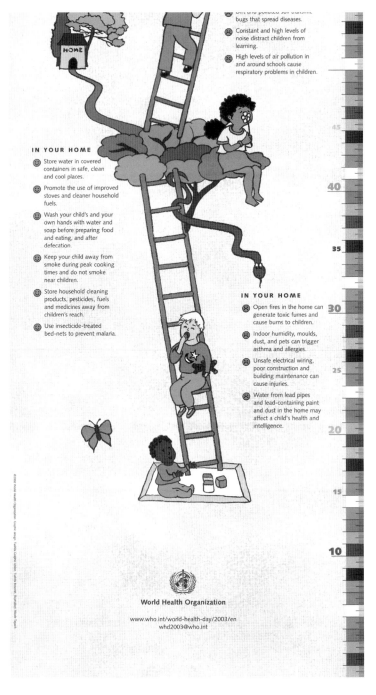

- Dirt and polluted soil transmit bugs that spread diseases.
- Constant and high levels of noise distract children from learning.
- High levels of air pollution in and around schools cause respiratory problems in children.

IN YOUR HOME

- Store water in covered containers in safe, clean and cool places.
- Promote the use of improved stoves and cleaner household fuels.
- Wash your child's and your own hands with water and soap before preparing food and eating, and after defecation.
- Keep your child away from smoke during peak cooking times and do not smoke near children.
- Store household cleaning products, pesticides, fuels and medicines away from children's reach.
- Use insecticide-treated bed-nets to prevent malaria.

IN YOUR HOME

- Open fires in the home can generate toxic fumes and cause burns to children.
- Indoor humidity, moulds, dust, and pets can trigger asthma and allergies.
- Unsafe electrical wiring, poor construction and building maintenance can cause injuries.
- Water from lead pipes and lead-containing paint and dust in the home may affect a child's health and intelligence.

World Health Organization

www.who.int/world-health-day/2003/en
whd2003@who.int

Communities and local governments

Enforcement of environmental regulations, housing initiatives, school and hospital administration, disease surveillance and reporting, and other public services usually fall within the jurisdiction of local governments, offering many opportunities to make communities "child friendly" in the environmental health context. Local governments often serve as first-line response to environmental incidents and are the key communicators with the general public. Not only are they responsible for communicating about risk and public safety, they also are the intermediaries between national policymakers and citizens. They can take proactive and preventive steps by promoting community events, sponsoring poison control centres, and creating innovative ways to educate and protect the public, especially children.

National governments

The words of a head of state can generate attention, political will and funding. National governments can gear environmental protection systems and structures to improve children's environmental health, supporting decentralized initiatives and working to formulate regulations and comply with national mandates. National governments are the ultimate champions for children's environmental health, and should monitor it through data collection and analysis. They should support communication and national public awareness efforts, pilot actions, specific projects and more. In addition, national govern-

Community meetings lead to reduction in childhood asthma

Particulate matter and harmful fumes are by-products of the combustion process used in foundries that melt scrap iron. Residents of Sandwell, an urban area in the United Kingdom, became concerned about the respiratory health of their children, who attended schools close to such a foundry, and organized a public meeting to discuss the issue. The resulting measures taken by the foundry management led to a significant reduction in asthma-related hospital admissions of schoolchildren in the area (Case Study 19, page 342).

The G8 Declaration 1997

The United States Environmental Protection Agency ushered children's environmental health into the international arena, through its insistence on the importance of children's environmental health for discussion by environment leaders of the group of eight highly industrialized countries (G-8) in 1997. With the unanimous adoption of the Declaration of the Environment Leaders of the Eight on Children's Environmental Health, the world took notice that children, both in developing and industrialized countries, could be at more risk from environmental threats than had previously been assumed. Not only did the Declaration help focus the G-8 national governments on improving policies and efforts within their own borders, it also inspired other international bodies to call for actions to protect children's environmental health, heightening the awareness of other country leaders.

ments should contribute to international efforts that spread the message beyond their borders, promote collaboration and strengthen the agenda at home.

International and global efforts

Over recent years, the international agenda has given considerable attention to children's environmental health, setting a framework for action by individuals and entities worldwide. Recent examples of progress on the international front include the following:

- At the World Summit on Sustainable Development in Johannesburg, South Africa, September 2002, the World Health Organization called for a global movement to improve children's environmental health, motivating countries, United Nations agencies and non-governmental organizations to create a "mass movement for children's environmental health". The organization has since taken steps to form a global Healthy Environments for Children Alliance to support countries as they strive to improve children's environmental health through national and local efforts (2). WHO programmes and regional offices have begun facilitating regional and national efforts to improve children's environmental health (5).
- The Commission for Environmental Cooperation of North America adopted an agenda for action on children's health and environment in June 2002 (4).
- In May 2002, the United Nations convened a General Assembly Special Session on children, which hosted side events on children's environmental health and resulted in a document that stressed the environment as an integral element of child health and welfare (5).
- Countries of South-East Asia and the Western Pacific were addressed by the International Conference on Children's Environmental Health: Hazards and Vulnerability, which took place in Bangkok, Thailand, in March 2002, resulting in the Bangkok Statement: a pledge to promote the protection of children's environmental health (see Chapter 1). The Statement urged the World Health Organization to support efforts in the region to improve children's environmental health.
- The United Nations Millennium Development Goals published in September 2001 called for a two-thirds decrease in the under-five mortality rate by 2015, which will require action to reduce illness and death from diarrhoeal disease and acute respiratory infections, two leading environment-related causes of death worldwide.
- The Budapest Conference held in 2004 focused on "the future of our children" and adopted, through its Declaration, a children's environmental and health action plan for Europe (CEHAPE).

　　　　　　　　　　　　　　SECTION V: TAKING ACTION

Ready . . . set . . . go!

From very small, local, community-based steps to dramatic international accords, children's environmental health continues to gain momentum, expand its audience and increase in significance. There is growing recognition that environmental health is both a right of children and the basis for sustainable development. Simple actions can improve the lives of children and give them the best possible opportunities.

With the goals of increasing public awareness, defining the roles and responsibilities of health professionals, and achieving government buy-in and policy change, four action areas have been defined: communication, education, advocacy and research. Efforts to inform people about children's environmental health have tremendous potential. As people become more informed, health professionals will need more knowledge to answer their questions. As health professional training changes to incorporate the recognition and management of environmental exposures and the particular vulnerabilities of children, health workers will add to the awareness and information sources of parents and of children themselves. As the competence of health professionals increases, they will begin to identify gaps in knowledge and research needs, make recommendations to policy-makers, and advocate for change to protect health and prevent disease. As people become more informed and health professionals more vocal, government officials will set policies that protect children from environmental harm. As governments champion country efforts, national movements will start that will serve to raise public awareness and improve professional education. Action targeted to any of these areas will result in positive effects all around.

Communication and public awareness

Communication and public awareness efforts involve a broadly based approach to inform people of all ages and functions, from children to heads of state, leading to an increased understanding of the importance of protecting children from environmental harm. Internet resources are powerful mechanisms to facilitate information exchange, allowing participation of individuals, communities and national groups in global efforts. Both formal and informal actions to raise public awareness have proven successful.

Education

Actions in the area of education aim to increase the competence of health professionals, especially those dealing with children. They need to learn how to recognize and manage the health effects of environmental exposures, and to break the cycle of exposure, illness, treatment and re-exposure. Physicians, nurses, midwives and other health professionals are in the front line of children's environmental health, and can use their clinical experience, scientific expertise and research efforts to work closely with children of all ages, their parents, families and carers. Increasing competence of health professionals in children's environmental health can have significant influence, leading to greater public understanding and awareness, improved diagnosis and treatment of environmentally related diseases, and extended advocacy efforts to promote policies that protect environmental health. The general outline of courses offered by WHO is presented in the box below.

Children's environmental health for health care provider
Contents of a training course

1. New knowledge on the vulnerability of children to environmental hazards
  a Why are children more vulnerable than adults?
  b The developing child and the effects of neurotoxicants (lead, mercury, manganese, PCBs)
  c Lung development and the effects of environmental pollutants
  d Vulnerability to pesticides: new data and growing concern
  e Genes as a target for environmental toxicants, malnutrition, micronutrients and toxic effects (including methylmercury, arsenic)
  f The effects of UV radiation on eyes, skin and the immune system
  g Other examples.

2. How, when and where does exposure occur? Environmental threats in specific settings and circumstances, *in utero* and during childhood and adolescence: "children growing in an adult-size world"
  a The poor home: particular risks (shanty towns); living near waste sites; polluted urban areas; rural areas; street children; parental exposure
  b Where the child plays: playgrounds (outdoors, indoors); recreational areas; hobbies
  c Where the child learns: child care centres; schools
  d Where the child works: cottage industry; factory; rural areas; street vendors; domestic workers; scavengers
  e Where the child is especially stressed: extreme and adverse climatic conditions (e.g. mountains, hot and cold weather); environmental and technological disasters (floods and droughts); war; conflict and postconflict circumstances; refugee camps
  f Exposure of parents: transgenerational effects.

3. Understanding the main environmental threats and setting the priorities for action
  a Access to safe drinking-water and sanitation
  b Indoor air pollution: open fireplaces indoors, environmental tobacco smoke (parents); solvents; moulds; pet dander; other
  c Ambient air pollution and the health of children from rural and urban areas: sulfur dioxide (SO_2); nitrogen oxides (NO_x); diesel fumes; fine particulate matter; lead; benzene; open burning (waste and other); other
  d Asthma and other respiratory diseases in children: role of the environment

e   Traffic-related paediatric pathology. Giving priority to children in township develop-
    ment planning: "child-size traffic". Rural traffic accidents
f   Non-intentional, intentional and environmental toxic exposures
g   Exposure to pesticides: acute and chronic effects
h   Endocrine disrupters
i   Drugs of abuse
j   The working child
k   Lifestyle changes influencing housing, transport and children's social surroundings

4. Assessing the global burden of environmental threats to the health of children

a   The concept of global environmental burden of disease (GEBD) in children
b   Harmonized procedures, tools and methodologies; guidance for assessing the GEBD
    in children; indicators of children's environmental health
c   Information available in developing and industrialized countries/regions; national
    profiles
d   Priorities identified (incl. main controversial issues)

5. Controversial issues, dilemmas and knowledge gaps in the area of children's environmental health (CEH)

a   The risks of living near hazardous waste sites, landfills and open burnings
b   Asthma: the contribution of indoor and outdoor environments
c   The potential effects of climate change (emerging infectious diseases and climate
    refugees)
d   Noise, hearing loss and other health effects in children
e   What is known about endocrine disrupters and CEH?
f   Cancer and environmental factors: how much do we know?
g   Birth defects, reproductive disorders and environmental factors
h   Is there a "safe" blood lead and mercury level in children?
i   The potential effects of exposure to low chronic radiation levels and electromagnetic
    fields
j   Problems posed by cyanobacteria in water and other contaminants
k   Parental exposure

6. Ensuring the appropriate risk assessment in developing children

a   Setting environmental guidelines and standards.
b   Considering variability in exposure and response
c   Critical windows of exposure
d   Special consideration of developmental effects
e   Cumulative toxicity/mixtures, multiple exposures
f   Recommendations for improved methodologies for exposure assessment and deter-
    mining health effects

7. Incorporating CEH issues in the work of child health professionals

a Recognizing the links between paediatric morbidity and environmental threats in the micro- and macroenvironments of children

b Clinical observations: harmonized case data collection and analysis

c Taking the paediatric environmental history: from symptoms to etiology to prevention

d Detecting emerging diseases and signals of environmental illness in the community

e Reporting and publishing observations

f Undertaking research studies

g Evidence-based interventions: illustrative cases

h Communicating with parents, teachers, the community, media, local authorities and decision-makers

Advocacy and public policy

These activities aim to improve the state of the environment and target policies towards children's health, so that local, regional and national governments act to improve both the environment and the health of children and those around them. In many countries, governments lead the effort. In other countries, policy-makers react to public and professional demands. All levels of society can advocate for children's environmental health and influence policy agendas. A global effort to develop children's environmental health indicators is under way, coordinated by the World Health Organization and the United Nations Children's Fund (UNICEF). Indicators of children's environmental health offer a tool to policy-makers for determining priorities and measuring progress towards set goals. Governments have the opportunity to join the global initiative on children's environmental health indicators by contacting WHO or UNICEF.

Research

Promotion of collaborative research in children's environmental health in developing and developed countries is essential if problems are to be addressed in their national and global contexts. The results of appropriate studies can be used in strategies for prevention, intervention, and remedial action, and as a foundation for evidence-based public health policies in countries. Collaborative activities would also result in technology transfer and capacity building, and in the development of a network of trained scientific collaborators throughout the developing world.

National profiles and indicators

WHO has developed indicators of children's health and the environment and other tools to assist countries in assessing the status of children's health and determining the readiness of governments to effect change. A format for doing rapid assessments that may help countries to prepare their national strategies is shown in the box below.

Outline for preparing national profiles on the status of children's environmental health

NOTE: please use the boxed headings as subheadings in the country/local profile you develop. Use the questions proposed as a guide for obtaining and collating information and developing an overall assessment of each area. These questions are intended to provide some orientation on the type of information that is relevant for assessing the status of children's health and the environment. Develop up to three paragraphs for each of the underlined headings, expanding even beyond the questions provided, as deemed necessary. Please take into account for each question the potential gender, rural/urban, cultural and ethnicity issues. Tables necessary to make a point can be annexed. The profiles should cover both existing situations, observations and ongoing activities as well as potential opportunities for actions that could be implemented at the country level. Profiles should be dated: once the **initial** profile is done, successive ones may be prepared on an annual basis to assess progress made and/or changes observed concerning the status of children's health and the environment in the country.

INTRODUCTION

Overview of children's environmental health in the country

Provide a general synopsis of the country's views and position on children's environmental health, for example, the awareness level of government officials (especially in the health and environment sectors) and the acceptance of this as a distinct issue.

Key environmental issues

WHO lists the following key environmental risks for children: unsafe water, air pollution (indoor/outdoor), poor food hygiene, poor sanitation and inadequate waste disposal, vector-borne diseases and exposure to chemicals (agrochemicals, industrial chemicals, persistent toxic substances, natural toxins and other). In addition, children's health is endangered by other environmental risk factors, such as: poor housing, environmental degradation and the the so-called "emerging" threats (e.g. global climate change, ozone depletion, radiation, exposure to endocrine-disrupting compounds, and others). Prioritize these for your country according to the impact they have on children's health, development and well-being. Add areas of focus if necessary. Propose a prioritized list of environmental concerns for children's health in your country.

Key causes of infant and under-five mortality/morbidity

This information is normally readily available from WHO websites or in the WHO representations in the country. List the top five causes of illness and death for children under one, for children five and under, for children up to 14 and for children as a whole. As the age groups of children vary somewhat from country to country, please define the age group that you are reporting (e.g. some use 18 and under, some 20 and under).

Burden of disease related to environment in children

WHO has some information available on its website (www.who.int/phe/health-topics, search for "environmental burden of disease") and at the WHO representation. WHO reports that environmental threats may cause up to one-third of the global burden of disease. What does the country report? Are there any significant differences between boys and girls or between rural and urban children? Has this issue been addressed at the country level or does it remain to be done?

ECONOMIC STATUS AND ETHNIC GROUPS

Economic spread between poorest and wealthiest

What is the percentage share of income or consumption for the wealthiest 10% of the population? What is the percentage share of income or consumption for the poorest 10% of the population?

Information on high risks/vulnerable groups and demographic profile of countries

Provide the approximate numbers or percentages of each ethnic population group in your country and the geographic areas they occupy. To what extent are environment and health statistics or any other statistics routinely desegregated by socioeconomic status or ethnicity? Do national environmental or other sectoral policies make specific reference to ethnic groups or to groups that are geographically isolated? Is there any evidence of the impact of ethnicity or socioeconomic status on the burden of disease related to environmental threats? Are there any activities on ethnic minorities (and their children) undertaken by international institutions or nongovernmental organizations to which an environment and health component might be added?

NATIONAL GOVERNMENT ROLE

National policies

Are there specific national policies or stated priorities that support the protection of children's environmental health? Are there specific national policies or stated priorities that seem to run counter to the objectives of increasing protection of children from environmental threats (e.g. lax pesticide or toxic chemical regulations, persistence of lead in gasoline despite the proven health benefits of removing it)?

Health sector

How does the health sector address environmental health in general and children's environmental health specifically? Is there legislation to protect public health from environmental hazards and is this legislation well-implemented? Is there any action to protect vulnerable sub-populations or children in particular? Are the medical, nursing and health-care professional communities informed and/or trained on environmental threats to human and—more specifically—on children's health? Are there health facilities that promote environmental health or children's environmental health? Describe the differences in approaches to environmental health in rural and urban settings. In the specific area of chemicals, is there a Poisons Centre in your country or a toxicology or other unit that deals with toxic exposures in children? Where are poisoned children seen and treated? Are chronic, low-level exposures to chemicals in children being considered? Has any action been taken concerning the potential effects of persistent toxic substances (and POPs)?

Environment sector

Discuss the country's environmental legislation and its level of enforcement. Is human health considered by the environmental legislation and/or is protecting human health part of the mandate of the environment ministry? Are there any specific considerations concerning children? Are specific media, such as water, air, soil, food, or chemical safety covered by environmental legislation? If so, list which media are covered and list any gaps. Does the environment ministry coordinate well with other ministries, such as health or education and, if so, which ones? Has the country signed the international conventions/treaties dealing with toxic chemicals/pollutants (e.g. The Stockholm Convention on Persistent Organic Pollution, The Basel Convention on the Control of Transboundary Movements of Hazardous Wastes and their Disposal, and The Rotterdam Convention for Prior Informed Consent)? Have the actions taken in the context of these conventions/treaties considered the potential impact on children's environmental health?

Education

What is the level of literacy in the country? How many children go to school, and up to what levels? Is attendance in the schools required up to a certain age? Are there differences in male/female school attendance? For elementary school and for high school, what are the opportunities for health and environmental education? Is there an environmental or a health curriculum taught in these grade levels? If so, are these taught in both rural and urban schools? Would environmental health education through elementary schools be possible and/or acceptable in the school systems?

Other pertinent ministry/sector

If applicable, list other pertinent ministries or governmental agencies that deal with children's health and the environment (e.g. in certain countries some of the environmental issues may be regulated through the ministries of agriculture, industry, youth, social well-being or others). In many countries there are ministries of culture, science, education, welfare, and family and youth that may play a role in the protection of children's environmental health. What are the ministries or agencies at the national government level which would play a role in implementing a national action plan on children's environmental health? List and describe the role they play.

Communities

Do the governmental units at the community level (e.g. county seats, communal or city governments) play a role in the protection of environmental human health—and more specifically—children's environmental health? If not, what role could they play, or might they take, at a local level to better protect children from environmental threats? Do they have the ability to pass local legislation? Are they charged with enforcing national legislation? Could they be encouraged to carry out public information campaigns on children's environmental health?

Nongovernmental organizations (NGOs)

Do NGOs play a strong role in building stakeholder input and public participation? What are the key NGOs (both national and international) involved in activities aiming at the protection of children's environmental health, organizing national campaigns on children's environmental health or promoting children's chemical safety? If none has been doing this, which one could eventually be interested in this area? What roles might they play?

Professional associations

Do professional associations play a strong role in building stakeholder input and public participation? What are the key professional associations (both national and international) that would become involved in children's environmental health? (e.g. paediatric, medical, toxicological, family doctors, occupational medicine, nursing, primary health care, and any other societies). What roles might they play?

Academia

What academic institutions (e.g. academies, post-graduate schools) could promote children's environmental health through research, advocacy, publications, medical education (of medical and postgraduate students and continuing medical education), development/use of children's environmental history taking, and development/use of indicators? What role would each play?

Private sector

Are there any private companies that would likely be interested in promoting the safety and health of children in the country? For example, pharmaceutical, hygiene and cosmetic products companies, agricultural chemical companies, water companies, food and beverage producers? What roles could the private sector take—considering after all ethical aspects involved—in the different areas (e.g. financing activities, public advertisements, educational campaigns, or advocating in favour of national legislation)?

SCIENCE

State of the science in the country (in relation to children's environmental health)

Has anyone in the country conducted research and published results on topics related to environmental health or children's environmental health (e.g. on the risk factors mentioned above, on children's settings, on specific topics such as chemical safety and poisonings)? Name the country's science ministry or unit in the government that conducts research and publishes findings. Is environment or health legislation based on scientific findings?

Capabilities to conduct research

What institutions promote science and research in the country? Does the national government invest in research and development? What type of scientific publications are released in the country? Is financing available to support research at universities, hospitals, laboratories or other facilities? Which institutions would most likely be interested in research on children's environmental health?

Research needs

List the top priority research needs around the topic of children's environmental health in the country. Is research on these topics under way? Are there barriers to conduct this research and, if so, what would help overcome the barriers? What are the needs? What are the top three ways in which an international organization or other countries or organizations could support research?

DATA AND REPORTING

Information systems and centres

Does the country have a centralized information gathering function on children's health data (e.g. health surveillance system, clinical case recording)? Does the country have national or private information centres, for example on health, demographics or environment? Does the country require reporting of certain paediatric diseases to support public health surveillance and disease prevention and, if so, how is that information gathered and where? Are there poison control centres in the country and, if so, do they record incoming and outgoing information in a harmonized manner? Does the country report indicators on environment or health? Does the country put out regular reports on disease, public health or environmental conditions? If so, how are they accessed by the public?

Data quality

The WHO national offices are most likely involved in data gathering on health, and local UNICEF and UNDP offices probably work on information collection systems, as well. Do these offices judge data quality as good enough to be useful and representative? Are there other entities that collect data on health, environment or status of children in the country? Can the national work on Millennium Development Goals help to clarify and address barriers to data quality in the country?

COMMUNICATION

Avenues of communication

What are the most effective means for disseminating information in the country (e.g. television, radio, newspaper, and role-playing)? Are these the same for both rural and urban settings? If not, list by rural and urban. What are the most effective means for communications through schools, adult literacy programmes, country or local governments? Are there other innovative means of communication, for example through local libraries, street theatres, radio/TV educational "soap operas", fairs or other local events?

Success stories in communication
Do you know of any local success stories in widespread communication on important topics related to health and the environment? (e.g. use of radio-based literacy programmes targeting children in rural areas may increase adult and child literacy and lead to a decrease in child agricultural workers and improve matriculation in rural schools). Could these successes be repeated, this time carrying a message for children's environmental health?

CONCLUSION

Summary of the country status of children's environmental health and opportunities for action
Given your findings, in a page or less, summarize your assessment of the country's potential, capacity and interest to take action to improve the environmental health of its children. What specific actions in this area are recommended? What are the areas/issues for natural success? What are the areas/issues where urgent actions are required? What are the key barriers or areas that need to be addressed to achieve success? Who (individuals and organizations) are the key players?

Annexes. Please provide any samples of useful or illustrative materials, such as educational, awareness building, information gathering, data collection forms, educational programmes, photographs, maps, charts, other.

A special invitation for nongovernmental organizations

Nongovernmental organizations (NGOs) have excellent opportunities to promote awareness of environmental hazards to children. They can use radio, television, newspaper advertisements, street theatre, health fairs, and other innovative ways to improve public awareness, increase training for health care professionals, enhance access to information and advocate better policies. The information era affords enormous potential to broadcast messages, reaching urban and rural areas alike. Religious leaders can also have a strong impact, reaching receptive audiences who want to take actions that benefit children.

Many NGOs actively promote activities that support the environment, from nature conservation to sustainable development, but there are relatively few in the field of environmental health or environmental medicine, particularly dealing with the special vulnerability of children. Two organizations that have reacted to the realization that children are particularly susceptible to environmental risks are the International Society of Doctors for the Environment (ISDE; www.isde.org) and the International Network for Children's Health and Environmental Safety (INCHES; www.inchesnetwork.net). Some countries have national networks for children's environmental health, such as the United States Children's Environmental Health Network (CEHN; www.cehn.org), the Canadian Institute for Child Health (CICH; www.cich.ca) and the German Network for Children's Health and Environment (www.kinder-agenda.de). The web sites of these national networks are rich in information resources and links.

Conclusion

Pollution and other environmental threats do not recognize borders. Action is required at all levels: even local, community-based activities may end up having great influence around the world. The history of children's environmental health demonstrates how local actions may have a global impact: a non-governmental organization with a clear mission convinces a minister of environment, who motivates an international declaration, boosting children's environmental health into the mainstream international agenda. Not only do actions at the different levels affect those in the immediate area, they also create energy for public good with worldwide benefits. Everyone at every level can do something to improve children's environmental health and advance sustainable development while contributing to the health, increased productivity and well-being of children around the globe.

References

1. *Tips to protect children from environmental risks.* US Environmental Protection Agency, 2004 (http://yosemite.epa.gov/ochp/ochpweb.nsf/content/tips).
2. *Healthy environments for children alliance.* Geneva, World Health Organization, 2003 (http://www.who.int/heca/en/).
3. Children's environmental health. Geneva, World Health Organization, 2004 (http://www.who.int/ceh/en).
4. Commission for Environmental Cooperation of North America. *Cooperative agenda for children's health and the environment in North America.* Montreal, 2002 (http://www.cec.org/files/pdf/POLLUTANTS/Children_coop_agenda-en.pdf).
5. *A world fit for children.* New York, United Nations, 2002 (http://www.unicef.org/specialsession/wffc/index.html).

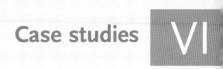
Case studies VI

CHAPTER 21

Case studies

1. THIOMERSAL IN CHILDREN'S VACCINES— THE RESPONSE OF THE UNITED STATES

C. J. Clements

Expanded Programme on Immunization, Department of Vaccines and Biologicals, World Health Organization, Geneva, Switzerland

Thiomersal is an organic mercurial compound that has been used for over 60 years as an antimicrobial agent in vaccines and other pharmaceutical products to prevent unwanted bacterial and fungal growth in the opened vaccine vial. When vials contain multiple doses of vaccine, the rubber stopper has to be punctured several times to withdraw doses; the liquid vaccine is thus exposed to the possibility of contamination. To avoid this, thiomersal is used in multidose presentations of vaccines such as diphtheria-tetanus-whole cell pertussis (DTP) and tetanus toxoid (TT), as well as certain formulations of diphtheria-tetanus-acellular pertussis (DTaP), hepatitis B and *Haemophilus influenzae* type b (Hib) vaccines, but not in live bacterial or viral vaccines. Vaccine preservatives, including thiomersal, have probably prevented illness and death in countless infants over the years by reducing the risk of contamination of opened multidose vials. In certain vaccines, thiomersal is also used during the manufacturing processes.

Although the mercury-containing preservative is known to cause local skin reactions when applied topically, it has been considered safe and highly effective when used in vaccines. However, in mid-1999, the chemical came under public and professional scrutiny because of its presence in certain vaccines that are included in childhood immunization schedules (*1*).

Questions regarding the safety of thiomersal in vaccines have arisen primarily because of recent studies suggesting adverse effects in children from *in utero* exposure to methylmercury (a similar organic mercury compound) at levels previously considered safe (*2, 3*) and the reduction by the US EPA of the recommended limits on methylmercury exposure (*4*).[1] Data on human health

---

[1] WHO, the US Environmental Protection Agency (EPA), the US Agency for Toxic Substances and Disease Registry (ATSDR), and the US Food and Drug Administration (FDA) have developed recommendations for safe exposure to methylmercury in the diet. These range from 0.7 µg/kg of body weight per week (EPA) to 3.3 µg/kg of body weight per week (WHO) and include a safety margin. Applying these guidelines to a female infant in the lowest 5th percentile of weight between birth and 14 weeks, the period during which most infant vaccines are given, results in limits of safe total methylmercury exposure of between 34 µg (EPA) and 159 µg (WHO). Application of these guidelines to thiomersal, which is metabolized to ethylmercury, assumes that the toxicity of ethylmercury is the same as that of methylmercury (still an unresolved question).

Table 21.1   Mercury exposure from thiomersal in typical immunization schedules

AGE OF INFANT	VACCINES[a]	HEPATITIS B (HB) VACCINE		MERCURY DOSE (µg)	
		SCHEME A	SCHEME B	SCHEME A	SCHEME B
Birth	BCG, OPV 0	HB 1		12.5	
6 weeks	DTP 1, OPV 1, Hib 1	HB 2	HB 1	62.5	62.5
10 weeks	DTP 2, OPV 2, Hib 2		HB 2	50	62.5
14 weeks	DTP 3, OPV 3, Hib 3	HB 3	HB 3	62.5	62.5
9 months	Measles, yellow fever				
Total potential exposure of infants				**187.5**	**187.5**
Women of childbearing age, and especially pregnant women	TT1—as soon as possible in pregnancy or as early as possible in the childbearing years				25
	TT2—at least 4 weeks after TT1				25
	TT3—at least 6 months after TT2				25
	TT4 and TT5—at least one year after the previous TT dose				50
Total potential exposure of women through TT					**125***

[a]OPV = oral poliovirus vaccine; DTP, diphtheria, tetanus, pertussis; BCG, bacille Calmette-Guérin; Hib1, Haemophilus influenzae type b; HB, hepatitis B; TT, tetanus toxoid.

effects of low level exposure to ethylmercury, the metabolite of thiomersal are lacking. Nonetheless, the tolerance of the public for risk without obvious benefit to the individual has diminished (5). The combination of these factors has led to an altered perception of mercury-containing products. As a result, the gradual removal of the preservative from vaccines is being supported by the US Public Health Service (USPHS), WHO, and industry (6, 7). At present, however, scientific investigation has not found conclusive evidence of harm from thiomersal in vaccines. In June 2003 experts convened by the Food and Agriculture Organization of the United Nations (FAO) and WHO reviewed additional information on methylmercury and recommended a reduced provisional tolerable weekly intake (PTWI) of 1.6 µg per kg of body weight, in order to protect the developing fetus (this new recommendation replaces the prior one of a dietary limit of 3.3 µg per kg of body weight per week).

Management and intervention

The addition of new vaccines to the recommended childhood immunization schedule during the past decade has increased the potential exposure of infants to mercury from vaccines. In July 1999, an FDA review found that some infants might receive more mercury from vaccines than was considered safe according to certain national guidelines (8). The USPHS and American Academy of Pediatrics (AAP) issued a joint statement concerning thiomersal in vaccines (6) and the AAP released an interim report to clinicians (9) recommending that thiomersal be removed from vaccines as soon as possible, while encouraging maintenance of efforts to ensure high vaccination levels. These events prompted international debate about preservatives and their safety as well as controversy over immunization recommendations for thiomersal-containing vaccines. One recommendation in the joint statement and interim report to clinicians was deferral of hepatitis B vaccination until 2–6 months of age for infants born to mothers at low risk of hepatitis B disease. An editorial in the *Journal of the American Medical Association* soon followed suggesting that the authorities should express a preference for thiomersal-free DTaP and Hib vaccines for infants (10).

The USPHS and various US vaccine advisory bodies, including the AAP, Advisory Committee on Immunization Practices (ACIP), and the American Academy of Family Physicians, continue to recommend the policy of moving rapidly to vaccines that are free of thiomersal as a preservative (2, 11), citing the desirability to minimize human exposure to mercury from all sources (1). With the approval in the United States of a single antigen thiomersal-free hepatitis B vaccine in August 1999, the ACIP recommended that the birth dose of hepatitis B vaccine be resumed for all infants (12). The FDA approved an additional preservative-free hepatitis B vaccine in March 2000 and a preservative-free DTaP vaccine in March 2001. In the USA, additional proposals to remove thiomersal as a preservative from other vaccines have been announced by manufacturers, and new vaccines under development are not being formulated with thiomersal.

Wider implications

In the USA, recent progress in reducing exposure to thiomersal in vaccines has relied mainly on reformulation of thiomersal-containing products into single-dose vials that do not require a preservative. This is not feasible in many developing countries for a number of reasons. For many vaccines there is no obvious alternative preservative, thus leaving many local producers with the option of either producing the vaccines in multidose containers without a preservative (greatly increasing risk of contamination) or in single-dose preparations (too expensive in terms of manufacture, storage and delivery). The cost of switching to single doses is high; the cold chain does not currently have the capacity to cope with the increased volume, and local vaccine producers could not easily adjust to increased demands on the manufacturing process caused by conversion to single-dose containers.

The theoretical risk from exposure to thiomersal has to be balanced against the known high risk of having no preservative in vaccines. Therefore, WHO (13), UNICEF, the European Agency for Evaluation of Medicinal Products (EMEA), and other key agencies continue to recommend the use of vaccines containing this preservative because of the proven benefit of vaccines in preventing death and disease and the lack of data indicating harm. Additional studies are planned or under way to address the gaps in knowledge on the potential health effects of thiomersal in vaccines.

Acknowledgements

This article draws on material published in *Drug Safety* and is used with permission (Clements CJ et al. Thiomersal in vaccines — is removal necessary? *Drug Safety*, 2001, 24:567–574).

References

1. *US Pharmacopeia 24*. Rockville, MD, US Pharmacopeial Convention, 1999:1644.
2. Centers for Disease Control and Prevention. Recommendations regarding the use of vaccines that contain thimerosal as a preservative. *Morbidity and Mortality Weekly Report*, 1999, 48:996–998.
3. Grandjean P et al. Cognitive deficit in 7 year old children with prenatal exposure to methylmercury. *Neurotoxicology and Teratology*, 1997, 6:417–428.
4. Environmental Protection Agency. *Integrated risk information system*. Cincinnati, OH, EPA Office of Health and Environmental Assessment, Environmental Criteria and Assessment Office, 1994 (*http://www.epa.gov/iriswebp/iris/index. html*).
5. Covello VT, Sandman PM, Slovic P. Guidelines for communicating information about chemical risks prospectively and responsively. In: Mayo DG, Hollander D, eds. *Acceptable evidence: science and values in risk management*. New York, Oxford University Press 1991:66–90.
6. Centers for Disease Control and Prevention. Notice to readers: Thimerosal in vaccines — A joint statement of the American Academy of Pediatrics and the Public Health Service. *Morbidity and Mortality Weekly Report*, 1999, 48:563–565.
7. World Health Organisation. Thiomersal as a vaccine preservative. *Weekly Epidemiological Record*, 2000, 75:12–16.
8. Ball LK, Ball R, Pratt RD. An assessment of thimerosal use in childhood vaccines. *Pediatrics*, 2001, 107:1147–1154.
9. American Academy of Pediatrics. Committee on Infectious Diseases and Committee on Environmental Health. Thimerosal in vaccines — an interim report to clinicians. *Pediatrics*, 1999, 104:570–574.
10. Halsey NA. Limiting infant exposure to thimerosal in vaccines and other sources of mercury. *Journal of the American Medical Association*, 1999, 282:1763–1766.
11. Centers for Disease Control and Prevention. Summary of the joint statement on thimerosal in vaccines. *Morbidity and Mortality Weekly Report*, 2000, 49:780–782.
12. Centers for Disease Control and Prevention. Availability of hepatitis B vaccine that does not contain thimerosal as a preservative. *Morbidity and Mortality Weekly Report*, 1999, 48:780–782.
13. *Children's vaccines — safety first*. Geneva, World Health Organization (Note to the press No. 18, 9 July 1999).

2. SILICOSIS AMONG CHILDREN IN THE AGATE INDUSTRY

H. N. Saiyed

National Institute of Occupational Health, Indian Council of Medical Research, Ahmedabad, India

Agate is a hard, semiprecious stone, a variety of chalcedony, with striped or clouded colouring and containing a large quantity of free silica (>60%). It is used to make cheap jewellery and various articles of decoration (Figure 21.1). Processing of agate stone comprises several steps, including chipping, baking, grinding, polishing, and drilling. Dust is generated mainly during the grinding process. A small quantity of dust is also generated during chipping. The agate industry is located in Khambhat (also known as Cambay) town and surrounding villages of Gujarat State and Jaipur city of Rajasthan State in Western India, and employs about 50 000 people. Grinding of the stones is carried out indoors or under open shade, on an electric emery. The machinery is primitive and the health and safety of the workers is usually disregarded. Dust generated during grinding pervades the work environment as well as the community. Children may be exposed in the community, when they accompany their mothers to work (Figure 21.2), or when they themselves are employed in the industry.

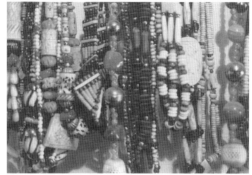
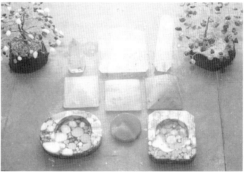

Figure 21.1 Jewellery and decorative articles made from agate

Silicosis and silicotuberculosis

Silicosis is the most common and ancient of all occu-

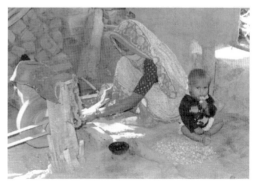

Figure 21.2 Grinding of agate stone under open shade

pational diseases of the lungs and, even today, it is among the most serious occupational diseases. It is an irreversible fibrosis of the lungs caused by repeated inhalation over a long period of time of fine particles containing free silica. Repeated exposure to silica dust results in fibrosis of the lungs. The disease is characterized by insidious onset of shortness of breath followed by cough, with or without expectoration. Exposure to silica dust also impairs the defence mechanism of the lungs against infection, in particular tuberculosis. A high incidence of tuberculosis is common among the working population exposed to silica.

Diagnosis of silicosis

The diagnosis of silicosis is based on the occupational history combined with typical radiological features consisting of fine bilaterally symmetrical nodular shadows on chest X-ray. To promote reproducibility and uniformity in reporting, the International Labour Organization (ILO) has devised the International Classification of Pneumoconiosis Radiographs for coding of radiological abnormalities (1). The abnormal shadows due to pneumoconiosis are coded as p, q, or r, depending on size and shape, and as 0, 1, 2, or 3 according to their density or profusion. Category 0 means no pneumoconiosis and 1, 2, and 3 correspond to increasing numbers of opacities per unit area, and usually reflect the severity of pneumoconiosis. These four categories are further subdivided into twelve subcategories 0/−, 0/0, 0/1, 1/0, 1/1, 1/2, 2/1 . . . 3/3 and 3/+. The categorization is made by comparing the chest radiograph of the patient with the standard radiographs supplied by ILO.

Silicosis is not confined to the developing countries, although the situation there is alarming. For example, according to the American Lung Association (2), about 1.6 million workers in the USA are at risk of silicosis, and 60 000 are expected to suffer from it.

Prevalence of silicosis and tuberculosis in children

Normally, silicosis does not occur in the general population in the absence of occupational exposure. However, a high prevalence of non-occupational pneumoconiosis due to exposure to free silica has been reported from a residential area in India, close to the agate industry (3). To find out the prevalence of silicosis and silicotuberculosis in agate grinders and the surrounding community, the National Institute of Occupational Health (NIOH), Ahmedabad, recently carried out an environmental and epidemiological study in 2050 subjects who were exposed to silica dust, either occupationally or non-occupationally (unpublished report). The study population included 230 children, of whom 58 (25.2%) had worked for a period as agate grinders. The radiological findings of these 230 children are shown in Table 21.2.

A total of 28 children (12.1%) showed radiological evidence of silicosis of category 1/0 or 1/2. There were 27 (11.7%) cases of silicosis category 1/0 and one girl aged 17 years who was working as a grinder showed category 1/2 silicosis on X-ray.

Table 21.2 Distribution of cases of silicosis and tuberculosis in children exposed to silica dust

AGE GROUP	CATEGORY OF SILICOSIS				TUBERCULOSIS
(YEARS)	0/0	0/1	1/0	1/2	
<10	7/10 (70%)	—	3/10 (30%)	—	2/10 (20.0%)
11–15	121/148 (81.8%)	7/148 (4.7%)	20/148 (13.5%)	—	10/148 (6.8%)
16–18	61/72 (84.7%)	6/148 (8.3%)	4/72 (5.6%)	1	3/72 (4.2%)
Total	189/230 (82.2%)	13/230 (5.7%)	27/230 (11.7%)	1/230 (0.4%)	15/230 (6.5%)

The overall prevalence of tuberculosis as diagnosed from X-ray was 6.5%. This is much higher than the prevalence reported in other studies. For example a recent tuberculin survey in northern India in 4200 children below 14 years showed an overall infection prevalence of 2.4% (4). Similarly a radiological study of a population in the North Arcot district of South India showed a tuberculosis prevalence of 1.7% in subjects above 14 years (5). The high prevalence of tuberculosis among the children could be attributed to occupational and non-occupational exposure to silica dust from the agate industry. Moreover, in a previous study, a prevalence of tuberculosis of about 42% in adult men and women working as grinders in the agate industry was reported (6). This adult population, particularly working mothers, may act as a source of infection to children.

Prevention and control of silicosis and silicotuberculosis

In 1997, the Ministry of Health and Family Welfare of India initiated the National Silicosis Elimination Programme, a long-term scheme, for which NIOH, Ahmedabad, is the nodal agency. The programme consists of: (1) identification of high-risk small and cottage industries, through environmental and epidemiological surveys, including surveys of the surrounding community; (2) development of simple devices for dust control in the community and work environment; (3) treatment of workers who suffer from dust-induced diseases; (4) strengthening of regulatory mechanisms through technical support for dust monitoring; and (5) awareness programmes for workers, employers, medical officers and factory inspectors.

The agate industry is part of this programme. As mentioned earlier, an environmental epidemiological study has already been completed. The cases of silicosis and tuberculosis detected during the survey were referred to the local health authorities for appropriate management. The government health department has opened a special clinic for agate workers at Khambhat for diagnosis and management of silicosis and silicotuberculosis. A 300 mA X-ray machine and supplies of medicine have been provided to the centre for surveillance of silicosis and tuberculosis.

The major challenge was to develop an appropriate dust control device acceptable to the workers and the owners. Several models of a local exhaust system were tried. Our initial attempt was to incorporate an exhaust system into the grinding machine. These models were not accepted by the workers because they required changes in their working posture. Finally we have developed a model of an exhaust system that fits over the cutting machine. This model does not require the workers to change posture and has met with a positive response. The efficacy of the local exhaust in reducing dust levels is about 90–95% as shown by an industrial hygiene survey. Model exhaust systems have been installed in six units and have been working satisfactorily over a period of one year.

For the long term, the State Government plans to relocate the industry outside the town by providing land and other infrastructure. It is proposed to form a cooperative society for the workers and the owners to take care of the environmental and occupational health problems. In addition, education programmes for the workers and the community are organized to ensure successful implementation of the silicosis elimination programmes.

Conclusions

An environmental epidemiological study of the agate industry demonstrated the poor working conditions in this cottage industry, and the serious health problems not only among the workers but also in the surrounding community. Children are very vulnerable to silicosis and tuberculosis through direct and indirect exposure, particularly through their mothers. Identification of industries with high occupational and environmental exposure to silica is important. Commitment from all parts of society — factory owners, workers, factory inspectors, medical officers, people living in the surrounding area and government authorities — is essential. A silicosis elimination programme should be incorporated in the national tuberculosis elimination programme in developing countries where tuberculosis is still a major health problem.

References

1. International Labour Organization. *Guidelines for the use of ILO International Classification of Radiographs of Pneumoconioses*. Geneva, ILO, 1980 (Occupational Safety and Health Series, No. 22).
2. American Lung Association (www.lungusa.org).
3. Saiyed HN et al. Non-occupational pneumoconiosis at high altitude villages in central Ladakh. *British Journal of Industrial Medicine*, 1991, 48:825–829.
4. Pattanaik D et al. Prevalence of tuberculosis infection in children below fourteen years in rural Haryana. *Indian Pediatrics*, 2002, 39:70–74.
5. Datta M et al. Tuberculosis in North Arcot district of Tamilnadu. A sample survey. *The Indian Journal of Tuberculosis*, 2000, July:47.
6. Sadhu SG et al. A follow up study of health status of small scale agate industry workers. *Indian Journal of Industrial Medicine*, 1995, 41:101–105.

3. PROTECTION AGAINST THE SUN IN SCHOOLS

S. Harper
School of Nutrition and Public Health, Deakin University,
Victoria, Australia

The problem

Australia has the highest incidence of skin cancer in the world — one out of two Australians will develop some form of skin cancer during their lifetime.

There are three forms of skin cancer — basal and squamous cell carcinomas (or common skin cancers) and melanoma. The annual incidence of common skin cancers, which comprise about 78% of new cancer cases in Australia each year, is 1000 per 100 000 people (*1*). Melanoma incidence is 30 per 100 000 people per year (*1*), and most of the 1200 skin-cancer-related deaths occurring annually result from melanoma. Excluding common skin cancers, melanoma is the third most common cancer in women and the fifth most common in men — it is also the most common cancer in people aged 15–44 years (*2*). Skin cancer is Australia's most costly cancer — direct costs of treatment have been estimated at US$ 5.70 per person per year (*3*). Yet it is almost totally preventable through sensible behaviour to protect against the sun.

Exposure to ultraviolet (UV) radiation from the sun, particularly during childhood and adolescence, is the most significant risk factor for development of skin cancer in later life (*2, 4*). It has been estimated that up to 80% of total lifetime exposure occurs during childhood (*4*). Both short, sharp shocks of sunburn and cumulative exposure over a number of years increase skin cancer risk. Although melanoma can develop during late adolescence, skin cancer is not usually seen in people under 40 years of age.

Australia receives high levels of UV radiation as a result of its proximity to the equator. The incidence of common skin cancers is related to latitude, and is highest in northern Australia (*5*). Fair-skinned people, who make up the majority of the population, are most at risk. Australians enjoy an outdoor lifestyle, and since the early 1900s there has been a belief that suntanned skin looks attractive and healthy.

Management and intervention

Because children are at school five days a week during the period when UV levels are at their peak, schools can directly influence the UV radiation exposure of their students. In addition, schools are ideally placed to educate students and the wider community through curriculum programmes and role models. Development of good habits during childhood can contribute to sensible behaviour in the sun later in life.

The SunSmart Campaign of the Anti-Cancer Council of Victoria has four sub-programmes — schools, media and public education, community support and sponsorships (6). The campaign has a strong empirical base — ongoing research and evaluation determine its direction and content. This multifaceted approach, which ensures that the messages promoted through schools are re-inforced at the broader community level, has been a major factor in the success of the programme. The Schools Program also has the endorsement of the Department of Education and other key educational and health bodies.

The SunSmart Schools Program emphasizes a whole school approach to protection against the sun (see Box). The key element is policy development, which as far as possible involves the whole school community — this increases the likelihood of broad support for and long-term sustainability of the chosen strategies. With the possible exception of shade development, most strategies can be implemented quite easily and at low cost to the school and to parents.

Schools implementing an approved policy can apply for accreditation as a SunSmart School. Successful schools receive a large (60 cm × 90 cm) metal *SunSmart School* sign, which both recognizes and promotes the school community's commitment to sun protection. A small joining fee partially covers the cost of producing and distributing the sign, and every school that applies, whether successful or not, receives a free copy of a teacher resource book, which can be used as the basis for development of curriculum programmes in sun protection.

Changes in staff and priorities can influence the level of support for the pro-gramme. However, growing awareness of what the *SunSmart School* sign rep-resents has raised parental expectations and encouraged schools to maintain their commitment to protection.

A SunSmart school day

Liam, aged 8 years, is a Grade 3 student at a SunSmart School. A typical school day might be as follows.

Before Liam leaves home, he applies SPF 30+ sunscreen and checks his school bag to ensure that he has packed his broad-brimmed school hat, sunscreen and swimming gear. After being dropped off, he walks into the school grounds past the SunSmart School sign on the front fence.

Liam's first class is physical education, in which students practise for the next day's swim-ming sports. The school conducts outdoor classes early in the morning whenever possible to avoid the period when the UV level is at its highest. Students who did not apply sunscreen before coming to school are given some from the school supply. The students and their teacher wear hats on the way to the swimming-pool, and at all times while out of the water. Some students wear special protective "sun suits", and those who do not are required to put on a T-shirt when not in the water. At the end of the session, students are reminded to reapply their sunscreen.

During the morning break, Liam helps to water the new trees the students planted recently to provide more shade and improve the school environment. Students raised the funds to purchase the trees and selected them themselves as part of the school's health and environmental studies programme.

Later, Liam's class discuss the results of their homework assignment, in which they were required to watch the television news or look in the newspaper and record maximum temperatures and UV levels and the times of day at which they occurred. The class then discusses what this means in terms of the times of day it is safest to be outside, and what precautions they should take. Students are asked to produce a poster showing what they have learnt—these will be displayed in the local pharmacy as part of a promotion for sun protective merchandise.

Shortly before the lunch break, Liam's teacher reminds the class to reapply their sunscreen and demonstrates how to do it properly. Students eat their lunches in their classrooms before going outside. Teachers wear broad-brimmed hats while on playground duty, and students without approved hats are required to stay in a special shaded area. Five students who are considered to have been particularly SunSmart receive tokens that they later give to their teachers. These tokens contribute to class points and at the end of the term the most SunSmart class is rewarded with a special treat, such as an excursion.

Following afternoon classes, there is a brief assembly, where students are reminded about the arrangements for the twilight swimming carnival the next day. There will be no school in the morning and the event is to begin at 3 pm. A prize will be awarded to the most SunSmart team and students are reminded to bring their hats, sunscreen and clothing to cover up between events. A newsletter, explaining the arrangements to parents, inviting them to attend and encouraging them to wear protective clothing is distributed before students are dismissed for the day.

Evaluation and follow-up

Over 70% of Victorian primary schools have become *SunSmart Schools* since the programme began in 1994. The following comments from three school principals reflect some of the outcomes achieved in participating schools and the advantages of the whole-school approach.

"It's wonderful to see the 'growth' in children's/parent's awareness since we first became a SunSmart school."

"We continue to see it as an important part of our school culture and curriculum."

"Children respond positively and have incorporated good habits in personal sun/skin care."

Baseline data regarding protection practices in a sample of Victorian schools were collected in 1998, with a follow-up study scheduled for 2001 and subsequently every three years. Unpublished data indicate significant improvements in policy and practices since the introduction of the programme.

It is too early to evaluate the programme's impact on skin cancer rates, which in any case cannot really be assessed independently of the broader campaign. However, there is evidence of changes in frequency of sunburn and in attitudes and behaviour relating to wearing a hat and using sunscreen (7). Recent trends in skin cancer rates also suggest that education campaigns may be beginning to have an effect (8).

However, the Schools Program does face some challenges. Because skin cancer does not usually develop until later in life, it can be difficult to convince people that protection is important. This applies especially to adolescents, for whom the desire for a suntan is often driven by a more immediate need for peer acceptance. Furthermore, protective clothing is generally perceived by young people as unfashionable. Also, the majority of skin cancers are not life-threatening, and in a society with relatively good access to medical services, there can be a tendency to believe that because suspicious spots are easily removed, skin cancer is not a serious problem. This is exacerbated by the fact that political priorities focus on funding treatment as opposed to prevention.

Application to other health problems and settings

Protection against the sun is a relatively easy issue (compared, for example, with issues such as tobacco, drugs, HIV/AIDS) for schools to begin with when attempting to implement a whole school approach to health, as exemplified by the Health Promoting Schools Framework (9). It is important however, that schools focus on strategies that are realistic and achievable in the context of their own school community; endorsement by key educational bodies is particularly important.

Recognition of good practice is essential, but while accreditation has been a successful element of the SunSmart Schools Program, it may not always be appropriate. For example, it is generally less relevant for Australian secondary schools, where differences from the primary school setting and adolescent attitudes towards sun protection necessitate a different approach.

A national programme based on the Victorian model was implemented in Australia in 1998 (10), and the principles of the SunSmart Schools Program can be readily applied in other institutional settings such as child care centres and pre-schools. Elements of the SunSmart Schools Program are now also being adopted in other countries with high skin cancer rates, such as the United States.

References

1. Australian Institute of Health and Welfare (AIHW) and Australasian Association of Cancer Registries (AACR). *Cancer in Australia 1995: Incidence and mortality data for 1995 and selected data for 1996.* Canberra, Australian Institute of Health and Welfare, 1996 (Cancer Series No. 10).

2. Khlat M et al. Mortality from melanoma in migrants to Australia: variation by age at arrival and duration of stay. *American Journal of Epidemiology*, 1992, 135:1103–1113.

3. Carter R, Marks R, Hill D. Could a national skin cancer primary prevention campaign in Australia be worthwhile? An economic perspective. *Health Promotion International*, 1999, 14:73–82.

4. Marks R et al. The role of childhood exposure to sunlight in the development of solar keratoses and non-melanocytic skin cancer. *Medical Journal of Australia*, 1990, 152:62–66.

5. Giles GG, Marks R, Foley P. Incidence of non-melanocytic skin cancer treated in Australia. *British Medical Journal*, 1988, 296:13–18.

6. Sinclair C et al. From Slip! Slop! Slap! to SunSmart: a profile of a health education campaign. *Cancer Forum*, 1994, 18:183–187.

7. Hill D et al. Changes in sun-related attitudes and behaviour and reduced sunburn prevalence. *European Journal of Cancer Prevention*, 1993, 2:447–456.

8. Staples M, Marks R, Giles G. Trends in the incidence of non-melanocytic skin cancer (NMSC) treated in Australia 1985–1995: are primary prevention programs starting to have an effect? *International Journal of Cancer*, 1998, 78:144–148.

9. WHO Global School Health Initiative. *Health promoting schools.* Geneva, World Health Organization, 1998.

10. Dobbinson S et al. A national approach to skin cancer prevention: the National SunSmart Schools Program. *Medical Journal of Australia*, 1998, 169:513–514.

4. PREVENTION OF ASBESTOS-RELATED DISEASES—THE FINNISH APPROACH

A. Karjalainen
Finnish Institute of Occupational Health, Helsinki, Finland

Asbestos has been widely used in modern societies. In Finland, some 250 applications and products containing asbestos have been identified in the construction industry. The main asbestos-containing products are construction sheets and thermal, fire and acoustic insulation materials (sprayed asbestos or asbestos laggings). Further uses include asbestos blankets, ropes and yarns, flooring materials, bitumen felts, adhesives, putties, plasters, ceramic tiles, paints, and friction materials (e.g. car brakes). In Finland, the use of asbestos-containing construction materials continued into the 1980s but was especially common from the 1950s to the 1970s. Owing to its physicochemical structure, asbestos is an extremely stable substance. All stages in the use and handling of asbestos products may release asbestos fibres that pose a risk to the workers and the entire population through the general environment and consumer products.

Asbestos is known to cause mesothelioma, lung cancer, lung fibrosis (asbestosis), pleural plaques, pleural effusions and fibrotic lesions of the visceral pleura. In addition, asbestos is suspected to increase the risk for malignant diseases of the larynx and some gastrointestinal organs. Prevention of asbestos-related diseases relies on elimination of exposure to asbestos-containing dust. The heaviest exposures occur in occupational settings, and preventive strategies therefore focus on the protection of the working population. In Finland, 120–130 cases of asbestos-related cancer, 120 cases of asbestosis, and 350 cases of asbestos-related pleural disease were reported as occupational diseases each year during the late 1990s. For Western Europe, the number of male deaths from mesothelioma alone is expected to almost double from 5000 in 1998 to about 9000 in 2018 (1).

While the risk of disease is highest among those with heavy exposure, a safe level of exposure does not exist. Even low environmental exposures in domestic or public buildings, in outdoor environments, or from consumer products containing friable asbestos pose a potential risk. Asbestos-related diseases have a latency time of 20–40 years from the onset of exposure to the occurrence of disease. This makes children, whose remaining life expectancy is long, an especially vulnerable group for asbestos hazards. Children also breathe more air per kilogram of body weight per day. Little is known about the possible long-term consequences of low-level asbestos exposure during childhood. However, cases of mesothelioma have been reported among the grown children of asbestos workers (2). In some areas, uncontrolled environmental exposures starting during childhood contribute significantly to the total burden of asbestos-related disease (3, 4).

In Finland, legislative measures to gradually restrict exposure to asbestos started in the mid-1970s. However, in the mid-1980s society became increasingly concerned about the sufficiency and scale of the measures planned and implemented. In response, the Ministry of Social and Health Affairs requested the Institute of Occupational Health to prepare a proposal on how to tackle the problem. Consequently, a nationwide Asbestos Programme was carried out in 1987–92 in close cooperation between government authorities, labour market organizations, occupational health and labour protection personnel, other interest groups and the mass media, with the common goal of preventing all exposure to asbestos, both occupational and non-occupational (5). The legislative and administrative actions of the programme were set out by the national Asbestos Committee in its final report (6). The committee report lists 27 measures falling under the responsibility of six ministries. The two main sets of measures proposed were a total ban on all new use of asbestos and asbestos-containing products, and improved control and stricter regulations concerning removal of existing asbestos. These measures gained widespread support and were rapidly incorporated into the Finnish legislation.

The Committee also proposed more stringent measures to ensure a safe living environment for children and the general population. The Committee estimated that two-thirds of all the asbestos used in Finland was still in place in buildings in the late 1980s, and that one-third of all buildings still had some asbestos-containing materials. This proportion was estimated to be higher for public buildings than for domestic dwellings. Consequently, the following was agreed on:

In 1989, the National Board of Health issued recommendations on asbestos abatement in schools, kindergartens, hospitals and other public buildings. These recommendations underlined that before any removal work, the buildings should be inspected for possible release of asbestos fibres. In case of such a possibility, the abatement work should be performed during school or kindergarten holidays. The recommendations also addressed the isolation of the work site from remaining facilities, appropriate ventilation during the abatement work, cleaning, and measurements necessary to assess the effectiveness of cleaning. These principles were integrated into the regulations concerning asbestos abatement work.

In 1990, the guidebook on the maintenance of houses published by the National Board of Health determined less than 0.01 fibres/cm³ as a standard for airborne asbestos in dwellings. This limit value is 30 times lower than the current standard for occupational exposure. During normal activities, the observed concentrations in domestic dwellings, schools and other public buildings were clearly below the limit. In situations, where asbestos materials were processed or demolished, the limit value was commonly exceeded even in adjacent parts of the building.

A total ban on the use of asbestos has been in force in Finland since 1994 and only licensed companies using special techniques and trained personnel are allowed to remove asbestos. The remaining challenge for the prevention of asbestos-related diseases is to ensure that the special asbestos abatement techniques are always applied. The State Asbestos Committee recommended that all buildings that are likely to contain asbestos, as a result of their age and type, should be systematically inspected and any asbestos-containing materials marked. If these are intact, closed and do not release asbestos fibres, they can be left in place and should be properly removed when the building is next renovated. If the asbestos-containing materials are friable and release asbestos fibres, they should be immediately removed or securely covered. The State Council Resolution on Asbestos Work (1380/94) further emphasizes that the constructor is obliged to ensure that materials to be demolished do not contain asbestos. If this is not ensured, the demolition work has to be carried out according to regulations concerning asbestos abatement work.

In addition to a solid legislative background, the prevention of asbestos hazards relies on a widespread public awareness. The national asbestos programme initiated an intensive information campaign to guarantee that potential asbestos hazards are always identified and appropriate measures taken to eliminate them (5). On several occasions, alert environmental protection personnel, school and kindergarten personnel, or parents have identified potentially dangerous situations in schools or kindergartens with friable or broken asbestos materials, or even outdoor environments located close to asbestos-producing or manufacturing facilities.

References

1. Peto J et al. The European mesothelioma epidemic. *British Journal of Cancer*, 1999, 79:666–672.
2. Anderson HA. Family contact exposure. In: *Proceedings of the World Symposium on Asbestos, Montreal, 25–27 May 1982*. Montreal, Canadian Asbestos Information Centre, 1982: 349–362.
3. Dumortier P et al. The role of environmental and occupational exposures in Turkish immigrants with fibre-related disease. *European Respiratory Journal*, 2001, 17:922–927.
4. Luce D et al. Environmental exposure to treolite and respiratory cancer in New Caledonia: a case-control study. *American Journal of Epidemiology*, 2000, 151:259–265.
5. Huuskonen MS et al. Finnish Institute of Occupational Health Asbestos Program 1987–92. *American Journal of Industrial Medicine*, 1995, 28:123–142.
6. Asbestos Committee. [*Final report 66/1989.*] Helsinki, Ministry of Labour, 1990 (in Finnish, English summary).

5. INFORMAL MARKETS OF TEGUCIGALPA, HONDURAS: ADOLESCENT PARTICIPATION IN MARKET CLEAN-UP CAMPAIGN

D. C. Kaminsky
Fundación Desarollo, Amistad y Respuestas (FUNDAR),
Tegucigalpa, Honduras

Description of the problem

Project Alternatives, a nongovernmental organization, introduced an integrated approach to the provision of primary health care and education services for a population of working street children and adolescents and their families in the informal market sector of the capital city of Honduras, Tegucigalpa.

Most of the children assist their family (usually a working single mother) in selling goods at a small stall or while walking through the markets and the surrounding streets. The goods vary from vegetables and fruits to candies, women's stockings, etc. Thousands of children and adolescents are found in the six markets. Multiple interventions included health education, primary health care, recreation activities, youth clubs and a "school for parents". The integrated approach was taken in order to address the multiple risks and interactions that determine the health and well-being of the children and young people. Also, there was a desire to provide a menu of activities whereby the beneficiaries could select those most interesting and important to them at different points in time.

Youth clubs were established in each market. Usually the clubs were composed of 25–50 adolescents and met once a week. This organization scheme provided the opportunity for the young people to have a voice in planning and conducting the various activities of the project, allowed a space and time for recreational activities for those who usually did not have this opportunity, and provided an organizational scheme for health education sessions, other training sessions and special activities.

In the informal markets, regular waste disposal was almost non-existent. Waste was thrown on the ground near the vending stalls and left to rot, attract flies, and occasionally be carried away to an open municipal dump nearby. Municipal control standards defining hygienic practices applied but were not enforced. The exposed population group was the adult vendors, their working children and their customers. Cholera and other diarrhoea problems are endemic in the country, thus the sanitary conditions of these markets provide the perfect setting for the development of an epidemic. Fortunately, there has not been an epidemic in these markets in recent years.

Project Alternatives introduced a waste management programme into its ongoing interventions as a special activity. Funds to support this special activity were taken from the general fund of the organization. The programme operated in six different market areas in various parts of the capital city. Some training activities were conducted in the open drop-in centre of the organization, which is five minutes walking distance from three of the six markets.

Management and intervention

The mothers of the working children, through the education activities of the School for Parents, were made aware of the potentially grave health consequences of the prevalent sanitary conditions of their workplace. Promotion of participation of children and adolescents was a cornerstone of the programme. Thus the conditions were right for the adolescents to take an active role in a market clean-up programme. At the same time as the mothers were talking with their children about the lack of proper waste disposal in the marketplace, the youth clubs from the six different market areas were forming a Youth Advisory Council with representation from all markets. The market waste disposal campaign was taken on by the Youth Advisory Council as the first joint project conducted under a common planning scheme for all markets. Besides the School for Parents, the Youth Advisory Council also coordinated mass clean-up campaigns of the Mayor's Office and the Fire Department when the markets would be closed for one day periodically and the firemen would wash down the streets with their fire hoses. The local Market Vendors' Associations also participated in the planning of all activities.

A formal plan of action was prepared by the Youth Advisory Council. Activities included health education sessions for the adult market vendors, and for the first time the placing of waste barrels in the markets. The barrels were painted with a message and the name of Project Alternatives. Carts were provided for carrying away the waste to the common disposal area, from where the municipal garbage disposal trucks transported it to a landfill outside the city. Health education posters were created by the young people and hung in various stalls and passageways of the markets. The young people also went through the markets collecting the waste, to serve as an example of the conduct they were promoting. The administrators of the market encouraged the vendors to use the newly placed barrels. The vendors reacted favourably and were receptive to these new ideas. The youth clubs of each individual market were responsible for the activities in their area and Council members monitored the activities. Approximately 100 young people were involved in the campaign. All the work was facilitated, planned and introduced under the guidance of the street education staff of Project Alternatives. The timetable for the intervention was as follows: one month before the mass campaign, health education activities were carried out in the markets both with groups and at the individual stalls; during this same time the barrel posters were purchased and painted; close to the campaign, coordination was established with the Mayor's office and the firemen. The campaign was carried out on a different day in each of the markets.

Follow-up and reference to other settings

The barrels were painted two more times at 6-week intervals in order to keep them looking new and attractive. During the 6 months following the mass campaign, young people made weekly visits to the stalls and conducted related health education activities, with the objective of reinforcing the use of the barrels for waste management in the markets and of promoting recognition of health risks related to an inadequate waste disposal system.

The factors that contributed to the success of this intervention included the role played by the mothers, who brought the situation and the need for a control programme to the attention of the young people. They allowed the young people to leave their selling activities in order to participate in the campaign, and they attended the group and individual health education orientation sessions. The coordination with official sectors of the city and the markets, and the Youth Advisory Council, were also important. Project Alternatives enjoyed an excellent reputation and working relationship with the municipal authorities and the market administrators through its permanent presence and activities in the markets, so that it was not difficult to obtain the cooperation and assistance of these entities.

6. ARSENIC EXPOSURE AND CHILD HEALTH

M. Rahman
Public Health Sciences Division, ICDDR, B Centre for
Health and Population Research, Dhaka, Bangladesh

Introduction

Historically, surface waters in Bangladesh have been contaminated with bacteria, causing a significant burden of acute gastrointestinal diseases. In the 1970s and 1980s, tube-wells were installed throughout the country to provide an alternative safe water source, resulting in a decrease in the incidence of diarrhoeal diseases. However, a major proportion of the tube-wells contain levels of arsenic that far exceed WHO's guideline limit of 10 µg/l, and even the less stringent standard of 50 µg/l set by the Government of Bangladesh. Since 1993, the occurrence of arsenicosis, a term used to describe the symptoms associated with chronic ingestion of arsenic, has been marked and widespread. Today, an estimated 97% of the rural population use tube-well water for drinking, cooking, and irrigation, and a recent report from the World Bank estimates that 20 million inhabitants of Bangladesh rely on arsenic-contaminated drinking-water. Young children are now also showing signs of chronic arsenic poisoning.

Review of the impact of arsenic on child health
Health effects of arsenic exposure

Arsenic is an enzyme poison that affects almost all organ systems. Characteristic skin lesions and skin cancer represent the most important

Table 21.3 ***Characteristics of Bangladesh and the extent of arsenic contamination of tube-well water***

CHARACTERISTICS	
Total area (km²)	148 393
Total number of districts	64
Total population (million)	120
Total children <14 years (million)	44.4
Number of districts with arsenic in tube-well water > 50 µg/l	42
Area of arsenic-affected districts (km²)	92 106
Population in affected districts (million)	79.9
Number of districts with identified patients with arsenic-induced skin lesions	25
Children in affected districts <14 years (million)	29.5
Children in affected districts <4 years (million)	7.4
Children in affected districts <9 years (million)	16.7

Source: refs 1 and 2.

health effect of chronic ingestion of inorganic arsenic. A cross-sectional survey of four rural villages revealed a 29% prevalence of arsenic-related skin lesions among Bangladeshis over 30 years of age. Furthermore, Milton et al. (3) reported an association between chronic arsenic ingestion and "chronic bronchitis" among 94 individuals with arsenic-associated skin lesions in three Bangladeshi villages. The mean concentration of arsenic in drinking-water was 614 µg/l.

Effects on reproduction

There is some evidence that arsenic exposure is associated with adverse reproductive and developmental outcomes. Women working in highly exposed jobs in a Swedish copper smelter had higher rates of abortion (28% versus 14%), and gave birth to babies of lower birth weight than nearby residents (3.087 versus 3.394 kg). In addition, smelter employees who worked during pregnancy had higher rates of congenital malformations than employees who did not work during pregnancy. In Hungary, exposure to drinking water containing more than 100 µg/l of arsenic was associated with increased rates of spontaneous abortion and stillbirths. In Chile, rates of fetal, neonatal, and postnatal infant mortality were all elevated with high arsenic exposure.

Effects of arsenic in children

Limited information exists on possible health effects among exposed children. A study on child growth and intellectual ability in Thailand revealed that chronic arsenic exposure as assessed by arsenic concentrations in hair was related to a decrease in intelligence quotient. The possible impact of arsenic on children has not received sufficient attention to date, but the collective evidence from human and laboratory studies suggests a large potential for adverse effects on child health and development.

Safe water options

Both governmental and nongovernmental organizations have recognized an urgent need to provide safe drinking-water to arsenic-affected areas of Bangladesh. Four potential sources of arsenic-free drinking-water have been identified, namely: (1) treated surface water, (2) rainwater, (3) treated groundwater, and (4) deep aquifers. Once a safe water source has been made available, continuous monitoring of its operation and maintenance is necessary over several months, to ensure that people do not return to using tube-well water.

Treated surface water

Filtering pond surface waters through a large tank filled with sand and gravel — the community-based pond sand filter — can remove bacteria and provide safe water for drinking and cooking.

Rainwater harvesting

Rainwater harvesting is already being introduced in arsenic-affected areas and can supply enough water for drinking and cooking throughout the dry season. The harvesting system uses a tin rooftop or plastic sheet to collect rainwater, which is then transferred into large cement tanks, where it can be stored indefinitely without bacterial contamination.

Deep aquifers

The deep aquifer of the underground water table is arsenic-free in most areas of Bangladesh, and may provide a good alternative water source to replace the arsenic-contaminated shallow aquifer.

In many regions of Bangladesh, especially in the southern part of the country, the alternative water sources currently in place, i.e. treated surface water, arsenic removal technologies and rainwater harvesting, are not viable throughout the year or are beyond the reach of the poor communities. The Government of Bangladesh, with financial support from the World Bank and the Danish and Swiss Development Agencies, has recently initiated the Bangladesh Arsenic Mitigation Water Supply Project (BAMSWP) to provide one deep tubewell for each group of 50 families.

Treatment of groundwater

Treatment of groundwater is also a potential option in rural Bangladesh. The following arsenic removal techniques are available:

Three Kolshi filter

This filter is normally used to remove arsenic at the household level. It is simple to construct out of materials that rural people are familiar with, and is based on a technology that is endogenous in Bangladesh. However, the flow-rate of water through the system is low and the amount of water produced is small. Despite these limitations, it is cost-effective, convenient and frequently used in rural communities.

Alcan/Buet-activated alumina

This method of arsenic removal is commonly employed at the community level. Technically, the system is very effective, at least in the short term and, because it is easy to use, is well accepted. Filtration rates are good in terms of serving the demand of the community. Although the initial cost is very high, the method is cost-effective in long-term use and in rural communities.

Steven/Tetrahedrons method

The Steven/Tetrahedrons method is also used at the community level to remove arsenic but is less effective than the Alcan/Buet-activated alumina method.

Communication and awareness raising

Bangladesh is divided into six divisions, 64 districts, 464 *upazillas* and several thousand unions. Supportive health campaigns and awareness raising at the *upazilla* and union level form an essential part of any approach to mitigate arsenic-related health problems. A baseline survey needs to be conducted throughout the affected *upazillas* to assess knowledge, attitudes and practices regarding arsenic contamination of tube-wells, patterns of water use in the community, the prevalence of arsenicosis, and the availability of local resources. Various governmental and nongovernmental stakeholders should be involved in raising awareness with a special focus on improving children's health.

Sensitization meetings

Sensitization meetings at the *upazilla* and union levels should be held to raise awareness and generate commitment among key stakeholders, and to mobilize the rural community, especially women and children.

Courtyard meetings

In Bangladesh, water for domestic purposes is mostly collected and handled by women. Courtyard meetings could serve to disseminate important information on the health hazards of arsenic and the importance of safe drinking-water, and could ultimately inspire women to implement arsenic-free safe water options at their own cost.

Tea stall sessions

Men usually attend the local weekly bazaar to buy necessary goods and to exchange information in tea stalls. These tea stalls provide an opportunity to disseminate health messages to men, who dominate the decision-making process at the household level.

School health programmes

Children can successfully convey messages to their families and ultimately bring about changes in the family environment. Young adolescents should be provided with information on arsenic, safe drinking-water and sanitation through a variety of teaching methods and classroom activities. A rally could be organized by students, teachers and community leaders to raise awareness in the community.

Training of traditional medical practitioners

In Bangladesh, there is one physician per 4866 population (4), which is grossly inadequate. As a result, a large number of people seek medical services from rural traditional medical practitioners, who form an essential part of Bangladesh's health care system, especially in the rural community. These traditional healers can play a crucial role in disseminating information about arsenic.

Conclusions

An increase in adverse health effects and more widespread knowledge about the gravity of the situation has led to panic in many affected communities. Children suffering from arsenicosis are often isolated by their school mates, illustrating that arsenicosis is not only a major health hazard but also a large psychosocial burden. Arsenic-related problems must be addressed through an integrated, comprehensive approach to mitigate the sufferings of the affected population.

References

1. Chowdhury UK et al. Groundwater arsenic contamination in Bangladesh and West Bengal, India. *Environmental Health Perspectives,* 2000, 108:393–337.
2. *Health and demographic surveillance system.* Matlab, ICDDR, B, 2001 (http://202.136.7.26/org/orgunits.jsp?idDetails+58&searchID=58).
3. Milton AH, Rahman M. Respiratory effects and arsenic contaminated well water in Bangladesh. *International Journal of Environmental Health Research,* 2002, 12:175–179.
4. Bangladesh Bureau of Statistics. *Statistical pocketbook.* 2000 (www.sdnpbd.org/sdi/statisticapocketbook/index.htm).

7. HOUSEHOLD WATER TREATMENT: A SUCCESS STORY

J. T. Macy
R. E. Quick
Safe Water System, Centers for Disease Control and Prevention, Atlanta, GA, USA

Description of the problem

Diarrhoeal diseases, which are frequently transmitted by contaminated water, are a leading cause of illness and death among children under 5 years old in developing countries. Human or animal faeces often contaminate unprotected sources of surface water (such as rivers, lakes, or springs) and groundwater (such as shallow wells). Piped water can become contaminated through cracks or unofficial connections in water lines. Also, if piped water is not adequately treated, the water delivered to the tap may be contaminated. Water can become contaminated during transport if carried in dirty containers or touched by dirty hands. Stored water can become contaminated if it is stored in a dirty or uncovered container, removed with a dirty cup, or touched by soiled hands.

Worldwide, over 1.1 billion people lack access to protected water supplies. Rural villages in Nyanza Province in western Kenya provide a good example of a population without access to safe water. The communities rely on unprotected surface water sources. In 1999, a survey conducted by CARE, an international nongovernmental organization, revealed that 66% of the population in this impoverished region lacked access to improved water supplies, and 47% of children younger than 5 years had experienced diarrhoea in the preceding 2 weeks. The populations of most of the surveyed villages did not have access to health care. When a child is sick with diarrhoea, the mother treats the child at home, usually with traditional remedies, and is unable to earn money for the family.

Management and intervention

In response to the problem of lack of access to safe water, the United States Centers for Disease Control and Prevention (CDC) and the Pan American Health Organization/World Health Organization (PAHO/WHO) developed the Safe Water System, a household-based water quality intervention (www.cdc.gov/safewater). The intervention has three main components: (1) point-of-use treatment with locally produced sodium hypochlorite solution; (2) safe storage through the use of containers with a narrow mouth, tight-fitting lid, and a spigot for removing water; and (3) behaviour change techniques, such as social marketing, community mobilization, motivational interviewing, and hygiene education. In projects in Africa, South America, and Central Asia, families who used the Safe Water System had 44–85% fewer episodes of diarrhoea than families who did not.

The CARE-CDC Health Initiative, which was created through a grant from the Woodruff Foundation to foster increased collaboration between the two organizations, awarded a grant to CARE Kenya in October 1999 to implement the Safe Water System in Nyanza Province. A total of 72 communities with a population of 45 000 people were selected for the project on the basis of having very limited or no access to protected water supplies. The different sectors and organizations involved in planning and implementing the intervention included CARE, CDC, a private company that produces sodium hypochlorite solution, and management committees at the local level that used participatory hygiene and sanitation transformation (PHAST) methods. Formative research conducted by CARE revealed that 91% of households stored drinking-water in open-mouthed clay pots and that these pots were preferred over plastic jerry cans. Laboratory and village-based studies determined that contaminated surface water treated with an adequate dose of sodium hypochlorite retained free chlorine residuals greater than 0.2 mg/l for 24 hours and had no detectable bacterial contamination.

Responding to the preference for storing water in clay pots, the project worked with the Oriang Women Pottery Group to produce improved pots with narrow mouths, fitted lids, and spigots. Point-of-use water treatment was promoted through the use of 1% sodium hypochlorite solution that was manufactured in Kenya and packaged in a bottle with an 8-ml cap that served as a dosing device.

The behaviour change techniques used in this project included community mobilization and social marketing. The disinfectant solution was sold under the brand name Klorin at a price affordable to the target population. Promotional activities included puppet shows, skits, dancers dressed in Klorin bottle costumes, a truck with a loudspeaker system, soccer tournaments, public demonstrations of the product, and Klorin quizzes with prizes. Village health promoters received T-shirts, water vessels, or Klorin bottles as incentives for meeting sales targets. To encourage improved water storage, the modified clay pots were subsidized and packaged with a free bottle of Klorin during the promotional period.

The project encountered difficulties. Daily power blackouts of up to 18 hours hindered product procurement and delayed implementation by 3 months. In addition, poor road conditions and large distances between communities made product distribution difficult. Despite these challenges, the project was ultimately successfully implemented.

Evaluation, follow-up and relevance to other settings

Six months after introducing the Safe Water System, product adoption was monitored in a random sample of 20% of households in 12 project villages. Water stored in 58 (33.5%) of 173 households had detectable free chlorine levels, indicating use of Klorin, and 32 (18.5%) of 173 households were using the modified clay pots.

To evaluate the health impact of the intervention, active diarrhoea surveillance, which consisted of weekly home visits by field workers trained by CARE to ask about diarrhoea episodes in children less than 5 years old in the preceding 7 days, was conducted for 8 weeks in 12 intervention and six comparison communities. Klorin use was also measured weekly by testing stored water for free chlorine. The surveillance data were analysed to determine adherence to Klorin use and the effect of various factors on diarrhoea rates. During the 8 weeks, 37–60% of households in intervention communities had free chlorine levels over 0.2 mg/l in their water. Overall, there was a 74% lower risk of diarrhoea in intervention communities than in comparison communities. Households using Klorin had a 58% lower diarrhoea risk than households not using Klorin, and households with latrines had a 45% lower diarrhoea risk than households without latrines.

Several factors contributed to the success of this intervention. First, CARE conducted thorough formative research to identify the local knowledge, attitudes, and practices related to water and diarrhoeal disease. Second, CARE obtained support early in the project from Kenyan government officials, community management committees, and leaders of women's groups. Third, CARE used a participatory approach to mobilize the community, which motivated and empowered the population. Fourth, the local community identified poor water quality and diarrhoea as their highest priority problems, so they were motivated to adopt the Safe Water System. Fifth, because the Safe Water System is a simple and inexpensive intervention, it was adopted by a large percentage of the target population. Sixth, social marketing activities conducted by CARE helped make the disinfectant solution and improved clay pots accessible.

To build on the momentum of these successes, the project is looking for opportunities to expand. In particular, CARE will engage the private sector by recruiting commercial establishments to sell Klorin at the current low price. To address the issue of economic sustainability, a Kenyan economist is conducting a cost-effectiveness study of the Safe Water System in this setting. In addition, further research on behaviour change strategies will be done to determine the approach that is most effective in motivating sustained use of the Safe Water System. The Safe Water System is relevant in any developing country setting where water quality is a problem. Successful projects in countries other than Kenya have demonstrated the intervention's practicality and usefulness. In Zambia, a pilot social marketing trial in a periurban slum rapidly expanded in response to a cholera epidemic and is now national in scope. The number of bottles of disinfectant sold has grown every year, and sales exceeded 1 million bottles in 2001. In Madagascar, CARE, Population Services International, and CDC launched a Safe Water System project in 30 poor neighbourhoods in urban

Antananarivo during a cholera epidemic, which immediately led to expansion beyond the project site. A series of three cyclones over a 9-week period accelerated demand to the point where the project grew to national scale in less than a year. These experiences demonstrate that there is a need, desire, and market for point-of-use water quality interventions in diverse communities throughout the developing world.

8. CONTAMINATED WATER DISTRIBUTION: AN INTERVENTION STRATEGY TO SOLVE A PUBLIC HEALTH PROBLEM

J. C. Semenza
School of Community Health, Portland State University,
Portland, OR, USA

Description of the problem

Extensive irrigation of cotton fields has depleted water resources along the Amudaria River leading to increased salinity and decreased fish population in the Aral Sea. Uzbekistan has been disproportionately affected by the Aral Sea crisis: along with declining socioeconomic status, the overall health of the population has deteriorated as a consequence of this environmental degradation.

To examine the health impact of this environmental crisis, we collected passive surveillance data from the Sanitary Epidemiologic Services (SES) in Nukus, a city of 200 000 residents, located 250 km south of the Aral Sea. While rates of cancer and other chronic diseases were stable over the past decade (with the exception of anaemia in women), we noted a marked seasonal pattern in the occurrence of diarrhoea and dysentery each year. There was a tenfold increase in diarrhoeal diseases during the summer months, with up to 180 cases a month. The problem disproportionately affected children under five years of age. Furthermore, the actual number of enteric cases was probably much higher, because the SES data only reflect cases that were treated in hospital.

Exposure to gastrointestinal pathogens can arise from several sources, such as surface water, household water containers, foods and drinks, poor personal hygiene and sanitation, or municipal water supplies. In order to improve the situation and take public health action to create a healthy environment for children, the most significant route of transmission had to be identified.

Management and intervention

We examined food-handling practices, personal hygiene and sanitation in the city of Nukus, but were not able to identify a significant overriding problem. In fact, personal hygiene practices, such as hand-washing before eating, appeared to be better than in the United States. We also evaluated the chlorination procedures at the water treatment plants in Nukus and concluded that, theoretically, the two-step chlorination procedure was adequate.

The pathway for diarrhoeal infections can be determined by establishing a reference population. One possible source of exposure, such as the water supply, is eliminated in this reference population and the impact on diarrhoeal rates is monitored. By creating such a reference population, which differs in only one respect (i.e. the water supply), conclusions can be drawn regarding the mechanism of disease transmission. If the intervention does not have an impact on diarrhoeal disease rates, the water supply is not contaminated; conversely, if the rates are reduced considerably the water supply is the likely source of the contamination.

We conducted a randomized intervention study involving a total of 240 households, each with at least one child under five years of age, 120 with and 120 without access to municipal piped water (1). The intervention consisted of providing a narrow-necked water container with a spout that prevented recontamination once the water had been disinfected with chlorine. Of the 120 households without access to piped water, 62 households received the intervention and were monitored for diarrhoea for 9½ weeks during the summer months (when the highest rates were observed), along with two control populations: households with and without access to piped water.

A group of local interviewers visited the households in the study twice a week and asked an adult family member about diarrhoea or dysentery among the family members. Intervention and no-intervention households were surveyed in an identical manner.

The intervention was conducted as a collaborative effort between scientists from the Centers for Disease Control and Prevention (CDC), SES, US Agency for International Development (USAID), and local physicians and municipal officials.

Evaluation and effectiveness of intervention

In the intervention households we found a dramatic reduction in childhood diarrhoeal rates. Children with access to disinfected water through their water container were three times less likely to suffer from diarrhoea or dysentery than the control group (42.2 episodes per 1000 children per month versus 127.7 episodes). Despite the fact that children in this intervention group did not have piped water at home and thus were of considerably lower socioeconomic status, they were half as likely to have diarrhoea as children in households with access to piped water (84.4 episodes per 1000 children per month). These data indicate that the deteriorating water distribution system in the city was contaminated, since children who drank tap water were more likely to get sick than children in the intervention group. We also found that 30% of the households with piped water lacked detectable levels of chlorine residues in their tap water, increasing the risk for diarrhoea, in spite of the two-stage chlorination procedure. In at least 42% of the households, water pressure had been intermittent in the two days prior to the interview.

On the basis of these epidemiological data we were able to implicate the water distribution system as the main source of disease transmission: lack of water availability (due to the Aral Sea crisis) and low water pressure allow contaminated water to be drawn into the drinking water lines where it depletes chlorine residues. This cross-contamination explains why subjects who drink tap water with inadequate residual chlorine are more likely to develop diarrhoea.

It also explains why subjects who have access to household water treatment suffer from fewer diarrhoeal episodes than those who drink tap water.

Conclusions

On the basis of these findings, with the support of USAID, city engineers increased water availability, allowing water pressure to be maintained in the distribution system. Leaks and water losses were minimized and chlorination was closely monitored by municipal officials. These relatively inexpensive modifications are expected to reduce diarrhoeal rates in Nukus and to have a positive impact on children's health, in contrast to other costly measures such as reverse osmosis technology. Installing reverse osmosis technology to purify drinking-water would have minimal impact on water quality since cross-contamination would introduce gastrointestinal pathogens into the drinking-water.

Since the neighbourhoods without access to piped water were permanent and long-standing rather than temporary, this intervention demonstrated the feasibility of providing disinfected water to a disenfranchised population. The intervention was well accepted by participants who realized the positive impact it had on their health. Bleach, as a source of chlorine, and water containers are readily available on local markets. However, the water containers used for this study suffered from leaks and punctures suggesting the need for a more durable type of container. Furthermore, the price of locally available water containers was more than the study participants were willing to pay. Therefore, access to these water containers remains a hurdle for widespread implementation of household water treatment (see also Case Study 7).

This simple community intervention provides evidence for a cost-effective public health solution that can be adapted in other settings where deteriorating water treatment facilities and distribution systems pose a threat to children's health. Furthermore, this case study in Uzbekistan illustrates how field epidemiology can be used as an analytical tool to address a children's environmental health problem and to guide public health policy decisions.

Reference

1. Semenza JC et al. Water distribution system and diarrhoeal disease transmission: A case study in Uzbekistan. *American Journal of Tropical Medicine and Hygiene*, 1998, 59:941–946.

9. A FLUOROTIC VILLAGE

E. Dahi
Environmental Development Co-operation Group, Soborg,
Denmark

The village

Ngungongare is a village of 2000 inhabitants in northern United Republic of Tanzania. It lies at the foot of Mount Meru, within the Rift Valley, which constitutes a large part of the African "fluoride belt", stretching from the Syrian Arab Republic and Jordan through Egypt, Sudan, Ethiopia, Kenya, and the United Republic of Tanzania down to South Africa. Natural weathering of the volcanic and sedimentary rocks releases the fluoride ion from its complex compounds into the natural waters.

Fluorosis

In Ngungongare, about 80% of adults and 95% of children are affected by *dental fluorosis*. The adults who are not affected usually grew up in a low-fluoride area. Healthy children are usually newcomers or still have milk teeth.

Nine-year-old Rebecca is a typical fluorotic child of Ngungongare, where she was born and has lived throughout her life. Her severe *dental fluorosis* is illustrated in Figure 21.3. Her parents, however, are "immigrants", with healthy, regular, white teeth. Rebecca tries to avoid smiling and, when she does, she covers her teeth in shame. All her teeth are affected, and some show deep black erosions. Rebecca says that her teeth cause her pain when she has cold or hot drinks or eats hard food.

Rebecca's arms and legs seem to be quite normal, with slight swelling at the joints. So far she does not feel *huma*, as the early signs of fluorosis associated with rheumatic fever and pain in the joints are called in Swahili. Rebecca and her parents do not know that it is only a question of time before she suffers from *non-skeletal fluorosis* and that in the long term she may suffer disability. She is still too young to understand that this irreversible disability may be detrimental for her future social life and working opportunities.

But Rebecca is more fortunate than others. Some children of her age already have deformities in their extremities, as shown in Figure 21.4. For example, Richard's elbows, knees and ankles are enlarged and

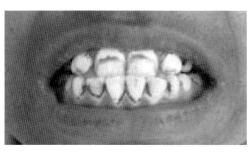

Figure 21.3 Dental fluorosis

rigid. He suffers from the first stage of *skeletal fluorosis* but is still capable of moving around and herding cattle. Up to 10% of the children of primary school age suffer from skeletal fluorosis; these children are at very high risk of *crippling fluorosis* later in life. Skeletal deformities, rigidity and pain in the joints, in addition to *huma* and teeth discoloration and decay, are common among the elderly in the village.

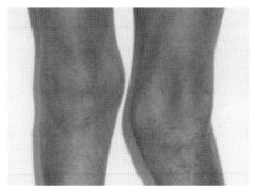

Figure 21.4 Skeletal fluorosis

The water

When Rebecca is asked if she knows the reason for her teeth discoloration and deterioration, she answers *"ni maji"*: it is the water. In a fluorotic village like Ngungongare, not only the water, but also air, soil and crops contain fluoride at concentrations well above normal. Furthermore, the local people tend to use *magadi*, a carbonate/bicarbonate salt that contains high concentrations of fluoride, as a food additive. In some countries, industrial and air pollution, especially due to the burning of coal, may also cause fluorosis. However, for a typical fluorotic village like Ngungongare, research has shown that exposure through drinking-water and water used in cooking is far more significant than all other exposures taken together.

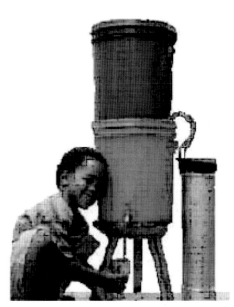

Figure 21.5 A domestic defluoridation filter

For decades, the villagers have been using the water from surrounding springs whose fluoride concentrations vary between 2 and 8 mg/l. In recent years, some families have started to collect rainwater for drinking during the few months of the year when this is possible. A piped water scheme has been made available to meet the increasing demand for water. However, this does not solve the fluorosis problem but, on the contrary, worsens it, in part because the piped water contains higher fluoride concentrations (of 12–21 mg/l), and in part because the villagers now obtain less water from the springs and rain, as the tap stands are easily accessible.

Similarity to arsenic

Fluoride shares some of its unfortunate properties with arsenic. In both cases the water is usually without colour, turbidity, smell or taste, yet it contains the agent at highly toxic levels. In both cases, equipment, chemicals and skilled personnel are needed to measure the agent in the water. In both cases, the effect on health does not appear immediately but with delay, and is irreversible. The appropriate technology to remove both toxic agents from the water is available, but experience with implementation is limited. And in both cases, the health problems prevail mainly in developing countries with severe socioeconomic constraints.

Mitigation

It has been estimated that more than 100 million people in the world suffer from one or more types of fluorosis. As in Ngungongare, the fluorosis problem is increasing, mainly as a result of general improvements in life expectancy and the increased use of groundwater. Providing piped supplies of safe water to fluorotic areas is often not possible. In these cases, the only solution to the problem is to install community or domestic defluoridation units for treatment of the water to be used for drinking and food preparation.

Any reduction in fluoride exposure would be beneficial, but to ensure healthy teeth for newborn children, the concentration of fluoride must be brought down to about 0.5 mg/l, i.e. far below what has been considered the "maximum allowable" and "optimum recommended" levels. Defluoridators are simple, workable and affordable and can be made using local materials and manpower. Figure 21.5 shows such a domestic defluoridator. It can be based on bone char, activated alumina or any other fluoride sorption medium. But such units can only be sustained if the family is disciplined and motivated and if capacity-building, logistic support and professional services are provided. An alternative solution is shown in Figure 21.6, a community unit ensuring that the water is taken only for drinking and cooking.

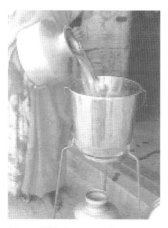

Figure 21.6 A community defluoridation plant

Mitigation of fluorosis will be a great challenge for nongovernmental organizations and donors in the decades to come.

10. CARBON MONOXIDE POISONING IN CHILDREN IN FRANCE

M. Mathieu-Nolf
Poison Control Centre, Lille, France

Description of the problem

Carbon monoxide (CO) is a tasteless, odourless, and non-irritating gas produced by the incomplete combustion of organic materials. The most common sources of CO include improperly maintained and poorly ventilated home or water heating systems (unvented or defective gas/coal/wood/fuel stoves and fireplaces, kerosene space heaters, water heaters), cooking devices (gas burners, barbecues), car exhausts, and cigarette smoke. Most of these sources are found indoors, where young children spend most of their time.

CO poisoning is a leading cause of accidental and fatal poisonings in many countries. In France, between 5000 and 8000 poisonings occur every year (10–15 cases per 100 000 inhabitants) with about 25% affecting children under 15 years of age. Up to 400 people die from CO poisoning every year, of whom 16.4% are children.

When inhaled, CO is readily absorbed from the lungs into the bloodstream and prevents oxygen uptake by binding to haeminic proteins. In addition to hypoxaemic hypoxia, CO poisoning induces histotoxic hypoxia. Carboxyhaemoglobin dissociation begins as soon as the patient is removed from the CO environment. Beyond the high risk of immediate death during intoxication, moderate to severe poisonings can lead to long-term effects including memory impairment, personality alterations, signs of parietal dysfunction and, more rarely, motor symptoms (hemiplegia, akinesia). In children, temporary cortical blindness and involuntary movements have also been reported. To date, there is little information about the risk of delayed neurological sequelae in infants with CO poisoning. Generally, the long-term consequences of CO poisoning in children are likely to be underestimated.

The frequency of CO intoxication varies between different regions depending on local heating or cooking habits, the socioeconomic situation, and weather conditions. For example, the morbidity incidence rate varies between 17.5 per 100 000 inhabitants in the Paris area and 24 per 100 000 inhabitants in the northern region. The high incidence in the north is a likely consequence of the coal mining industry, which was active until 1980, the high rate of unemployment and frequent fog.

As almost 30% of CO poisoning cases are misdiagnosed at first, the risk of inadequate treatment is high. Despite efforts to improve prevention, medical education and public information, intoxication remains frequent and severe, and is too often overlooked. Early recognition and correct treatment and follow-up of CO poisoning in children are crucial for the prevention of recurrence and long-term health effects.

Management and intervention

Considering the high incidence of CO poisoning in the north of France, a systemic approach was adopted to act on the multiple factors responsible for CO poisoning.

Decreasing risk of CO exposure

A continuous surveillance system was set up by the regional poison centre (PC) in 1986. This toxicovigilance programme follows up every case of CO poisoning that results in hospitalization. Data are collected from a network involving the Critical Care Unit and Hyperbaric Centre of Lille University Hospital, every emergency department, paediatric unit and critical care unit of the regional and general hospitals, medical rescue services, fire-fighters and environmental health engineers at regional and departmental public health services. CO poisonings are classified as certain, probable, suspected, not related, or unknown. For every case, a systematic follow-up is carried out by medical staff of the poisons centre by telephone or visits at 1, 3, 6 and 12 months after the poisoning occurred. To obtain information on deaths outside hospitals from CO poisoning (82% of victims are found dead at home or die before reaching hospital) the poisons centre set up a complementary surveillance programme to record all deaths, using other sources of information, such as forensic departments.

The two surveillance systems are used to monitor the frequency, severity and mortality from CO poisoning, and to identify high-risk circumstances or populations. When the surveillance system detects a sudden increase in the incidence of CO poisoning an alert is sent to health, environment and consumer authorities, and to the general public via the media. For example, a rapid increase in the incidence of CO poisoning in the north of France was detected in 1989 related to the introduction of kerosene space heaters. National health authorities and the consumer council were alerted, and as a result manufacturers were obliged to equip heaters with CO detectors and other safety devices. During the following four years, only one case of CO poisoning was recorded. However, after a change in regulations, six new cases were recorded in 1994 and the incidence of CO poisonings has been increasing ever since. New technical preventive measures are currently under investigation.

Increasing awareness and skills of health professionals

Training and continuous education programmes for medical students, physicians and paramedics were developed aimed at preventing complications and sequelae. The programme emphasizes the risk of misdiagnosis and inadequate treatment. Health professionals are encouraged to pay particular attention to high-risk populations such as pregnant women and children.

Data on CO poisoning in 140 children and 774 adults, collected at the Lille University Hospital, illustrated the risk of misdiagnosis in infants. While headache, nausea, and coma were less frequent in children than adults, uncon-

sciousness, convulsions, and lethargy were more frequent. Neurological examinations found fewer abnormal plantar responses and more flaccidity in children than in adults. Many of the early manifestations of CO poisoning are
difficult or impossible to observe in infants. Especially in neonates and toddlers,
CO poisoning is frequently interpreted as gastroenteritis.

The training courses were reformulated and improved to take into account
the particular difficulties of correct diagnosis and treatment in children.

Decreasing the recurrence rate

CO intoxication frequently recurs if no preventive measures are taken. The
Hyperbaric Centre and Emergency Department of Lille University Hospital and
public health engineers developed a programme to decrease the rate of recurrence. Information on the reasons for CO poisoning and preventive measures
is given to patients by medical staff just before the patient is discharged from
hospital, when he or she is most likely to be receptive to the health message.
Furthermore, the physician proposes that a public health engineer should visit
the patient's home to identify sources of CO and other factors relevant to CO
poisoning. Since the implementation of this programme in 1986, the surveillance system has recorded a progressive decrease in the recurrence rate from
4.5% in 1993 to 1.5% in 2000. While this trend is encouraging, efforts must be
maintained.

Evaluation, follow-up and relevance to other settings

The implementation of a surveillance system prior to preventive action has
been the key factor for success. The system monitors data on CO poisonings
with a short-response time to provide up-to-date information to consumer associations and other bodies. As it allows vulnerable subpopulations and risk
behaviours to be identified, prevention messages can be focused on these
groups and have greater impact.

A large multidisciplinary and highly motivated group consisting of physicians and other health professionals, firemen, social workers, manufacturers,
heating professionals, and consumers was essential to raise awareness and
improve skills in relation to CO poisoning among health professionals and the
general public. Use of intermediary persons to convey the message was found
to be very effective.

Despite a multifaceted prevention programme the number of CO poisonings remains high. However, improved information dissemination, regulatory
measures and the implementation of specific social aids could further reduce
the incidence.

Conclusion

The approach to CO poisoning described can be taken as a model for an
efficient toxicovigilance system to monitor other environmental poisons and

pollutants, such as lead. The evolution in data collection from simple data recording via telephone calls to the active collection of representative and meaningful data is essential for preventive action, and points to a much wider role and responsibility for poison centres.

11. CHILDREN DESERVE A SMOKE-FREE WORLD

A. M. David
S. A. Tamplin
Tobacco Free Initiative,
WHO Regional Office for the Western Pacific, Manila,
Philippines

S. Pineda-Mercado
Philippines Department of Health, Department of Health
Promotion and Health Education, University of the
Philippines, Manila, Philippines

Tobacco use contributes significantly to premature mortality and the burden of chronic disease and disability in the Western Pacific Region. While the health impact of the tobacco epidemic on smokers is well documented, the effect on children exposed to second-hand smoke is less frequently recognized. Nevertheless, a growing body of evidence points to second-hand smoke as an important risk factor for sudden infant death syndrome, asthma, and pulmonary and middle ear infections in children (1).

The Philippines has 76 million inhabitants; about 40% are under the age of 15. One in three adults smokes, and an estimated 60% of households have at least one smoker (1). Therefore, the number of children potentially at risk from exposure to second-hand smoke in the home is considerable. In addition, before 1999, no national legislation existed to ensure smoke-free public places.

The influential lobby of the tobacco industry and the tobacco farmers' association from the northern provinces presented a barrier to policy changes regarding tobacco control and provisions for smoke-free public places. A strong and unequivocal message was needed to demonstrate that support for tobacco control would be in the interest of the majority of the population, particularly vulnerable groups such as children.

Working in partnership with the Philippine Department of Health, UNICEF and a private advertising company, WHO developed a communications and advocacy strategy with the aim of empowering nonsmokers to speak up and defend their right to clean, smoke-free air. The precampaign survey indicated that, while most tobacco control advertising focused on health risks to the smoker, nonsmokers believed that they were also at risk. In addition, the nonsmoking survey respondents reported feeling annoyed and resentful when exposed to tobacco smoke, but were reluctant to speak up, even in areas designated as nonsmoking.

WHO created three television advertisements, set in the family environment, the workplace and a coffee bar, carrying the message: "It's OK to say you mind." These focused on the dilemma nonsmokers face when persons near them light up, and their hesitation to address the issue. In all three advertisements, the individuals who find the courage to speak up for themselves are surprised to find that smokers, even teenagers, are responsive and willing to stop smoking when asked.

One of the advertisements attempted to relate the nonsmoker's right to clean air with the high value Filipinos give to their children's welfare. Filipinos treasure their offspring, and this is even reflected in national policy. The Declaration of Policy of the Child and Youth Welfare Code states: *"The child is one of the most important assets of the nation. Every effort should be exerted to promote its welfare and enhance its opportunities for a useful and happy life."* Filipino parents are willing to sacrifice much for their children's sake. Thus, when made aware that they are unintentionally exposing their children to a health hazard, many parents will give up their hazardous behaviour. The advertisement illustrates this by depicting a family with three young children and a father who smokes at the dinner table. After hearing one of the children coughing in the background, the eldest son gently speaks up and asks his father not to smoke. The father is momentarily taken aback, but realizing that his smoking is adversely affecting his children, he apologizes and puts out his cigarette.

All three advertisements were run on national television from October 1999 to January 2000 using commercial and public television stations. A postcampaign survey to assess the impact of the communications campaign was carried out in February 2000. This survey showed that the advertisement featuring the smoking father and his children was the best remembered among both smokers and nonsmokers (Table 21.4), and that the visual elements and message were the most recognized (2). Graduate students at the College of Mass Communications of the University of the Philippines evaluated locally produced tobacco control-related TV advertisements from 1992 to 2000, based on visual attractiveness, audience recall, cultural relevance and overall impact. This particular advertisement was considered to be one of the most effective in conveying the powerful health message to refrain from tobacco use.

While a child's right to a safe and healthy environment is not yet anchored within the Convention on the Rights of the Child, the Philippines' Child and Youth Welfare Code states clearly that *"every child has the right to live in a*

Table 21.4   Audience recall of television advertisements

TELEVISION ADVERTISEMENT	AUDIENCE RECALL (%)	
	SMOKERS ($n = 81$)	NONSMOKERS ($n = 75$)
1: Family at dinner	31%	23%
2: Peer group	1%	11%
3: Workplace	9%	12%

community and a society that can offer him an environment free from pernicious influences and conducive to the promotion of his health and the cultivation of his desirable traits and attributes." Partly as a result of the media exposure generated by the television campaign, both the public and the private sector started to show interest in tobacco control as a means to protect the rights of children to a clean and healthy environment. For example, the Philippine Paediatric Society and the National Asthma Movement started to include sessions on tobacco as an environmental hazard to children in their various conferences and national congresses. The National Institutes of Health and the Department of Health held a research forum for the media and academia on the effects of involuntary exposure to tobacco smoke among infants and children. The Department of Health chose the theme of protecting children from tobacco smoke in its tobacco control campaign. On World No Tobacco Day 2000, they organized a Youth Congress where young people from each of the political districts held a symbolic session at the National Congress to pass tobacco control legislation. These young people gave impassioned speeches on why it is critical for the government to speak up on behalf of all Filipino children and take action to preserve their right to a clean, tobacco-free environment.

The Philippine Clean Air Act, ratified in 1999, has been in the process of implementation since 2000. It includes a provision for smoke-free enclosed public places and public transport. While enforcement needs to be improved, it represents significant progress towards ensuring a healthy indoor environment for children. A new alliance of government and nongovernmental organizations is continuing political advocacy for tobacco control using the issue of safeguarding children's health as a major theme.

Emphasizing the hazardous effect of exposure to second-hand smoke on children's health can also serve as a means to broaden the audience for tobacco control advocacy. By demonstrating the consequences of indirect exposure to tobacco smoke, nonsmokers — who form the majority of the population but are often left out of typical tobacco control messages — can be engaged in tobacco control. Policy leaders and legislators may not always be receptive to the health arguments for controlling tobacco use. However, these key political leaders are sensitive to issues that involve infringement of the rights of vulnerable groups, particularly children. Framing tobacco control as a means of protecting children's rights to clean air and a healthy environment can be a potent tool towards mobilizing support for tobacco-free environments.

References

1. *International Consultation on Environmental Tobacco Smoke (ETS) and Child Health, 11–14 January 1999.* Geneva, World Health Organization, 1999 (background papers).
2. Taylor Nelson Sofres Philippines. *Campaign effectiveness survey, 2000.* Manila, 2000.

12. IMPROVEMENT IN RESPIRATORY SYMPTOMS IN CHILDREN AS A RESULT OF POLLUTION CONTROL STRATEGIES IN A DISTRICT OF THE CITY OF SÃO PAULO, BRAZIL

H. Ribeiro
School of Public Health, University of São Paulo, Brazil

São Paulo, Brazil, an urban sprawl of 1051 square kilometres and 16.7 million inhabitants, is one of the biggest cities in the world. Over 40 000 potentially polluting industries and 5.7 million vehicles are currently registered.

During the 1970s, emissions from factories had an important influence on health problems as industrial activities of a diverse nature dominated the economy of the region until the 1980s. The installation of industrial plants close to residential areas was common and, in several cases, this resulted in severe health risks. Respiratory diseases were the second largest cause of death in São Paulo in 1980. The process of industrialization and land occupation, together with meteorological conditions unfavourable to the dispersion of pollutants (frequent low altitude thermal inversions during winter in a topography formed by a floodplain surrounded by mountains in the north and north-east, receiving predominant winds from the ocean in the south-east) resulted in the deterioration of air quality.

The average concentration of sulfur dioxide and particulate matter in air in the metropolitan area for 1973–1984 was mapped by this author. A survey was conducted at seven schools of the government school system in three neighbourhoods of São Paulo, to assess the influence of air pollution on respiratory symptoms of children between 11 and 13 years of age. The three neighbourhoods had a similar family income but distinct pollution levels reflecting different types of land use. The first district, which was used as a control area, was a watershed protection area surrounded by parks; the second was a blue collar worker's district with more modern industrial plants and medium pollution level, close to the air quality standard limits of the national Environment Bureau (CETESB) (1); the third showed very high levels of pollution throughout the year. The age group was chosen because children are more sensitive to air pollution, do not smoke and are not affected by occupational pollution. Children may receive a higher dose of outdoor pollutants than adults because they have a higher minute ventilation per unit body mass, are generally more physically active, and spend more time outdoors than adults (2). The research tool employed was a questionnaire developed by Ferris and a team from the Pulmonary Disease Division of the US National Heart, Lung and Blood Institute in the Epidemiology Standardization Project (3). Between 100 and 150 questionnaires were completed in each of the three neighbourhoods.

The area where pollution levels were highest was Tatuapé, an old industrial district with mixed land use: workers' houses located among large factories, some built before 1920 and others in the 1940s and 1950s, with little or no pollution control. A dense population and a significant number of children were exposed to pollution levels that largely surpassed the national primary standards for annual average concentrations limit of $80\,\mu g/m^3$. In Tatuapé, the average annual concentration of sulfur dioxide was $124\,\mu g/m^3$, and of particulate matter $127\,\mu g/m^3$ during the period 1973–1986 (Fig. 21.7). A strong correlation was found between levels of sulfur dioxide and particulate matter and respiratory symptoms in children.

Management and intervention

Air quality management in São Paulo started in 1976, when air quality standards and emission standards were set for stationary sources. Initially, standards were set for four major pollutants — particulate matter, carbon monoxide, sulfur dioxide and photochemical oxidants — with levels similar to the primary standards of the US Environmental Protection Agency (USEPA). In 1990, these were revised and the new air quality standards incorporated primary standards for the protection of public health, and secondary standards for the protection of the environment and for human well-being in relation to suspended particles, inhalable particles (PM_{10}), smoke, sulfur dioxide, carbon monoxide, nitrogen dioxide and ozone.

In addition to the standards, regulatory mechanisms, improved technology, and the transfer of many heavy industries to other parts of the state and of the country have reduced industrial sources of air pollution to the point where vehicles are the main sources of air pollution in the city. At first, control programmes were initiated by the State Government, in part as a response to growing international pressure following the UN Conference in Stockholm in 1972, and were financed by State Government, private and public industries, and the World Bank. In 1980, a law was passed to regulate industrial zoning for the areas where pollution problems were acute. These policies and increased media coverage contributed to increased awareness among the general public in the 1980s and 1990s. This was also greatly influenced by the preparations for the UN Conference on Environment and Development which took place in Rio de Janeiro in 1992. Nongovernmental organizations, universities and research institutes played an important role in awareness raising and in training professionals and local authorities to face the problem.

Sulfur dioxide concentrations fell as a result of the industrial pollution controls adopted in 1982, lower limits for sulfur levels in fuel oil, and the substitution of fuel oil by natural gas. In Tatuapé, sulfur dioxide levels dropped from $124\,\mu g/m^3$ in 1973–1983 to $40\,\mu g/m^3$ in 1990–1998 (Fig. 21.7) (4, 5). The concentration of particulate matter also decreased significantly in the district, as many industries moved to other areas, making room for residential land use. Levels of particulate matter dropped from $127\,\mu g/m^3$ in 1973–1983 to $65\,\mu g/m^3$ in 1991–1992. From 1992, smoke levels were also monitored. Between 1992 and

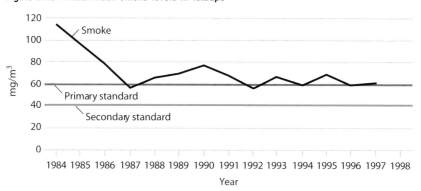

Figure 21.7 Annual mean levels of sulfur dioxide in Tatuapé

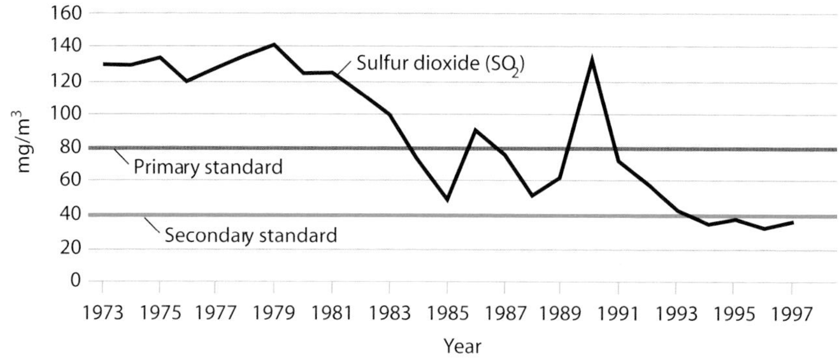

Source of data: ref. 4.

Figure 21.8 Annual mean smoke levels in Tatuapé

Source of data: ref. 5.

1997, smoke concentrations were on average $61 \mu g/m^3$, close to the primary air quality standard limit of $60 \mu g/m^3$ and above the secondary air quality standard limit of $40 \mu g/m^3$ (Fig. 21.8).

Effect of pollution control on children's health

The first survey, conducted in 1986, indicated that symptoms of respiratory disease tended to increase with higher pollution levels. In Tatuapé, there was a higher prevalence rate of 26 of the 35 symptoms studied (72.2%) than in areas with lower pollution levels.

Twelve years later, in 1998, a second survey was undertaken (3) to evaluate the impact of pollution management programmes on pollution levels and respiratory symptoms among children. In 1998, Tatuapé had a higher prevalence of only 12 of the 35 symptoms (34%) studied when compared with the other

SECTION VI: CASE STUDIES

two areas. The prevalence of symptoms in the other two neighbourhoods increased between 1986 and 1998; pollution control programmes were less effective there and largely neutralized by the higher number of cars in the streets. In Tatuapé, the prevalence of 19 indicators decreased: cough with cold (by 6.3%); phlegm with cold (12.3%); phlegm on most days (6.2%); congested chest more than one week per year (6.7%); wheezing with cold (3.2%); chest illness which caused lack of activity for more than three days a year (0.7%); chest illness with more phlegm (3%); measles (12.4%); sinus trouble (1.5%); pneumonia (1.8%); whooping cough (2.3%); frequent ear infection (age group 0–2 years: 5.2%; age group 2–5 years: 1.3%; above 5 years: 2.9%); surgical removal of tonsils or adenoid (9.3%); asthma diagnosed by doctor (1.4%); having to take medicine for asthma (0.3%); heart problem (2.9%).

Conclusions

Public policies and programmes to control air pollution and for industrial zoning have proved to be important tools in reducing health risks. Levels of most air pollutants, with the exception of ozone, decreased and are below or close to the acceptable limits. Respiratory diseases fell from second to fourth leading cause of death in São Paulo. Nevertheless the effectiveness of the programmes is unequally distributed in the urban area. It is important that, in addition to emission control programmes and industrial zoning, an environmental plan, which incorporates health, traffic, public transportation and housing sectors, is elaborated and put in practice with community support.

References

1. Companhia de Tecnologia de Saneamento Ambiental (www.cetesb.sp.gov.br).
2. Committee of the Environmental and Occupational Health Assembly of the American Thoracic Society. Health effects of outdoor air pollution. *American Journal of Respiratory and Critical Care Medicine*, 1996, 153:3–50.
3. Ferris BG. Epidemiology standardization project. *American Review of Respiratory Disease*, 1978, 118:1–120.
4. Ribeiro H. Air pollution and respiratory disease in São Paulo (1986–1998). *Ninth International Symposium in Medical Geography. University of Montréal, Canada,* 2000.
5. Companhia de Tecnologia de Saneamento Ambiental (CETESB). *Relatórios de qualidade do ar no estado de São Paulo.* São Paulo, CETESB 1980 to 2000.

13. AIR POLLUTION AND PREGNANCY OUTCOME

R. Sram

*Laboratory of Genetic Ecotoxicology, Institute of
Experimental Medicine, Academy of Sciences of the Czech
Republic, Prague, Czech Republic*

There is widespread concern over the health effects of ambient air pollution. Support is growing for the idea that several adverse pregnancy outcomes may be the result of maternal or paternal exposure to airborne pollution. A consistent relationship between maternal exposure to fine particles in early gestation and intrauterine growth retardation (IUGR) was recently observed in a highly polluted district of Northern Bohemia in the Czech Republic. One possible explanation for this finding is that, not the particles themselves, but some associated co-pollutants, such as polycyclic aromatic hydrocarbons (PAH), may interfere with fetal development.

The Teplice district is one of four mining districts in Northern Bohemia, where power plants produce approximately 50% of the electricity for the Czech Republic. These power plants burn brown coal that is rich in sulfur and, together with glass production, chemical manufacturing and the petrochemical industry represent a major contributor to air pollution. In 1988, Northern Bohemia produced 47% of the sulfur dioxide emissions and 39% of the nitrogen oxide emissions in the Czech Republic.

This pollution significantly affects the health of the approximately 500 000 inhabitants of the region, leading to decreased life expectancy, increased incidence of cancer, cardiovascular diseases, and immune deficiencies in children, and a number of reproductive and behavioural abnormalities. In November 1990, the Czech Government initiated the Teplice Programme to provide scientifically valid information on environmental health problems in the Northern Bohemian mining districts.

Management and intervention

A population-based study of pregnancy outcomes evaluated the impact of air pollution and lifestyle on the outcome of all pregnancies delivered in hospital, using biomarkers as a measure of exposure. The study group included all 7800 single births in the Teplice and Prachatice (control, without pollution) districts between 1994 and 1998. Only full-term births of mothers of European origin were included.

Low birth weight (LBW; defined as below 2500 g), premature birth (less than 37 weeks) and intrauterine growth retardation (IUGR) were chosen as the main reproductive outcomes. IUGR is an important predictor of neonatal morbidity and mortality as well as of diseases later in life, such as non-insulin-dependent diabetes, hypertension and coronary heart disease. Two basic approaches were combined:

- In a prospective cohort study, the simultaneous effects of air pollution and several other factors on pregnancy outcomes were analysed, and critical windows of exposure considered for different outcomes.
- In a nested case–control study a sample of cases with diverse adverse outcomes and systematically selected controls were studied.

To evaluate the exposure, response and state of the mother and her child, selected biomarkers were determined in venous blood, cord blood and placenta. Different metabolic genotypes were also determined to estimate the magnitude of the variation in genetic susceptibility to exposure to air pollution.

A considerably higher prevalence of all adverse outcomes was found in the highly polluted district of Teplice than in Prachatice; this difference remained significant even after adjustment for ethnic and social composition and smoking habits. A significant and dose-dependent relationship between risk of fetal growth retardation and levels of fine particles (PM_{10}, $PM_{2.5}$) was observed in Teplice region. IUGR risk increased 1.19 times with every $10 \mu g/m^3$ increase in PM_{10} exposure during the first month of gestation. No similar association was observed in Prachatice. On the other hand, a strong dose-related association between IUGR risk and concentration of carcinogenic polycyclic aromatic hydrocarbons was found in both Teplice and Prachatice. IUGR risk increased 1.22 times with every $10 ng/m^3$ increase of PAH in early pregnancy. These findings suggest that the first gestational month is a critical period for the effects of air pollution on fetal growth. This is in agreement with the current hypothesis that IUGR is triggered by an abnormal reaction between the trophoblast and uterine tissues during the first week of pregnancy. Also, IUGR is one of the most common consequences of mutagenic exposure around the time of implantation.

PAHs are mostly adsorbed on the surface of fine particles. The above results suggest that PAHs rather than the particles themselves primarily influence fetal growth. PAHs are known to inhibit epidermal growth factor receptors and to alter early trophoblast proliferation. In this way fetoplacental exchange of oxygen and nutrients may be reduced and fetal growth could be impaired. The main source of PM_{10} and PAHs is local heating, especially using coal. Air pollution increasing IUGR is probably present in all large towns in the Czech Republic during the winter season.

The impact of exposure to environmental tobacco smoke (ETS) was analysed in the same cohort of mothers; it was shown that passive smoking reduced the birth weight of infants delivered by nonsmoking mothers and also increased the risk of delivery of low-birth-weight infants by nonsmoking mothers 1.5 times. On the basis of the study, it was estimated that every year approximately 470 babies are born with low birth weight caused by the exposure of non-smoking mothers to ETS. ETS exposure also contributed to birth weight reduction in babies of smoking mothers.

Conclusions and relevance to other settings

Spurred by the results of the Teplice Programme, the Czech Government invested US$ 200 million in Northern Bohemia to replace coal heating by gas, using modern technology. As a result, atmospheric concentrations of sulfur dioxide and suspended particulate matter in the year 2000 had fallen to approximately 15% of the levels in 1990. This substantial decrease in air pollution is a major success story of the recent introduction of an environmental policy in the Czech Republic.

The Teplice Programme showed for the first time that air pollution may adversely affect human reproductive outcomes, including fetal growth. The induced changes appear to include not only observable birth defects but also subtle functional changes affecting their carriers throughout their lives. From their conception, children's complex development is vulnerable to environmental hazards as well as being affected by their mothers' lifestyle such as cigarette smoking or poor diet.

The adverse impact of air pollution on reproductive health is a topic of increasing public health concern. The information presented in this case study should provide new inputs for prenatal care worldwide. This new understanding about children's vulnerability to air pollution should be disseminated to medical professionals and should be included in postgraduate medical education for gynaecologists and paediatricians. We are slowly reaching an understanding of how important the first month of pregnancy is for the future health of the child.

14. ASTHMA CASE STUDY

G. W. K. Wong

Department of Paediatrics, Chinese University of Hong Kong, China, Hong Kong Special Administrative Region

Asthma is one of the most common chronic disorders affecting children in the developed and developing world (1). The prevalence of asthma in children varies widely from less than 5% to more than 30% in different countries. Environmental pollution is one of the important factors contributing to asthma. Environmental pollution, in general, is a more significant problem in the developing world. Most of the outdoor pollutants, including ozone (O_3), sulfur dioxide (SO_2), and nitrogen dioxide (NO_2), are related to combustion of fossil fuels.

In Hong Kong SAR, childhood asthma is a common disorder (2). The main sources of outdoor pollution include automobile exhaust and burning of fossil fuels by various factories. Exposure to SO_2 has been linked to the development of airway inflammation and bronchial hyperresponsiveness (BHR). The level of atmospheric SO_2 is highly dependent on the sulfur content of the fuel used in the community. An increasing level of atmospheric SO_2 is associated with an increasing rate of hospitalization of Hong Kong children for asthma (3). There have been several studies investigating the effect of SO_2 on children's lung health in different districts in Hong Kong SAR. Kwai Tsing district has more than 8000 industrial outlets and air pollution is known to be a big problem. The Southern district is primarily residential and the level of pollution is low.

Table 21.5 shows the dramatic differences between the air quality in these two areas in 1989. Pollutants, including SO_2, NO_2 and respirable suspended particulates (RSP), were significantly higher in the Kwai Tsing district (4). Children from primary schools from the two districts were invited to participate in a ques-

Table 21.5 *Air quality, respiratory symptoms and bronchial hyper-responsiveness in two districts in Hong Kong SAR*

	SOUTHERN	KWAI TSING
Air quality ($\mu g/m^3$)		
SO$_2$	9	117
NO$_2$	21	40
RSP	30	54
Respiratory symptoms	$n = 1486$	$n = 2027$
Wheezing	4%	100%
Doctor-diagnosed asthma	3%	6%

RSP, Respirable suspended particles.

Table 21.6   Results of histamine challenge in children

| | PERCENTAGE SHOWING BHR | | |
	1990	**1991**	**1992**
Southern district	22.6	15.8	10.9
Kwai Tsing	27.4	24.2	12.2

BHR, Bronchial hyperresponsiveness.

tionnaire survey and bronchial challenge test. Symptoms of wheezing and BHR were significantly more common in the Kwai Tsing district.

In July 1990, new government fuel regulations were implemented and the sulfur content of fuel was restricted to a maximum of 0.5%. This resulted in a rapid reduction in atmospheric SO_2 level by more than 80%. A follow-up study of the cohort was performed yearly for two years after the implementation of the new regulation. For children from the polluted Kwai Tsing district, the percentage with BHR decreased significantly from 27.4% to 12.2% (Table 21.6) (4). Such reduction in atmospheric SO_2 should also reduce morbidity in asthmatic children, such as asthma attacks and hospitalization (3).

These sequential analyses of children for BHR demonstrated the effect of successful environmental control on the level of outdoor air pollution. The health benefits were objectively documented by the significant reduction of BHR in schoolchildren.

References

1. The International Study of Asthma and Allergies Steering Committee. Worldwide variation in the prevalence of symptoms of asthma, allergic rhinoconjunctivitis, and atopic eczema: ISAAC. *Lancet*, 1998, 351:1225–1232.
2. Wong GWK et al. Prevalence of respiratory and atopic disorders in Chinese children. *Clinical and Experimental Allergy*, 2001, 31:1225–1231.
3. Wong GWK et al. Temporal relationship between air pollution and hospital admissions for asthmatic children in Hong Kong. *Clinical and Experimental Allergy*, 2001, 31:565–569.
4. Tam AYC et al. Bronchial responsiveness in children exposed to atmospheric pollution in Hong Kong. *Chest*, 1994, 106:1056–1060.

SECTION VI: CASE STUDIES

15. INFANT EXPOSURE TO ORGANOCHLORINE CONTAMINANTS IN BREAST MILK

G. C. Moy
Food Safety Department, World Health Organization, Geneva, Switzerland

Description of the problem

Although its benefits are beyond question, breastfeeding should not be seen as necessarily free of risk (1). Many contaminants are found at elevated levels in breast milk and most of these arise from the mother's consumption of contaminated foods. Few of the chemicals employed in agriculture and industry have been thoroughly investigated for their potential toxicity to animals and humans. Information is particularly scant about their long-term effects on infants and children. In general, the risk assessment and emergency planning that underpin the regulation of environmental contaminants and other chemicals in food have not considered the potential contamination in human milk and its public health dimension.

Risk assessment of exposure to organochlorine contaminants

Physiological factors may cause toxic effects in infants exposed to contaminants in their food (breast milk or formula) to be more serious than those in similarly exposed adults. As infants generally depend on only one source of food, the levels of contaminants in that food are of greater concern than when a variety of foods is consumed in the diet (2).

Organochlorine compounds gained prominence about 50 years ago, particularly as pesticides. Their use was subsequently curtailed as their negative effects on non-target species became known. Initially believed to have low mammalian toxicity, organochlorine compounds are now known to have a range of toxic effects, including immunotoxicity, carcinogenicity, neurotoxicity, reproductive disorders and interference with infant and child development. Because of their stability and fat solubility, many of these compounds accumulate in the environment, especially in long-lived species at the top of the food chain, such as polar bears and humans. Breast milk contaminants arising from food may include food additives, residues of pesticides, residues of veterinary drugs used in food-producing animals, and environmental pollutants.

Twelve organochlorine compounds — dioxins and related dibenzofurans, dieldrin, endrin, heptachlor, hexachlorobenzene (HCB), hexachlorocyclohexane, mirex, polychlorinated biphenyls, toxaphene, and DDT (dichlorodiphenyltrichloroethane isomers and degradation products) — were the initial focus of the 2001 Stockholm Convention on Persistent Organic Pollutants (POPs). The Convention is intended to protect human health and the environment by phasing out the production and use of these compounds. All these POPs have been found in breast milk to different degrees. Two of them, DDT and HCB, will be discussed here for illustrative purposes. More detailed assessments of POPs in breast milk are available elsewhere (3, 4).

One of the best known POPs, DDT was widely used in agriculture and public health in many countries. Because its use was discontinued some time ago in the majority of developed countries, mean DDT intake in breast milk is well below the tolerable daily intake (TDI).[1] In contrast, many developing countries and some European countries, report DDT levels in breast milk above the current TDI. However, mean concentrations in the population have declined in much of the world as a result of the restrictions on the use of DDT. No confirmed adverse health effects have been reported in infants exposed to DDT while suckling, even in communities where the reference level was frequently exceeded (4).

Only a few countries have reported levels of HCB in human milk to GEMS/Food.[2] There are wide deviations in the observed HCB levels, some of which exceed the TDI many times. There is, moreover, no clear pattern between industrialized and developing countries. HCB contamination of breast milk cannot necessarily be expected to decrease as long as inadequately controlled synthetic processes result in continued production and dispersion of HCB as a product of the chemical industry and waste disposal operations.

Considerations for risk management

Human breast milk is the natural and best food for infants, has the optimal composition to meet their nutritional needs in early life, and provides immunological, psychological and economic advantages (5–9). As a general rule, WHO recommends that all infants should be fed exclusively on breast milk from birth up to 6 months of age (10).

The health benefits of breastfeeding are especially great where the family situation is suboptimal, which frequently occurs in developing countries or in disadvantaged subgroups in developed countries (11). Hence, any advice to reduce breastfeeding on grounds of contaminant-mediated harm to the child is only appropriate if the risk to the child's health is sufficiently great to outweigh the benefits of breastfeeding.

In a number of countries, groups of mothers with known or suspected high levels of a contaminant in their breast milk, caused by either acute intoxication or low levels of sustained exposure, have been advised by health professionals

---

[1] Standard reference intakes such as the acceptable daily intake (ADI), the provisional tolerable weekly intake (PTWI), and the tolerable daily intake (TDI) are jointly established by WHO and the Food and Agriculture Organization of the United Nations (FAO).

[2] GEMS/Food is an international data collection and assessment activity undertaken by WHO to examine the health significance of levels and trends of chemicals in food and the diet, including breast milk.

and public health authorities to reduce exposure to their nursing infants. For example, lactating women involved in mass intoxications and occupationally exposed pregnant women have been advised not to breastfeed at all, or to do so for a limited time.

Some governments have advised women who are pregnant, lactating, or plan to become pregnant in the near future not to eat fish of several species harvested in particularly polluted areas. This recommendation was based on concerns not only about organochlorine compounds, but also mercury. Sweden also recommended that breastfeeding women should not lose large amounts of weight abruptly, in order to avoid release of contaminants stored in fat (12). A similar recommendation against weight loss had been issued by a consultation convened by the WHO Regional Office for Europe (13).

In 1993, the US National Academy of Sciences/National Research Council called for improvements in the animal testing protocols used in regulatory decisions about suitability for use, including information about effects of lactation exposures (14). Subsequently, the Food Quality Protection Act of 1996 was enacted which requires that testing protocols for chronic toxicity and carcinogenicity be modified to include *in utero* exposure during the last trimester, lactation exposure, and post-weaning dietary exposure. Where these data are not available, the law stipulates that an additional safety factor of up to 10-fold be applied. Similar requirements to improve testing protocols to protect unborn and nursing infants are being considered by other countries and international organizations.

Perspective and concluding remarks

Few countries systematically assess levels of organochlorine components in human breast milk. In the light of suspected high levels of many contaminants in breast milk, the following considerations are offered to assist responsible authorities and relevant health and environmental professionals in responding to health concerns:

- Basic monitoring and assessment programmes for breast milk need to be established in all countries for at least the contaminants of priority concern. However, at present the routine screening of individual breast-milk samples to estimate the potential health risk to individual infants does not appear to be cost-effective.
- Responsible authorities should examine their food monitoring and control programmes to assess whether greater attention should be paid to foods known to be potentially high in breast milk contaminants, and whether tolerable residue levels in these foods should be changed to protect women of childbearing age.
- National response plans for large-scale intoxications, either through occupational exposure or highly contaminated foods, need to be

established or strengthened. Epidemiological studies linked to the monitoring of food and breast milk are urgently needed to assess the possible long-term health hazards from the intake of contaminated breast milk.

- If warranted, dietary recommendations may be formulated for lactating mothers and women intending to become pregnant based on levels of contaminants in national diets. These recommendations may include limiting consumption of heavily contaminated foods, such as certain fish and avoiding extreme weight loss during pregnancy and while breastfeeding.

- Primary preventive measures to control and reduce the introduction of organochlorine chemicals into the environment are the most effective way to minimize exposure.

References

1. International Programme on Chemical Safety. *Principles for evaluating health risks from chemicals during infancy and early childhood: the need for a special approach.* Geneva, World Health Organization, 1986 (Environmental Health Criteria No. 59).

2. FAO/WHO. *Food consumption and exposure assessment of chemicals. Report of a Joint FAO/WHO Consultation, Geneva, 10–14 February 1997.* Geneva, World Health Organization 1997 (unpublished document WHO/FSF/FOS/97.5).

3. *Levels of PCBs, PCDDs and PCDFs in human milk. Report of a second round of WHO-coordinated exposure study.* Copenhagen, WHO European Centre for Environment and Health, 1996 (Environmental Health in Europe No. 3).

4. *GEMS/Food international dietary survey: Infant exposure to certain organochlorine contaminants from breast milk — a risk assessment.* Geneva, World Health Organization 1998 (unpublished document WHO/FSF/FOS/98.4).

5. Kovar M et al. Review of the epidemiologic evidence for an association between infant feeding and infant health. In: Foege W, ed. *Report of the Task Force on the Assessment of the Scientific Evidence Relating to Infant-Feeding Practices and Infant Health. Pediatrics*, 1984, 74(Suppl.):615–638.

6. Jason J, Nieburg P, Marks J. Mortality and infectious disease associated with infant-feeding practices in developing countries. In: Foege W, ed. *Report of the Task Force on the Assessment of the Scientific Evidence Relating to Infant-Feeding Practices and Infant Health. Pediatrics*, 1984, 74(Suppl.):702–727.

7. Lawrence R. *Breastfeeding, a guide for the medical profession.* St Louis, MO, CV Mosby Co., 1989.

8. Rogan W. Should the presence of carcinogens in breast milk discourage breast feeding? *Regulatory Toxicology and Pharmacology*, 1991, 13:228–240.

9. Habicht J, Da Vanzo J, Butz W. Does breastfeeding really save lives, or are apparent benefits due to biases? *American Journal of Epidemiology*, 123:279–290.

10. *Global Strategy for Infant and Young Child Feeding.* Geneva, World Health Organization, 2001 (document A54/INF.DOC./4).

11. Macintyre UE, Walker ARP. Lactation — how important is it? *Journal of the Royal Society for Health*, 1994, 114:20–28.

12. Slorach S. Kvicksilver och andra främmande ämnen i fisk — åtgärder för att begränsa hälsoriskerna. [Measures to reduce health risks from mercury and other chemical contaminants in fish.] *Vår Föda*, 1992, 44:163–170 (in Swedish with English summary).

13. *PCBs, PCDDs and PCDFs in breast milk: assessment of health risks.* Copenhagen, WHO Regional Office for Europe, 1988 (Environmental Health Series No. 29).

14. National Academy of Sciences, National Research Council. *Pesticides in the Diets of Infants and Children.* Washington, DC, National Academy Press, 1993.

16. ESCHERICHIA COLI O157:H7 OUTBREAK IN JAPANESE SCHOOLCHILDREN

H. Toyofuku
Food Safety Department, World Health Organization, Geneva, Switzerland

F. Kasuga
Department of Biomedical Food Research, National Institute of Infectious Diseases, Shinjuku-ku, Japan

Escherichia coli O157:H7 infection can cause severe bloody diarrhoea and abdominal cramps. Usually, little or no fever is present, and the illness resolves within 5–10 days. However, in 2–7% of cases, particularly in children under 5 years of age and the elderly, the infection can lead to a complication called *haemolytic uraemic syndrome*, in which red blood cells are destroyed and the kidneys fail, sometimes causing death.

Description of foodborne outbreaks within the school system

In 1996, there were a large number of outbreaks of foodborne disease in Japanese schools (Table 21.7). Infections due to *E. coli* O157:H7 were of particular significance as these caused 8 of the 18 outbreaks (Table 21.8), and were responsible for five children dying. Comprehensive investigation results are available for two outbreaks. These cases illustrate the need for good hygiene practices during the preparation and distribution of school lunches. The identification of the source of contaminated food was important for the design of measures to prevent future incidents of a similar nature.

In July 1996, Sakai City experienced the largest outbreak of *E. coli* O157:H7 infection ever reported, causing three child deaths. Among the 47 643 schoolchildren in three Sakai school districts, 8355 displayed symptoms, and 398 had

Table 21.7   Foodborne outbreaks in Japan and within the school system

YEAR	TOTAL			SCHOOL LUNCH SYSTEM		
	NO. OF OUTBREAKS	NO. OF CASES	NO. OF DEATHS	NO. OF OUTBREAKS	NO. OF CASES	NO. OF DEATHS
1996	1217	46 327	15	18	11 651	5
1997	1960	39 989	8	8	2 325	0
1998	3010	46 179	9	8	3 901	0
1999	2697	35 214	7	8	1 503	0
2000	2198	42 568	4	5	547	0

Source: Based on Food Poisoning Statistics 1996–2000, Ministry of Health, Labour and Welfare, Japan.

Table 21.8 E. coli O157:H7 outbreaks in Japanese schools in 1996

AREA OF OUTBREAK	MONTH	CASES (DEATHS)	
Oku-town, Okayama Prefecture	May	468 (2)	Primary school
Tojo-cho, Hiroshima Prefecture	May	185	Primary school
Gifu City, Gifu Prefecture	June	395	Primary school
Sakai-town, Gunma Prefecture	June	138	Primary school
Niimi City, Okayama Prefecture	June	360	Primary school
Sakai City, Osaka Prefecture	July	7966 (3)	Primary school
Morioka City, Iwate Prefecture	September	121	Primary school
Obihiro City, Hokkaido Prefecture	October	158	Kindergarten

Source: Ministry of Heath and Welfare of Japan, 8 May 1998.

to be hospitalized (1). White radish sprouts from a single farm were the only uncooked food implicated in all meals.

At the end of September, Morioka City also experienced an outbreak of *E. coli* O157:H7 infection, involving more than 121 cases. Salad and seafood sauce prepared in the school kitchen were identified as the vehicles for transmission (2).

Management and intervention

The school lunch programme in Japan has been in operation since 1954. It represents a unique system in which the same menu may be prepared from the same raw materials for all schools in a given district. Individual school kitchens or the district's school lunch centre is responsible for the final preparation and distribution of the meals (3). This system increases the risk that many children may be infected simultaneously.

In the case of Sakai, the most likely source of contamination was identified to be the seed of white radish sprout. *E. coli* O157:H7 grow rapidly in radish seeds at the time of germination (4). Viable *E. coli* O157:H7 organisms have been demonstrated in the inner tissues of radish sprouts grown from experimentally contaminated seed.

During the investigation it became apparent that neither the distribution centre, nor the trucks used for delivery to the schools, nor the school kitchens had freezing or refrigeration equipment. Furthermore, there was no testing of random food samples for bacteria after food was delivered to distribution centres or school kitchens.

In the case of Morioka, baskets containing cooked food were left on the kitchen floor for up to two hours. As workers entered the kitchen without changing or disinfecting their shoes, the food may have become contaminated through splashes from the wet kitchen floor. The same sink was used for cooling the cooked food and thawing and washing the raw materials without any cleaning between the two operations. Furthermore, some ingredients of the salad were cooked for too short a time and at insufficient temperatures, and after cooking were left at ambient temperature (2).

School lunch is considered an essential part of education, and is therefore under the jurisdiction of the Ministry of Education, Culture and Science, rather than the Ministry of Health, Labour and Welfare. In April 1997, the Ministry of Education, Culture and Science published the *Standard of good hygienic practice in school kitchens*, which enforces the improvement of kitchen facilities, thorough cooking, and prevention of cross-contamination through the separation of raw and cooked materials (5). This standard was prepared in accordance with directives issued by the Ministry of Health and Welfare, including a hygiene control manual for large-scale catering facilities (including school kitchens and school lunch preparation and distribution centres), and a manual on foodborne outbreak investigation for inspectors.

The Ministry of Education, Culture and Science also started on-site inspections in selected school kitchens that had been affected by the outbreaks, to evaluate compliance with the standards. The results showed that, despite some improvements, further efforts were needed to educate kitchen workers on how to prevent growth of pathogens. Cooking time and temperature must be appropriately controlled. Cross-contamination and excessive storage time at room temperature should be avoided. High-risk foods, such as raw radish sprouts, should not be included in the school lunch menus until effective control methods can be implemented (3).

Since 1998, as a result of the many efforts to reduce the risk of foodborne infections, the number of cases has decreased (Table 21.7). Advocacy to promote essential food safety practices could improve the health situation in many countries. The five keys to safe food promoted by WHO are applicable throughout the world:

1. Keep clean.
2. Separate raw and cooked food.
3. Cook thoroughly.
4. Keep food at safe temperature (below 5 °C or above 60 °C).
5. Use safe water and raw materials.

References

1. Michino H et al. Massive outbreak of *Escherichia coli* O157:H7 in school children in Sakai City, associated with consumption of white radish sprouts. *American Journal of Epidemiology*, 1999, 150:787–796.
2. Shinagawa K et al. [Outbreak of *Escherichia coli* O157:H7 in school children in Morioka City, the responses and challenges.] *Bulletin of the National Institute of Public Health*, 1997, 46:104–112 (in Japanese).

3. Michino H, Otsuki K. Risk factor in causing outbreaks of food-borne illness originating in school lunch facilities in Japan. *Journal of Veterinary and Medical Science*, 2000, 62:557–560.
4. Hara-Kudo Y et al. Potential hazard of radish product as a vehicle of *Escherichia coli* O157:H7. *Journal of Food Protection*, 1997, 60:1125–1127.
5. Report on the improvement of hygiene practice in school lunch system. Tokyo, Ministry of Education, 1998 (in Japanese).

17. HEALTH HAZARDS OF PESTICIDE USE: STUDIES BY THAI SCHOOLCHILDREN

S. Wichanee
Khao Praya Sangkharam School, Kan Sak District, Thailand

M. Tianponkrang
Thai Education Board, Bangkok, Thailand

M. Jakiet
Thai Education Board, Bangkok, Thailand

H. Murphy
FAO Programme for Community IPM, Rome, Italy

The problem

Rural children in developing countries come into closer contact with pesticides than their urban counterparts because in many cases their families use pesticides in small-scale farming. Their playgrounds are the family field, and toys are made from anything lying around, including colourful pesticide containers. Children also frequently participate in agricultural practices, helping weed or harvest freshly sprayed fields. As the households of private land-owners are usually small, pesticides are frequently stored in living areas. Finally, pesticides decanted into smaller containers (e.g. beverage bottles) or recycled containers (for food or water storage) can lead to accidental poisonings (1). Children are more susceptible than adults to the toxic effects of pesticides because of their low body weight and rapid metabolism (2). As children's ability to detoxify and excrete pesticides is not yet fully developed, they are more vulnerable to long-term, adverse developmental effects (3). A total of 171 cases of pesticide poisoning among children between 0 and 14 years of age were reported to the newly expanded and centralized Thai Poison Control Centre in Bangkok in 2000 (4). Another 495 were reported in young adults (15–24 years of age). As nationwide coverage continues to be strengthened and standardized, these figures will no doubt increase in the future.

Thailand is the biggest consumer of pesticides in South Asia, spending over US$ 247 million on pesticides each year (5). Some 77% of its agriculture sector is made up of private landholders (6); 73% of imported pesticides are highly toxic to human health as categorized by the World Health Organization (5). These include class Ia (extremely hazardous) products, such as methyl parathion, mevinphos, and alachlor, and class Ib (highly hazardous) products, such as monocrotophos and methamidophos (7).

The Thai Education Foundation, with support from the community Integrated Pest Management (IPM) programme of the Food and Agriculture Organization of the United Nations has been testing an innovative strategy to raise awareness of these hazards among the rural population. Schools aim to identify the toxic pesticides available in the farming communities, and the hazardous ways of applying, storing and discarding them. The children also assess the acute health effects suffered by their parents by conducting a health history and examination before and after spraying. The goal is to raise awareness among children and their parents about the hazards of pesticides and to eliminate exposure and the resulting adverse health effects.

Management and intervention

The pilot test was conducted at the Khao Praya Sangkharam School in Kan Sak District, Utai Thani Province where a programme of integrated pest management was part of the science programme. Students learned about ecology and nonchemical pest control methods through experiments on crops growing within the school grounds. A health component was added to the programme, in which 27 eighth grade students gained a better understanding of the potential health effects of pesticides by conducting surveys among their farming parents.

Five topics were covered:

- classifying common pesticides by chemical family and WHO health hazard level;
- calculating the amounts sprayed per season;
- hazards of handling pesticides and routes of exposure;
- household storage and disposal hazards; and
- the signs and symptoms of pesticide poisoning.

One topic per day was presented in the classroom through games and practical exercises. Each afternoon and evening the students, as homework, gathered information on the topic from their parents and household. This included estimating the seasonal amounts of pesticide their parents used, observing spraying, taking a simple health history and examination, and recording the data on a body map, surveying their own household, and making a list of the pesticides used. The following morning, the data for each topic were analysed in the classroom, first in small groups then for the entire class. The findings were presented on posters and discussed with the parents in a community meeting.

Evaluation and follow-up

To evaluate the impact of their efforts, the 27 students repeated the survey 4 months later, at the end of the semester. In addition, the students themselves were tested and observed in discussion about what they had learned. In terms of the impact on parents, the students detected changes in household storage and disposal and spraying practices, and a reduction in adverse health effects.

Results of the second survey

Household pesticide storage and disposal practices improved. Initially, students identified that pesticides were stored in areas where children played (under their houses on stilts, in the garden, hanging from trees). After four months, the proportion of houses defined as "child unsafe" had decreased from 64% to 45%. Pesticide storage and disposal that were potentially contaminating food, water and livestock improved by 31%, 22%, and 20% respectively. Homes recycling pesticide containers diminished from 16% to 5%.

Students reported that their parents took greater care to protect themselves during spraying. All wore rubber gloves and boots and none smoked during the spray operation.

Of the 18 signs and symptoms of health effects initially reported by parents, all but two decreased in frequency. For instance during the first survey, 23% reported an episode of vomiting and 28% uncoordinated gait associated with a spray operation. The corresponding figures in the second reporting period were 0 and 6%.

In a written examination, all students were able to identify the most hazardous pesticide classification, 63% one sample product, and 81% the correct common and brand names. They were able to calculate correctly the amounts of pesticide used by their parents, and could correctly identify hazardous spraying, storage and disposal practices. The students' understanding was also clearly demonstrated by what they had to say at the end of the studies:

- "Chemical pesticides should be kept up high out of the reach of children. Recycling the containers should be prohibited and the empty containers must be buried, and must not be used as toys by the children."
- "There is a risk that kids may touch a chemical container before they eat or drink. This potential risk will only be reduced if pesticides are correctly stored."
- "If we do not stop using chemical substances in our village, the environment and especially our health will be affected."
- "I would like to make my parents and relatives realize how poisonous chemical substances are. Also, we would like the farmers in our village

to decrease or even stop using chemicals. The introduction of biological agents should be encouraged."

- "In Uthaithani and some other provinces, chemicals are still applied on a large scale, and some banned substances are still available. I will try to convince my parents and neighbours to avoid using chemicals in our village. I will also ask for help from the health agents to increase understanding about the chemicals."

One student and her teacher presented the class's findings to the governor. He was so impressed that he requested all the schools in the province to conduct similar studies. To date, 31 other schoolteachers have been trained in this methodology. Of the 11 schools that are planning studies, six have completed pilot tests, and another two have surveyed their entire community. The Thai Ministry of Education has also visited demonstration areas and will be adding an environmental education component to the curriculum, which will include these pesticide-related health studies.

Application to other health problems and settings

This is an example of nonformal discovery learning, which is highly relevant for children. This powerful educational method stimulates observation and communication skills, involves mathematics and art, and promotes critical thinking. Furthermore, students act as agents for change in the community as well as child-to-child and child-to-parent educators. Although the data are not validated by outside specialists, they illustrate the hazards of pesticide use in a rural farming community.

This methodology can be applied to a range of other public health issues that require change in behaviour based on community data. For instance, surveillance of diarrhoea incidence, with promotion of hand-washing or food safety, monitoring of indoor air, and immunization coverage or campaigns are activities in which schoolchildren could be involved.

References

1. Murphy HH, Sanusi A. *Pilot studies on the use and health effects of paraquat: Pasaman, Sumatra Barat.* Jakarta, FAO/IPM, 1998.
2. United States Environmental Protection Agency. *Protecting children from pesticides.* 2002 (www.epa.gov/pesticides/factsheets/kidpesticide.htm).
3. Landrigan PJ et al. Pesticides and inner-city children: exposures, risks, and prevention. *Environmental Health Perspectives,* 1999, 107(Suppl 3):431–437.
4. National Poison Control Center, Ministry of Health, Bangkok, Thailand.
5. *The pesticide industry.* Toxic Trail (http://www.toxictrail.org).
6. Ministry of Agriculture. Bangkok, Thailand (www.alro.go.th).
7. International Programme of Chemical Safety. *The WHO recommended classification of pesticides by hazard and guidelines to classification 1998–1999.* Geneva, World Health Organization, 1998 (WHO/PCS/98.21).

18. PSYCHOSOCIAL STATUS AND SOMATIC OUTCOMES AMONG THE YOUNGER POPULATION OF THE UKRAINE AFFECTED BY THE CHERNOBYL NUCLEAR PLANT ACCIDENT[1]

N. Korol
Research Laboratory for Population Health of Radiation
Exposed Children, Academy of Medical Science of Ukraine,
Kiev, Ukraine

On 26 April 1986 the largest disaster in the history of the nuclear industry took place at unit IV of Chernobyl's nuclear power plant. The radioactive fall-out led to the contamination of 2218 Ukrainian cities, towns and villages in an area of 50500 km^2, with a population of 17.5 million, including 2.5 million children under 7 years. The collective thyroid exposure dose for the Ukrainian population was estimated as 1300000 person-Gy (1). The magnitude of the collective effective exposure dose of the Ukrainian population is estimated at 50000 person-Sv over 10 years, excluding thyroid exposure.

Numerous epidemiological studies on children living in the contaminated areas confirmed that a dramatically increased thyroid cancer incidence was associated with exposure to radioactive iodine. From 1986 to 2000, 1900 cases of thyroid cancer were registered among people who were under 18 years of age at the time of the accident (2). While the incidence of thyroid cancer was 0.1 per 100000 in 1986, by 1990 it had increased to 1.5 per 100000. A maximum incidence of 5.2 per 100000 was observed in 1996 (1, 2).

Even though the accident occurred more than 15 years ago, it still affects many Ukrainians in all aspects of their life. Beside the direct health effects, such as childhood thyroid cancer, caused by exposure to ionizing radiation, psychological and social effects play an increasingly important role. As a consequence of evacuation, discrimination, confusion about safe dose limits, departure of people with high socioeconomic status, changes in lifestyles, and insecurity about the level of contamination of food, Chernobyl produced chronic stress in children and adolescents. The 3000 children who were evacuated from the immediate surroundings of Chernobyl in April 1986 received the highest doses of ionizing radiation and therefore form the highest risk group. Many of these children and adolescents personally remember the chaotic and poorly organized evacuation and grew up under psychological pressure in an environmentally aggressive society.

In Ukraine, investigations of health effects of the Chernobyl accident among young people are conducted by the Research Laboratory for Population Health

---

[1] Reviewed by **Dr Zhanat Carr**, Radiation and Environmental Health, WHO, Geneva, Switzerland.

which was set up in October 1986 at the Research Centre for Radiation Medicine (RCRM). Since then, the Laboratory has been collecting epidemiological data on health status of the affected children. A total of 3000 evacuated children and adolescents have been regularly examined at the RCRM since 1986. The clinical surveillance programme includes: physical examination, biochemical and haematological analysis, and ultrasound imaging of the thyroid gland and abdomen. For the psychological examination, a general health questionnaire (GHQ-12) was used.

A serious deterioration in the health status of the evacuated children has been observed. The number of children officially classified as healthy gradually decreased from 31% in 1987 to 4% in 2000. This index among the same age group in Kiev showed a similar trend but without any statistically significant difference (32% in 1987 and 26% in 2000). There are no data on pre-Chernobyl levels. The proportion of children officially classified as disabled is four times higher among those evacuated from Chernobyl than among other Ukrainian children. Furthermore, there appears to be an elevated prevalence of peptic disease, cardiovascular disorders, and nervous and immune system disorders. Psychological stress seems to be a major risk factor for these conditions.

Psychological and social examinations showed that these children have been under constant psychological stress since the Chernobyl accident. During the first few years, many children had fatalistic ideas, expecting to develop cancer themselves or that it would develop in members of their family. After 1997, the Government stopped providing social support for Chernobyl victims, such as extra housing, school and job opportunities. As a result, the psychological and social problems changed: anxiety is still very common, but its manifestation has changed. In 1987, Chernobyl children's role was emphasized as a role of victims, expecting social privileges. In contrast, by 1999, they attempted to downplay the fact that they belonged to the affected population, because they feared discrimination in education, work and marriage as "Chernobyl victims".

It appears that psychosomatic effects triggered by the Chernobyl disaster have a more significant impact on the population than radiation-induced cancer. While cancer has a dramatic impact on individuals, it only affects a small number of people, and there is little opportunity for population risk management. In contrast, public health interventions aimed at modifying psychosomatic effects can have a significant positive impact on the health and health perception of the whole population. Based on the outcomes of our study, the following directions have been proposed:

1. **Treatment:**
   treat chronic stress related to self-identification as a victim, as any other stress

2. **Information:**
   educate local communities and explain the nature of radiation effects and separate psychosomatic outcomes; explain any restrictions on physical or intellectual activity, and recommend appropriate nutritional diets.

3. **Training:**
   give basic training in mental health promotion, including the need for personal warmth, active listening, calm communication, and empathetic response.

4. **Counselling theory and practice:**
   group work, case management, group counselling, counselling children and families, and relationship consultation.

A further issue of increasing importance is the reproductive health of the younger population, especially teenagers. This mentally immature but physically developed group is at high risk because of their specific psychological profile. For example, many take the attitude: "We have all been exposed. We will die soon. Let us enjoy ourselves!" This leads to reckless behaviour, such as alcohol and drug consumption, smoking, and unsafe sex. Furthermore, it has been suggested that exposure to ionizing radiation may lead to alterations in immune response that may change personal resistance to virus infections, e.g. human papilloma virus (HPV), genital herpes and human immunodeficiency virus (HIV). The prevalence of sexually transmitted diseases (STDs) among Chernobyl victims is much higher than the average for Ukraine. Many married couples choose to have an abortion because of fear of congenital malformations or other inherited disease allegedly resulting from exposure to ionizing radiation. It is very important to develop educational reproductive health programmes for adolescents affected by the Chernobyl disaster, as well as for young married couples, pregnant women and parents concerned about the effects on their children of their exposure to ionizing radiation. These should include the following elements:

1. Identification of behaviours that put adolescents at risk of reproductive health problems, using questionnaires, psychological tests and voluntary anonymous screening for STDs; work with the parents of at-risk adolescents.
2. Educational literature and a website to inform adolescents about reproductive health, safe sex, and risks.
3. Training seminars for public health specialists and support groups, 24-hour hot-lines and counselling for adolescents including those adolescents with an STD or drug dependence.
4. Scientific and popular literature explaining biological effects of exposure to ionizing radiation; genetic counselling for young married couples.
5. Support centres for pregnant women and young parents, and information about prenatal and postnatal hygiene and child care.

6. Scientific and popular literature about psychological therapy, social orientation, life planning skills and legal counselling.

The experience of Chernobyl illustrates that neither the former USSR nor the international community were prepared to manage a nuclear disaster. It took 13 years for formal agreements to be reached between the governments of the affected areas and donor countries. While much attention has been given to the increase in thyroid cancer among children and adolescents, to date no international study has been conducted to investigate all long-term health effects in the aftermath of Chernobyl. From a public health point of view, psychological and reproductive health problems are likely to play a much bigger role than the observed increase in thyroid cancer rates, and there is an urgent need for effective health promotion programmes.

References

1. United Nations Scientific Commission on Effects of Atomic Radiation. Exposures and effects of the Chernobyl Accident. In: *Sources and effects of ionizing radiation. UNSCEAR 2000 report to the General Assembly.* New York United Nations, 2000, Annex J.
2. Tronko N et al. Thyroid cancer in children and adolescents of Ukraine having been exposed as a result of the Chernobyl accident (15-year expertise of investigations). *International Journal of Radiation Medicine*, 2002, 4:222–232.

19. HOSPITALIZATION FOR ASTHMA IN CHILDREN LIVING NEAR AN IRON FOUNDRY IN THE UNITED KINGDOM

B. Olowokure
Department of Public Health, Sandwell Health Authority,
West Bromwich, England

P. J. Saunders
Department of Public Health and Epidemiology, University
of Birmingham, England

R. C. Wilson
Department of Public Health and Epidemiology, University
of Birmingham, England

R. L. Smith
West Midlands Cancer Intelligence Unit, University of
Birmingham, England

Setting and background

Sandwell is an urban area in the heart of the West Midlands, England. Over a number of years the local department of public health has received complaints from a local community regarding emissions from a nearby foundry. The foundry is one of 30 in Sandwell and was established in 1936. It is surrounded by residential property with a number of schools within a few hundred yards. The foundry melts scrap iron and, although the principal by-product of the combustion process is ferrous fume and particulate matter, a complex mix of air pollutants that are incompletely characterized is produced.

Nearby residents have repeatedly complained of noise, unpleasant odours, visible smoke and a fine dust that covers windows and parked vehicles. However, the community was particularly concerned about the possible adverse effects of the emissions on the respiratory health of their children. Following a public meeting where residents voiced their concern to representatives of the foundry, the local council, and the local department of public health, it was agreed that the local department of public health would examine the communities' health concerns. Two studies were undertaken: the first examined hospital admissions for asthma from 1994 to 1996; the second was a questionnaire survey in 1995 of parents of 6–7-year-old children in three schools close to the foundry. Both showed that there were no significant differences between the "exposed" population and the rest of Sandwell with regard to respiratory health.

The intervention

In 1997 foundry management installed dry-bag filters on all emission points. Dry-bag filtration is a process that is primarily used to remove particulate matter and is considered best practice. A further study was therefore undertaken, using a geographical and epidemiological approach, to assess whether the children's respiratory health changed following the introduction of the intervention.

Evaluating effectiveness of the intervention

To define the study area and population a geographical information system was used to construct a series of three concentric 750-m bands centred on the foundry (Figure 21.9). A line was drawn through the foundry, from north to south, dividing the study area into two areas of probable exposure to air pollution, based on the prevailing wind direction. These were then designated as high-risk (downwind) and low-risk (upwind) areas. The impact of the intervention was then assessed by examining hospital admission rates for asthma in children under 15 years in the 2 years before the intervention, and in the 2 years after the filters had been operating for 1 year.

Figure 21.10 shows that, prior to the introduction of the intervention, hospital admission rates for asthma in the high-risk area (11.5/1000) were significantly higher than in the low-risk area (6.4/1000). After introduction of the filters, there was a threefold reduction in admission rates for children in the high-risk area (3.9/1000). There was also a fall in the low-risk area to 3.1/1000,

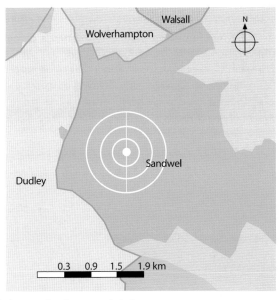

Figure 21.9 Study area showing area of study

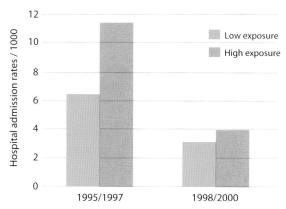

Figure 21.10 Hospital admission rates for asthma in children under 15 years before and after the intervention

and the difference between the areas was no longer statistically significant. In the high-risk area, the fall in admission rates was mainly due to a large and significant fall in admission rates for children under 5 years of age, with smaller reductions in those aged 5–9 years and 10–14 years. A similar but less dramatic fall was seen in those under 5 years in the low-risk area. Overall, statistically significant trends were not identified in relation to increasing distance from the foundry.

Conclusions

- The intervention had a positive impact on children's respiratory health in the exposed population.
- The methodology used in the study is relatively simple and provides a useful approach to examining environmental health problems, although there are limitations associated with this type of study.
- Responding to reported adverse health events perceived to be associated with a source of environmental pollution is a difficult but important part of the public health function.
- Communities should not suffer in silence but be advocates for the health of their children.

20. AN ENVIRONMENTAL EDUCATION AND RESEARCH LEARNING PROGRAMME: SOUTH TEXAS ENVIRONMENTAL EDUCATION AND RESEARCH (STEER)

The South Texas Environmental Education and Research (STEER) Center, a part of the University of Texas Health Science Center at San Antonio, Texas, USA, implements courses on environmental public health matters addressing medical students and residents and nursing and public health students. The team instructors are from the Health Science Center and the University of Texas-Houston School of Public Health, and include local educators, health professionals, engineers, sanitarians and community leaders. These professionals provide a hands-on approach to learning, so that trainees join in health fairs, meet local residents, and see living conditions on both sides of the Mexican-American border.

Part of a STEER student's training involves making an "environmental house call", which is described in the box below.

Environmental house calls

Families with children who have asthma volunteer to let the students into their homes. Under professional supervision, the students visit the family home three times. They learn about the relationship between illness and the environment.

"Before coming here, I would have never thought to do home visits to identify allergens in the environments of children with asthma," said Liz Lowenthal, a fourth-year student at Baylor College of Medicine. "Now I want to find a way to make such visits routine for my patients who have multiple hospitalizations for asthma exacerbations."

On the initial visit, students look for air contaminants that might contribute to asthma: mould, tobacco smoke, dust from unpaved roads, car and truck exhaust, combustion byproducts and allergens. On the second visit, students conduct selected testing for carbon dioxide, carbon monoxide, allergens, mould and airborne particulate matter.

On their third and final visit, the students and the host family members discuss exposures that concern them, ask questions, and consider ways to reduce irritants at home. The house calls are supported by the US Environmental Protection Agency and the National Environmental Education and Training Foundation. The goal is to develop a protocol for educational house calls that medical and nursing schools can use to teach their students.

Index

Allergies 247
  climate change and 209
  moulds 116
Amanita poisoning 167
American Academy of Pediatrics (AAP)
    276–277
Americas
  impact of climate change 206, 208,
    210
  unintentional injuries 178
  water quality 72
Ammonia 108
Anaphylactic reactions, hymenoptera
    stings 172
Angola 56
Animals
  aquatic 172–173
  domestic 35
  effects of endocrine disrupters 218
  as parasite hosts 136
  venomous 169–174
Ant stings 172
Antidotes, poison 157
Antioxidant supplementation 125
Apple juice 142–143, 150
Aquatic animals, venomous 172–173
Aquifers, deep 85, 296
Aral Sea 303
Armed conflicts *see* Wars and conflicts
Arsenic
  in air 108, 110
  health risks 77–78, 294–295
  in water 75, 77–78, 86, 294–298
Arsenicosis 294, 298
Asbestos 7, 108, 288
Asbestos-related diseases, prevention
    288–290
Ascariasis 97
Asia
  child labour 46
  food insecurity 208
  sanitation and hygiene 5, 95, 100,
    103, 104–105
  substance use 66
  unintentional injuries 181

vector-borne diseases 37, 210
venomous animals 171
water quality 71–72
Asthma 7–8, 42, 247
  air pollution and 7, 120, 121–122,
    123, 323–324, 342–344
  antioxidant supplementation and 125
  community measures to prevent 259
  environmental house calls 345
  in Hong Kong 120, 323–324
  household pets and 35
  near iron foundry 342–344
  solid fuel smoke exposure and 110
  tobacco smoke exposure and 112
Atomic bomb survivors 189–190, 191
Attention deficit disorder 9
Audiometry 198
Australia
  asthma 8
  sun protection 246, 253, 283–287
  unintentional injuries 178
  venomous animals 171, 173, 174
Autism 9
Ayurvedic remedies 163

Bacteria
  in breast-milk substitutes 144
  foodborne 136–138
  in water 76
Bacteriological quality, drinking-water
    guidelines 91
Bangkok Statement (2002) 11–14, 159,
    260
Bangladesh
  arsenic exposure 77, 78, 155,
    294–298
  floods 206
  unintentional injuries 179
Bangladesh Arsenic Mitigation Water
    Supply Project (BAMSWP) 296
Bee stings 172
Behaviour, history-taking 237–238
Belarus 190
Benzene 109, 164
Bhopal chemical disaster (1984) 155

Courtyard meetings, in Bangladesh
297
Crisis situations *see* Extreme stress
Critical periods in development 19,
23–24
Croatia 179
Crowding 30, 36
Cryptorchidism 219
Cultural history-taking 237, 242
Cyanide (CN) poisoning 161–162
Cycle helmets 183
Cyclones 58, 205
Czech Republic, air pollution and
pregnancy outcome 119,
320–322

Dampness 34
Data 269
DDE
(dichlorodiphenyltrichloroethylene)
218
DDT (dichlorodiphenyltrichloroethane)
141, 325–326
Deafness *see* Hearing loss
Deaths 4
cancer 8
diarrhoeal disease 5, 72
foodborne illnesses 135
poisoning/toxic exposures 153, 154
poor sanitation-related 97–98
unintentional injuries 7, 177, 178–179
vector-borne diseases 6
Debt bondage 50
Decibels (dB) 194
Declaration of the Environment
Leaders of the Eight on Children's
Environmental Health (Miami
1997) (G-8) 10, 259
Deferoxamine 165
Defluoridation, water 307, 308
Dehydration
treatment guidelines 83–84
weather disasters and 205
Dengue (and dengue fever) 6, 36, 37
climate change and 209, 210

Density, high population 30, 36
Dental caries 79
Dental fluorosis 306
Developed countries, sanitation and
hygiene 102
Developing countries
environmental history-taking
227–239
foodborne illnesses 135
sanitation and hygiene 5, 103
Developmental delay
climate change and 207–209
lead poisoning 43, 79–80, 166
Developmental disorders 9, 43
Developmental processes
critical or sensitive periods 19
psychological 51
susceptibility to disruption 4,
17–18
timing of exposure 18–24
windows of susceptibility 17–18
Developmental toxicity 20
Diarrhoeal diseases 5, 42
climate change and 205–206
foodborne 135, 138–139, 144–147
Kenya case study 299–302
treatment guidelines 83–84
Uzbekistan case study 303–305
water/sanitation-related 72, 97
weather disasters and 205
Diazinon 247–248
Dibenzofurans 141, 220, 325–326
Dichlorodiphenyltrichloroethane (DDT)
141, 325–326
Dichlorodiphenyltrichloroethylene
(DDE) 218
Dieldrin, in breast milk 325–326
Diesel automobile exhaust 119–120
Diet
breastfeeding mothers 327,
328
history-taking 236, 242
see also Food
Dietary supplements 143, 163
Diethylene glycol 162

Fetus
  foodborne hazards 144, 145–146
  radiation sensitivity 187, 192
  vulnerability to toxicants 154
  see also Prenatal exposures
Fiji 207
Filariasis, Bancroftian 97
Finland
  asbestos-related disease prevention
    288–290
  poisonings 153
  unintentional injuries 178
Fires
  burn injuries 180
  bush 58
  cooking *see* Cooking stoves/fires
  see also Fuel combustion emissions
First aid, poisonings 158
Fish
  in diet of breastfeeding mothers 327,
    328
  endocrine-disrupting chemicals 218,
    220
  mercury contamination 141
  protection from contaminated 255
Floods 54, 55, 58, 205
Fluoride 78–79
  health aspects 78–79
  in water 75, 78, 86, 307–308
Fluorine 110
Fluorosis 78, 79, 110
  case study 306–308
  crippling 307
  dental 306
  mitigation 308
  non-skeletal (huma) 306, 307
  skeletal 307
Food
  availability, climate change and
    207–209
  complementary 144–147, 149–150
  intake 3–4, 140
  safety 148, 332
  see also Diet
Food additives 143

Food and Drug Administration (FDA)
  (US) 275, 276, 277
Food Quality Protection Act 1996
  (USA) 327
Foodborne hazards 133–152
  breast- and bottle-fed infants 144,
    147, 325
  children/infants receiving
    complementary foods 144–148,
    149–150
  developing fetus 144, 145–146
  history-taking 236
  magnitude of problem 134–135
  risk analysis 135
  in schools 42, 330–332
  see also specific hazards
Formaldehyde 31, 108, 109, 115–116
France, carbon monoxide poisoning
  113, 309–312
Fruit consumption 22
Fuel combustion emissions (including
  smoke) 109–111, 205
  asthma and 110, 323, 324
  components 32–33, 109
  health effects 110, 203
  history-taking 241
  indoor air 31, 107, 109–111
  pregnancy outcome and 320–322
  routes of exposure 109
  in São Paulo, Brazil 317–318
  in schools 41
Fungi
  airborne 116–117
  poisonous 167
  see also Moulds; Mycotoxins
Furnishings, home 115

Gas cooking 109
Gasoline, leaded *see* Petrol, leaded
Gastroenteritis 134
  viral 138–139
  see also Diarrhoeal diseases
GEMS/Food 326
Gene–environment interactions
  23

German Network for Children's Health and Environment 271
Germany 197
Giardia lamblia 136
Glioma 8
Global efforts, environmental protection 260
Global environmental change 202–216
  effects on children's health 204–212
  pathways of health effects 203
  prevention options 212
Global warming *see* Climate change, global
Glycoside-containing plants 168
Gold mining industry 155
Governments
  assessing role 266–267
  environmental protection 259–260
Greece 8
Greenhouse gases 203, 212
Groundwater safety 85
Growth retardation 207–209

Haemolytic uraemic syndrome 137, 149, 330
Haemophilus influenzae type b (Hib) vaccine 275, 276, 277
Haiti 155
Hantavirus pulmonary syndrome 203
Headaches 247
Health problems, history-taking 238
Health professionals 261
  carbon monoxide poisoning and 310–311
  education and training 261–264, 345
Health protection, environmental *see* Environmental health protection
Health sector, national profiles 266–267
Healthy Environments for Children Alliance 10, 260
Hearing 194–195
  screening 198
  temporary threshold shift (TTS) 195

Hearing loss 195
  noise-induced *see* Noise-induced hearing loss
Heat stroke 205
Heat waves 203, 205
Heating devices
  carbon monoxide emission 113, 160, 310
  history-taking 241
  indoor air pollution 31, 107, 109
  see also Fuel combustion emissions
Helmets, cycle 183
Helminths (worms) 72, 97
Hemlock poisoning 168
Hepatitis A 134, 138–139
Hepatitis B
  cancer risk 8
  vaccine 275, 276, 277
Hepatitis C 8
Heptachlor, in breast milk 325–326
Herbal medicines 163
Hexachlorobenzene (HCB), in breast milk 325–326
Hexachlorocyclohexane, in breast milk 325–326
History, paediatric environmental *see* Paediatric environmental history
Hobbies 236–237
Holly berries 168
Home 29–39
  air pollution *see* Indoor air pollution
  audits 230, 231
  biological contaminants 34–35
  chemical contaminants 31–34
  crowding and density 36
  environmental history 232–233, 240–241
  indoor environment 31
  physical hazards 38
  toxic exposures 6, 36, 155
  unintentional injuries 36, 181
  water and sanitation 35
  water containers 300, 304, 305
  water treatment 72, 85, 299–302, 304–305

Respiratory illnesses (and symptoms) 247
  air pollution-related 110, 119, 121–122, 123
  environmental history 241
  mould allergies 116
  in poisonings 156
  prevention 254
  in São Paulo, Brazil 119, 316–319
  see also Asthma
Respiratory infections, acute (ARI) 6, 110, 121–122
Respiratory tract
  deposition of inhaled particles 119–120
  irritation 110, 115–116
Respiratory ventilation rates 3–4, 22
Risk-taking behaviour 42
Road traffic injuries (RTIs) 7, 179–180
  prevention 182–183
  risk factors 181
  schoolchildren 42
Rodents 42
Romania 8, 9
Rotaviruses 138–139
Rural areas
  child labour 46, 50
  indoor air pollution 107
  pesticide exposure 82, 154
  school environment 41
  unintentional injuries 179, 180, 181–182
  vector-borne diseases 6
  water supply/sanitation 5, 71–72, 101, 102–105
Russian Federation 8, 190

Safe Water System 299–302
Safety seats, child 182
Salicylate poisoning 168–169
Salmonella species (salmonellosis) 137
Sand pits 31
Sanitary Epidemiologic Services (SES) 303, 304

Sanitation 5, 35, 74, 95–106
  barriers to improving 98
  future perspectives 100–101
  global access 95, 96, 102–105
  health aspects 72–73, 95–98
  history-taking 233–234
  informal markets in Honduras 291–293
  recommendations for improving 99–100
  school 41, 99–100
  see also Hygiene; Water
Santeria 117
São Paulo, Brazil, respiratory illnesses 119, 316–319
Saudi Arabia 172, 181
Scalds 180
Schistosomiasis 6, 37, 72, 97
School(s)
  arsenic awareness raising 297
  asbestos exposure 289, 290
  child health protection 253–254
  foodborne disease outbreaks 330–332
  history-taking 233, 242
  hygiene education 101
  performance, noise exposure and 197
  pesticide education 335–337
  sanitation 41, 99–100
  sun protection 283–287
School environment 40–45
  health effects of adverse 42–43
  healthy 43, 44
  main threats 41–42
  need for safe 44
  physical, components 40
Science, national profile 268–269
Scopolamine-containing plants 168
Scorpion stings/bites 170, 171–172, 174
Selenium 80–81
  health aspects 81
  in water 75, 80–81, 86
Selenosis 81

Sensitive periods in development 19, 23–24
Sensitization meetings, in Bangladesh 297
Sewerage systems 95, 98, 99
Sex differences, unintentional injuries 181
Sexual abuse 52
Sexually transmitted diseases (STDs) 340
Silicosis/silicotuberculosis 279–282
    diagnosis 280
    prevalence in children 280–281
    prevention and control 281–282
Skeletal fluorosis 307
Skin cancer
    arsenic-related 294–295
    sunlight exposure and 211, 245, 283, 286
Skin lesions, arsenic-related 294–295
Slavery, child 50
Sleep deprivation, noise-induced 195
Smog, urban summer 121
Smoke see Fuel combustion emissions; Tobacco smoke
Smoke detectors 114
Smoking, tobacco
    cessation advice 112–113, 243–244
    control, Philippines 111, 313–315
    education materials 244
    history-taking 242–245
    parents 111–113, 242–243, 314
    passive see Environmental tobacco smoke
    prevention 112–113, 253
Snakebites 170–171
Society role, national profile 268
Socioeconomic status
    national profiles 266
    unintentional injuries and 181
    see also Poverty
Sodium hypochlorite 300
Soil ingestion 22, 30
Solanine poisoning 167
Solvent abuse 163–164

Solvent encephalopathy 164
Sound 194
    day-night average level (DNL) 199
    decibel ranges and effects 199–200
    see also Noise
South Africa, road traffic injuries 180
South-East Asia
    Bangkok statement (2002) 10–14, 260
    childhood cancer 8
    unintentional injuries 7, 178
    vector-borne diseases 6, 37
South Texas Environmental Education and Research Center (STEER) 231, 345
Spain, toxic cooking oil (1981) 155
Sperm counts 218–219
Spider bites 171, 174
Spores, fungal 108
Sports 237
Sri Lanka 154
Steven/Tetrahedrons method, arsenic removal 296
Stings, venomous 169–174
Stockholm Convention on Persistent Organic Pollutants (2001) 141, 325–326
Street children
    history taking 233
    substance use 66
Stress
    extreme see Extreme stress
    psychological see Psychological stress
    response, to noise 195, 197
Subclinical toxicity 5
Substance use 64–67
Sudden infant death syndrome 112
Sudden sniffing death 164
Suicide 153
Sulfur compounds, airborne 120
Sulfur dioxide (SO_2)
    asthma and 323–324
    indoor air 108, 109, 110
    outdoor air 120, 316, 317–318, 322

Ultraviolet (UV) radiation exposure
climate change and 211
history-taking 234, 245
protection measures 245–246, 255,
283–287
at school 41
UNICEF *see* United Nations Children's
Fund
Unintentional injuries 7, 177–186
causes 178, 179–181
child workers 48–50, 52
history-taking 239
home 36, 181
magnitude of problem 178–179
remedial action, prevention and
education 182–184
routes of exposure and risk factors
181–182
school children 42–43
terminology 177
see also Drowning; Road traffic
injuries
United Arab Emirates 180
United Kingdom
asthma 8, 342–344
carbon monoxide poisoning 33
environmental health protection 259
unintentional injuries 180, 182
United Nations 260
United Nations Children's Fund
(UNICEF) 10, 56–57, 264, 313
United Nations Environment
Programme (UNEP) 10
United States (USA)
air pollution 114, 115, 116, 122, 125
air quality standards 124, 125
asthma 7
child labour 47, 49–50
childhood cancer 8
clinical environmental history
240–249
developmental disorders 9
environmental education and
research 231, 345
environmental health protection 253

foodborne illnesses 135, 136, 138
lead poisoning 8–9
noise exposure 196, 197
noise protection guidelines 199
organochlorines in breast milk 327
poisonings 153–154
school environment 41
severe weather events 206
smoking cessation 112
thiomersal in vaccines 275–278
unintentional injuries 178, 181
vector-borne diseases 210
venomous animals 170, 171, 172
water-borne disease 83
Urban areas
air pollution 6, 121, 122
alcohol and drug use 64
asthma prevalence 7
child labour 46, 50
lead poisoning 9
school environment 40, 41
unintentional injuries 179, 181–182
water supply/sanitation 71–72, 99,
101, 102–105
US Agency for International
Development (USAID) 304, 305
US Public Health Service (USPHS)
276–277
Uzbekistan, contaminated water
distribution 80, 303–305

Vaccines, thiomersal in 275–278
Vector-borne diseases 6, 36–37
climate change and 203, 209–210
history-taking 235
housing quality and 36–37
in schools 42
water-related 73, 97
Vectors, disease 6
Venezuela 206
Venomous animals 169–174
Ventilation, home 116
Viet Nam 153
Violence, extreme situations 55, 56,
57